International Practices in Pancreatic Surgery

René Mantke • Hans Lippert
Markus W. Büchler • Michael G. Sarr
Editors

International Practices in Pancreatic Surgery

Springer

Editors
René Mantke
Department of Surgery
City Hospital Brandenburg
Brandenburg
Germany

Markus W. Büchler
Department of Surgery
University of Heidelberg
Heidelberg
Germany

Hans Lippert
Department of Surgery
Otto von Guericke University
of Magdeburg
Magdeburg
Germany

Michael G. Sarr
College of Medicine
Department of Surgery
Mayo Clinic
Rochester
Minnesota
USA

ISBN 978-3-540-74505-1 ISBN 978-3-540-74506-8 (eBook)
DOI 10.1007/978-3-540-74506-8
Springer Heidelberg New York Dordrecht London

Library of Congress Control Number: 2012953477

Printed on acid-free paper

Springer is part of Springer Science+Business Media (www.springer.com)

Contents

Introduction

This book, entitled *International Practices in Pancreatic Surgery*, represents the somewhat unique method of allowing high-visibility pancreatic surgeons from around the globe to discuss and compare their approaches to pancreatic cancer, cystic neoplasms of the pancreas, chronic pancreatitis, and acute pancreatitis. This book may serve as a code of practice for residents as well as specialized pancreatic surgeons in the clinical practice of pancreatic surgery. Diagnosis and subsequent management, from evaluation/staging to operative treatment, are described clearly, and the many forms of operative techniques are described, concentrating on the important details. The prevention and the treatment of common complications are included. Superb photos and drawings complement the comprehensive descriptions of the various surgical treatments for pancreatic cancer, cystic neoplasms of the pancreas, and chronic and acute pancreatitis. We specifically avoided needless theoretical information and discussions of the literature. This book was designed to be a practical guide, including information used on a day-to-day basis, for the surgeon, i.e., planning for resection, the instruments or sutures to be used, details of the possible reconstruction, the drugs required or that should be available, and perioperative management. Many well known experts from all over the world describe their individual techniques and thoughts about pancreatic surgery. This discussion is combined with the latest results in their departments and contrasts with the four basic chapters from the Otto-von-Guericke-University in Magdeburg and the Ruprecht-Karls-University in Heidelberg.

The concept of this book is unique and immediately relevant to the daily routine of a surgeon. We hope you find it interesting, and we believe that it will provide new insights into the diagnosis and management of the more common disorders that require pancreatic surgery.

Brandenburg, Germany — R. Mantke
Magdeburg, Germany — H. Lippert
Heidelberg, Germany — M.W. Büchler
Rochester, MN, USA — M.G. Sarr

Part I

Surgery of the Pancreatic Carcinoma

1 Basic Chapter

René Mantke and Hans Lippert

1.1 Carcinoma of the Pancreatic Head/Periampullary Adenocarcinoma

1.1.1 Relevant Basic Information, Indication and Contraindication

Periampullary adenocarcinoma includes cancer of the pancreatic head, ampullary cancer, distal bile duct cancer, and duodenal cancer. About 70 % are carcinomas of the pancreatic head. The operation procedure is essentially the same for all of these types of neoplasms. The frequency of lymph node metastases in patients with pancreatic cancer is associated with a 5-year survival rate of only 5 % or less. This very aggressive tumor biology is the rationale for an extended lymph node resection in pancreatic cancer. Another major problem with performing operations for pancreatic head carcinoma is also the frequent presence of perineural invasion; perineural involvement is also associated with a very poor prognosis. Because involvement of the mesenteric neural plexus is extensive, it is difficult to achieve a negative, retroperitoneal margin even with a radical resection.

Clinical symptoms (usually jaundice related to obstruction of the distal bile duct), computed tomography (CT), and endoscopic retrograde cholangiopancreatography (ERCP) or magnetic resonance imaging (MRI)/magnetic resonance cholangiopancreatography (MRCP) lead to the diagnosis of a periampullary carcinoma. We prefer a high-quality, multiphase, contrast-enhanced, thin-section, helical CT including angio-CT (Table 1.1). MRI requires more time to perform, is more expensive, less available, and more difficult to read, yet MRI is less "invasive" compared to CT and ERCP; moreover, CT is usually easier for a surgeon to interpret than MR images. Preservation of fat around the major peripancreatic vascular structures suggests a lack of direct tumor invasion and is consistent with the clinical prediction of "resectability". Isolated involvement of the superior mesenteric vein or the portal vein is not necessarily a contraindication for resection. We believe that circumferential vessel involvement by tumor, infiltration of the hepatic or mesenteric artery, or occlusion by the tumor of these vessels should be absolute contraindications for resection. We use ERCP and biliary stents only selectively. If the diagnosis is clear and the operation can be done in a short time window, we see no need for insertion of an endoscopically placed endo-biliary stent when the findings on CT or MRI/MRCP are unclear, we will often proceed to ERCP including cytologic investigation. In the case of cholangitis or bilirubin levels >300 μmol/l (>18 mg/dl),

R. Mantke (✉)
Professor of Surgery, Chair, Department of Surgery, City Hospital Brandenburg, 14770 Brandenburg, Germany
e-mail: mantke@klinikum-brandenburg.de

H. Lippert, M.D.
Professor of Surgery, Chair, Department of Surgery, Otto von Guericke University of Magdeburg, 39129 Magdeburg, Germany
e-mail: hans.lippert@med.ovgu.de

R. Mantke et al. (eds.), *International Practices in Pancreatic Surgery*,
DOI 10.1007/978-3-540-74506-8_1, © Springer-Verlag Berlin Heidelberg 2013

Table 1.1 Diagnostic in patients with suspicion of a periampullary carcinoma

Diagnostic method	Questions
Clinic	Jaundice, pain, vomiting, weight loss, glucose intolerance, new diabetes, gastrointestinal bleeding, steatorrhea, palpable abdominal mass
Laboratory evaluation	Standard parameters
Standard chest X-ray	Pulmonary lesions, metastases
Ultrasound	Pancreatic tumor, ascites, liver metastases
CT (high quality multiphase contrast enhanced, thin-section helical CT), Angio-CT	Size and location of the tumor, relationship to the mesenteric and portal vein and hepatic and superior mesenteric artery, liver or lymph node metastases, peritoneal metastases
ERCP	Strictures and obstruction of pancreatic or bile duct, endobiliary stenting, biopsy – cytologic investigations
Endoscopic ultrasonography	Size and location of the tumor, relationship to the mesenteric and portal vein and hepatic and superior mesenteric artery, local lymph node metastases, strictures and obstruction of pancreatic or bile duct
MRT + MRCP + Angio-MRI	*All-in-one procedure, size and location of the tumor, relationship to the mesenteric and portal vein and hepatic and superior mesenteric artery, liver or lymph node metastases, peritoneal metastases, strictures and obstruction of pancreatic or bile duct*
Diagnostic laparoscopy (in combination with the resection procedure – in one step)	*Small liver metastases (which are not seen with CT or MRI), peritoneal metastases*
Preoperative biopsy	*Histological confirmation of the tumor, only important for nonresectable patients*

Italic = optional tests for specification of the diagnosis

endoscopic papillotomy and stenting is indicated. In practice, we often get patients with suspected pancreatic cancer referred from other hospitals or gastroenterology departments with biliary stenting already performed for the treatment of jaundice. In contrast to some authors, we have not seen a greater rate of postoperative complications (fistulas, infections, mortality) in patients with endobiliary stents placed preoperatively.

Endoscopic ultrasonography is a relatively non-invasive diagnostic tool to investigate the primary neoplasm. If the CT or MRI is unclear, the patient will get an endoscopic ultrasonography to confirm or supplement the other diagnostic results. We see no need for a preoperative biopsy in potentially resectable patients because of high rates of false-negative biopsies and the risk of tumor seeding. Pancreas biopsy is usually only necessary in patients who will not be resected and palliative therapy will be done.

Staging: Operative resection only benefits patients with loco-regional disease. Preoperative imaging/staging should be undertaken to exclude distant metastases. There should be no evidence of involvement of the hepatic, celiac, or superior mesenteric arteries and no diagnostic evidence of occlusion of the superior mesenteric or portal vein. Extensive resection should be avoided in patients with occlusion of the superior mesenteric vein (SMV) or portal vein (PV) and collateralization because of a strong risk of bleeding and a high mortality. Segmental vein resection and reconstruction of the portal and/or the superior mesenteric veins in selected patients provided a complete resection can be achieved with this procedure. Candidates for resection of the pancreatic head should have a good functional status and physiologic reserve to withstand the resection procedure. Chronologic age alone should not be a contraindication for pancreatic resection.

General contraindications for pancreas head resection are (exceptions are possible):

- Liver metastases
- Peritoneal metastases (malignant ascites)
- Other distant metastases
- Tumor involvement of the superior mesenteric artery (SMA) or hepatic artery
- Circumferential tumor involvement or occlusion of the SMV or PV
- Patient in an unsatisfactory medical condition, other relevant diseases limiting expected survival

Table 1.2 Steps of a standard procedure (Traverso–Longmire)

Resection	
1	Exploration
2	Biopsy of liver or peritoneal metastases if necessary
3	Elevation of the duodenum and pancreatic head (Kocher maneuver)
4	Division of the right half of the gastrocolic ligament
5	Mobilization of the right colon flexure
6	Division of the gastrohepatic ligament
7	Division of the gastroduodenal artery and identification of the portal vein on the superior border of the pancreas (attention of a relevant stenosis of the common hepatic artery or atypical arterial perfusion of the liver)
8	Exposure of the SMV at the inferior border of the pancreas
9	Division of the postpyloric duodenum
10	Freeing of the gallbladder and transection of the common hepatic bile duct
11	Division of the jejunum distal the ligament of Treitz and delivery the jejunum and the distal duodenum to the right of the superior mesenteric vessels
12	Division of the pancreas
13	Freeing the uncinate process and division of the lateral branches of the SMV and SMA
14	Complete lymphadenectomy
Reconstruction	
15	Pancreaticojejunostomy
16	Hepaticojejunostomy (optional t-tube)
17	Duodenojejunostomy
18	Drainage and closure of the abdominal wound

1.1.2 Surgical Technique

Our preferred procedure for pancreatic head resection is the pylorus-preserving pancreatoduodenectomy described by Longmire and Traverso (Table 1.2). Long-term survival has not been influenced by pyloric preservation in several studies. The Longmire/Traverso procedure is faster than the classic Kausch-Whipple procedure and perhaps more physiologic because of the preservation of the pylorus.

The pylorus-preserving pancreatoduodenectomy is started with a bilateral subcostal incision with an extension more to the right side of the upper abdomen (Fig. 1.1). We regularly use a self-retaining retraction system for the costal margin (Fig. 1.1). The liver and the peritoneal cavity are first inspected and palpated to exclude the presence of metastases. A wide Kocher maneuver is performed to confirm that the tumor does not invade the vena cava, the retroperitoneum, or the superior mesenteric artery (Fig. 1.2). Using bimanual palpation anterior and posterior to the SMA, it is possible to exclude a gross tumor involving the SMA. Direct tumor invasion of the ligament of Treitz is a strong indicator for involvement of the SMA and a contraindication for resection.

Next the right half of the gastrocolic ligament is divided between ligatures or with the harmonic scalpel. The greater omentum is preserved on the transverse colon. Usually, the vascular supply to the greater omentum remains excellent after this procedure. At the end of the operation, the greater omentum is placed in the subhepatic space in front of the pancreatic anastomosis to cover this area to "protect" the pancreaticojejunostomy. Overall, well-vascularized omentum helps to control postoperative complications of the pancreatic anastomosis; omentum with a poor blood supply should be resected. The right colon flexure is then mobilized from the liver, the duodenum, and the anterior surface of the pancreatic head. The transverse mesocolon is detached from the pancreatic head down to the right lateral aspect of the superior mesenteric vein (Fig. 1.3). For optimal exposure of the infrapancreatic superior mesenteric vein and the anterior surface of the pancreatic

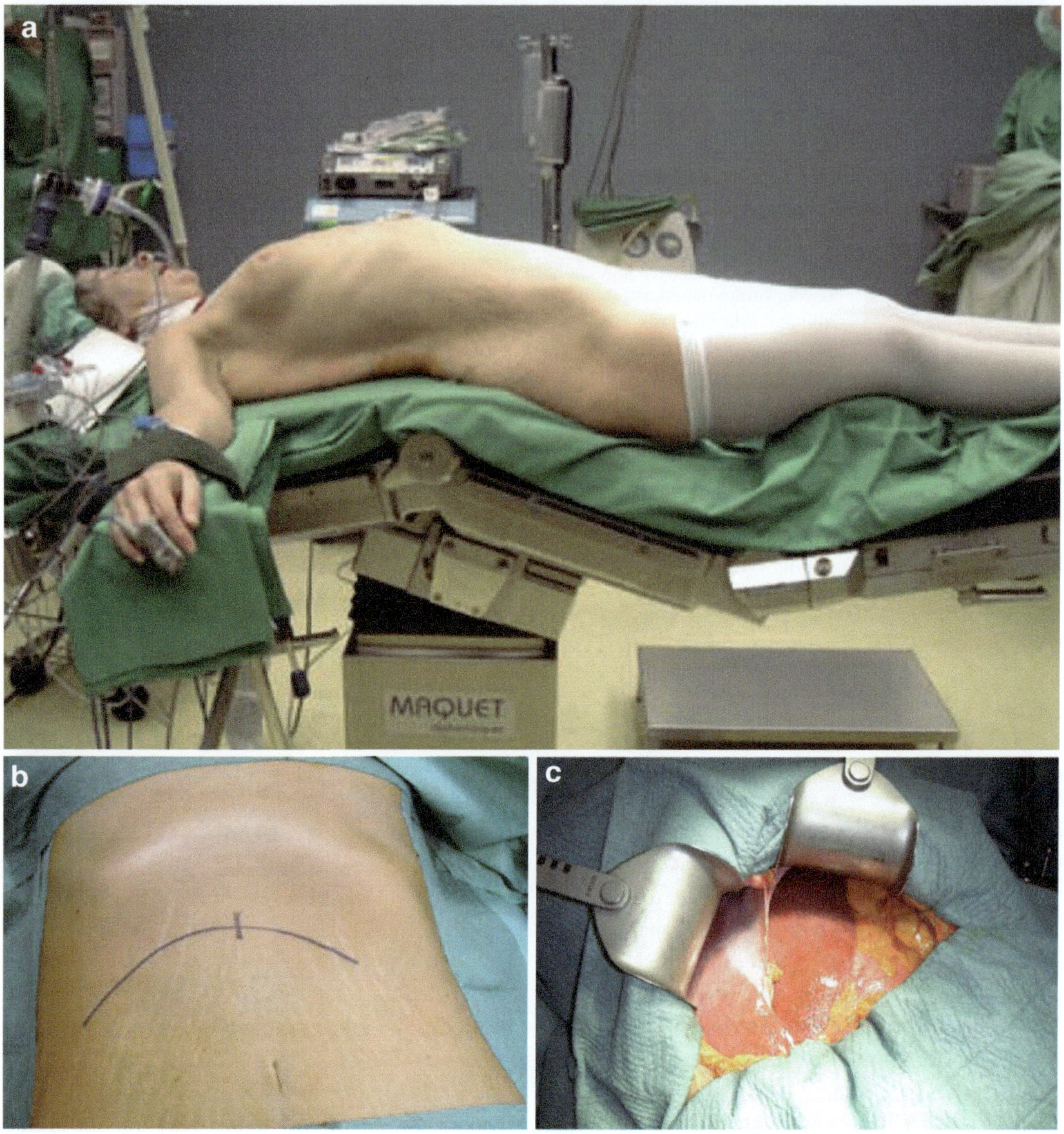

Fig. 1.1 Position of the patient (**a**), initiated incision for pylorus preserving pancreatoduodenectomy (**b**), and using a self-retaining retraction system after opening the abdomen (**c**)

head, it is necessary to divide the gastroepiploic artery and vein (gastrocolic trunk) (Fig. 1.3). The gastrohepatic ligament is then divided and the common hepatic artery, the gastroduodenal artery, and the suprapancreatic portal vein are identified (Fig. 1.4). Dividing the gastroduodenal artery is often necessary for a complete exposure and dissection of the suprapancreatic portal vein. The SMV is mobilized infrapancreatically by following the venous branches of the transverse mesocolon that drain into the SMV.

At this point, it is very important to confirm that the confluence of the superior mesenteric vein and the splenic vein with the portal vein is not invaded by tumor. Using a blunt clamp, the pancreatic tissue can be mobilized carefully from the anterior surface of the confluence of the veins (Fig. 1.5). If this mobilization is possible, this

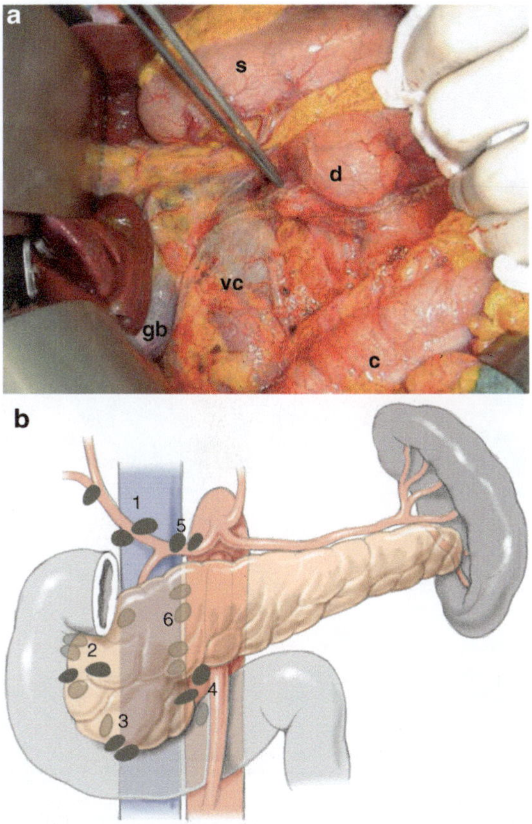

1 gastroduodenal and hepatic ln
2 superior pancreaticduodenal anterior and posterior ln
3 inferior pancreaticduodenal anterior and posterior ln
4 mesenteric ln (right side of the SMA)
5 suprapancreatic ln (hepatic artery and right side of celiac trunk)
6 aortointercaval ln

Fig. 1.2 (**a**) Mobilization by Kocher (not yet completed). A retropancreatic lymph node is marked by forceps (*c* colon, *vc* vena cava inferior, *gb* gallblader, *s* stomach, *d* duodenum). (**b**) Relevant lymph node stations for carcinomas of the pancreatic head. *Gray* nodes are located behind the pancreas (*1* gastroduodenal and hepatic lymph nodes, *2* superior pancreaticoduodenal anterior and posterior lymph nodes, *3* inferior pancreaticoduodenal anterior and posterior lymph nodes, *4* mesenteric lymph nodes, *5* suprapancreatic lymph nodes, *6* aortointercaval lymph nodes) (From O´Morchoe 1997). (Illustration by Reinhold Henkel, Heidelberg)

Fig. 1.4 (**a, b**) Identification of the common hepatic artery, the gastroduodenal artery and the suprapancreatic portal vein (*gb* gallbladder, *s* stomach, *d* duodenum, *p* pancreas over the venous confluence, *pv* portal vein suprapancreatic, *ch* common hepatic artery, *g* divided gastroduodenal artery, *b* bile duct)

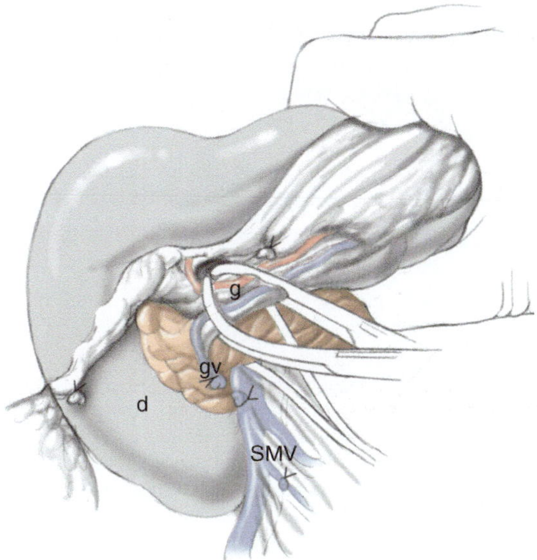

Fig. 1.3 The mesocolon transversum is detached from the pancreatic head to the right lateral aspect of the superior mesenteric vein and dividing the gastrocolic venous trunk (vena gastroepiploica dextra). The right gastroepiploic artery and vein are divided at the anterior surface of the pancreatic head (*g* right gastroepiploic artery and vein, *gv* divided gastrocolic venous trunk (vena gastroepiploica dextra), *SMV* superior mesenteric vein, *d* duodenum). (Illustration by Reinhold Henkel, Heidelberg)

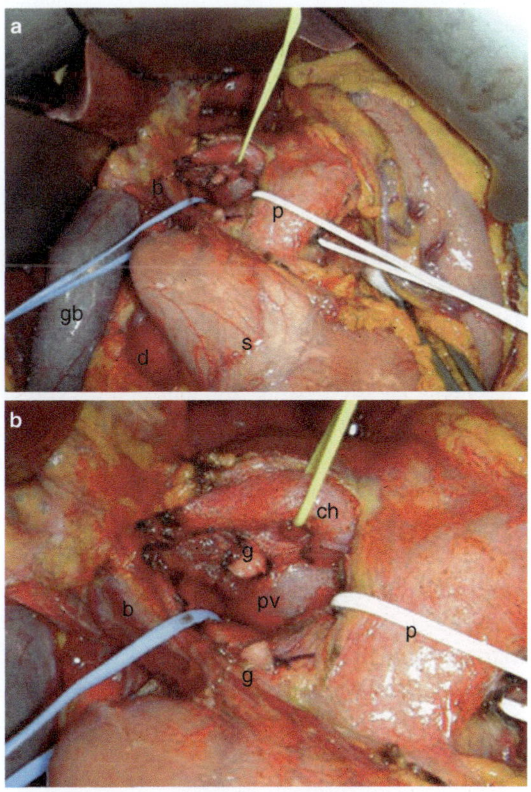

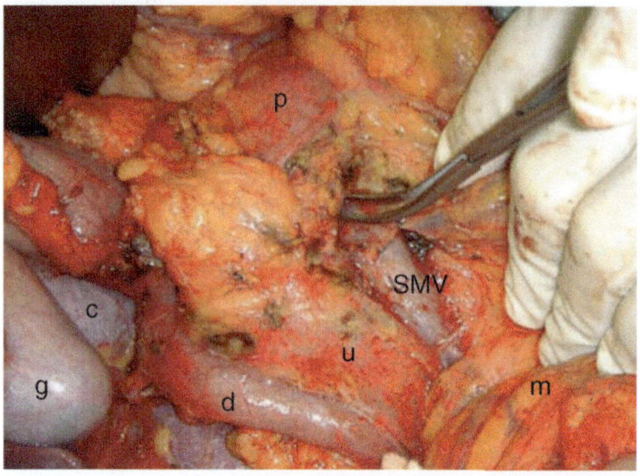

Fig. 1.5 Using a blunt clamp the pancreatic tissue can be carefully mobilized from the confluence of the superior mesenteric vein and the portal vein (*SMV* superior mesenteric vein, *p* pancreas, *d* duodenum, *u* uncinate process, *g* gallbladder, *m* mesocolon transversum, *c* vena cava inferior)

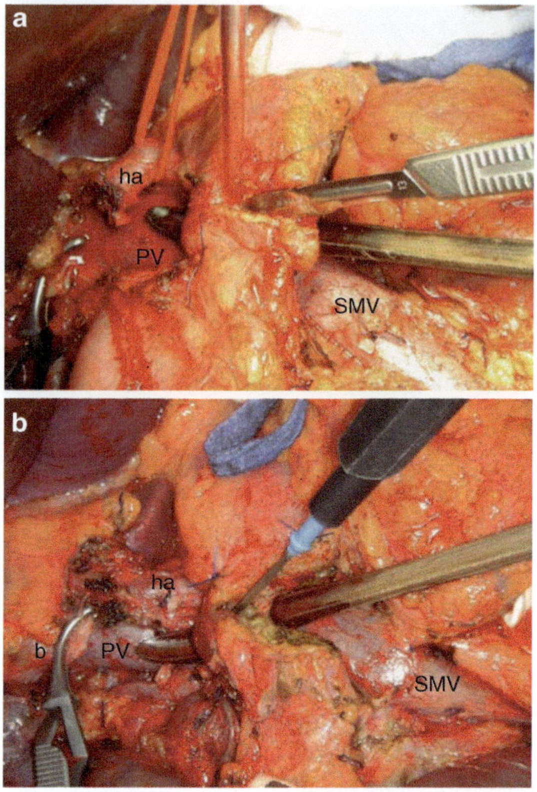

Fig. 1.6 (**a**, **b**) A special nonmetallic probe is placed in front of the venous confluence between the confluence and the pancreas and the pancreas is divided with a scalpel (using an electrocautery scalpel, cutting mode, low energy, a thermal necrotic zone on the specimen can complicate the diagnosis of a tumor free pancreatic margin by the pathologist) (*SMV* superior mesenteric vein, *b* bile duct, *PV* portal vein, *ha* hepatic artery)

maneuver confirms resectability of the pancreatic head. In the absence of gross tumor infiltration of the duodenum, and especially in the postpyloric portion of the duodenum, a pylorus-preserving pancreatoduodenectomy is usually possible. The duodenum is then divided about 2–3 cm distal to the pylorus using a linear stapler (Proximate 75 mm Linear Cutter®, Ethicon Endo-Surgery, Johnson & Johnson, Somerville, USA, blue magazine). The stomach is then mobilized into the left upper abdomen. The gallbladder is removed and the common hepatic duct is transected superior to the junction with the cystic duct. To avoid continuous leakage of bile into the abdomen, the hepatic duct is occluded using a nontraumatic vascular clamp. The jejunum is divided about 8–12 cm distal to the ligament of Treitz using a linear stapler (Proximate 75 mm Linear Cutter® Ethicon Endo-Surgery, blue magazine) and the mesentery divided using the harmonic scalpel (Generator 300®Ethicon Endo-Surgery, Johnson & Johnson); the harmonic scalpel offers excellent control of bleeding and saves time. After mobilizing the ligament of Treitz and the fourth portion of the duodenum, there is free communication between the left and the right side of the abdomen posterior to the superior mesenteric vessels. The fourth portion of the duodenum and the short segment of devascularized proximal jejunum are then drawn to the right side of the abdomen posterior to the superior mesenteric vessels through the bed of the duodenum. Before dividing the neck of the pancreas, we place single sutures on the superior and inferior rim of the pancreas (Prolene® 4/0, Ethicon) to control small vessels that often bleed during transection of the pancreas. A nonmetallic, special probe or a blunt clamp is placed anterior to the venous confluence but posterior to the neck of the pancreas, and the pancreas is divided with a regular scalpel (Fig. 1.6). When using an electrocautery instrument (cutting mode, low energy) to transect the pancreatic neck, the pathologist can encounter problems determining a tumor-free resection margin if the tumor has reached the thermal necrotic zone. Usually several bleeding points are evident after transection of the pan-

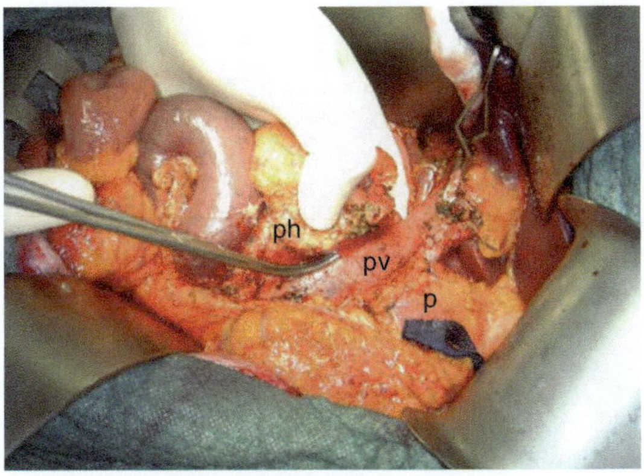

Fig. 1.7 The venous confluence will be exposed by a tension of the pancreas head with the left hand of the surgeon to the right. Small veins from the uncinate process to the superior mesenteric vein or in the portal vein were ligated selectively (*pv* portal vein, *p* pancreas corpus, *ph* pancreas head in the left hand)

creas. We use bipolar electrocautery for hemostasis of these bleeding points on both sides of the transected pancreatic tissue.

The venous confluence is now exposed. Rightward traction applied to the pancreatic head using the left hand is very helpful in this situation. Several small veins drain the uncinate process directly into the superior mesenteric vein or into the portal vein. Such branches are isolated and ligated selectively (Fig. 1.7). After this maneuver, the portal vein can be retracted medially. Sometimes, vascular involvement of the SMV or the portal vein is able to be seen only at the time of operation (a point of no return because the pancreas has been fully transected). Tumors in the uncinate process can be especially adherent to these vessels. Segmental vein resection and reconstruction of the portal and/or the superior mesenteric vein is possible if complete resection (RO) can be achieved with this procedure. Of course, those patients with vascular involvement also have a high rate of lymph node metastases and retropancreatic perineural infiltration. These facts limit the long-term survival independently of the RO vein resection. The long-term survival after RO resection including vein resection is, however, better than palliative surgery in several studies. Vein resection should be an individual decision in every patient.

Several types of vein resection are possible. The lateral wedge resection is the simplest procedure (Fig. 1.8). The vein is clamped using a "side-biting" vascular clamp laterally such that venous flow persists. The defect is closed over the vascular clamp with a continuous nonabsorbable 5/0 monofilament suture (Prolene®, Ethicon). The functional diameter of the SMV or portal vein should not be decreased significantly with this type of resection provided the lateral defect does not involve much of the circumference of the vein. For greater tumor involvement of the vein, a circumferential resection or venous patch reconstruction of the vein is a better oncologic procedure (Fig. 1.8). Venous reconstruction is possible with a primary anastomosis, an autologous vein graft (superficial femoral vein), or synthetic graft. We prefer to use an autologous vein graft, or a direct suture of the vein which ist often possible after a wide mobilization. The junction of the splenic vein and the SMV can be preserved by tangential excision of the SMV (Fig. 1.8). After dealing with the SMV and portal vein, attention is turned to resecting the uncinate process from the superior mesenteric artery. The superior mesenteric artery can and should be identified easily by palpation and visualization. The specimen is now only fixed by the retroperitoneal tissue around the SMA. Usually, many small lymphatic vessels are located in this tissue. This retroperitoneal margin of the specimen often shows invasion of tumor cells into the lymphatic vessels and perineural tissues which is the cause for the relatively high rate of local recurrence after resection of carcinomas in the pancreatic head. This tissue is divided on the right side of the SMA using individual ligatures or the harmonic scalpel. The inferior pancreaticoduodenal artery should be sought, isolated, and ligated selectively (Fig. 1.9). We send the complete specimen to the pathology department for frozen section analysis of the bile duct, pancreatic transection margin and, if necessary, the postpyloric duodenum. Positive resection margins need a further resection of the bile duct, pancreas, or stomach. Further resection in the area of the SMA (retroperitoneal margin) is usually not indicated or not possible, which is why we do not obtain a frozen section in this area.

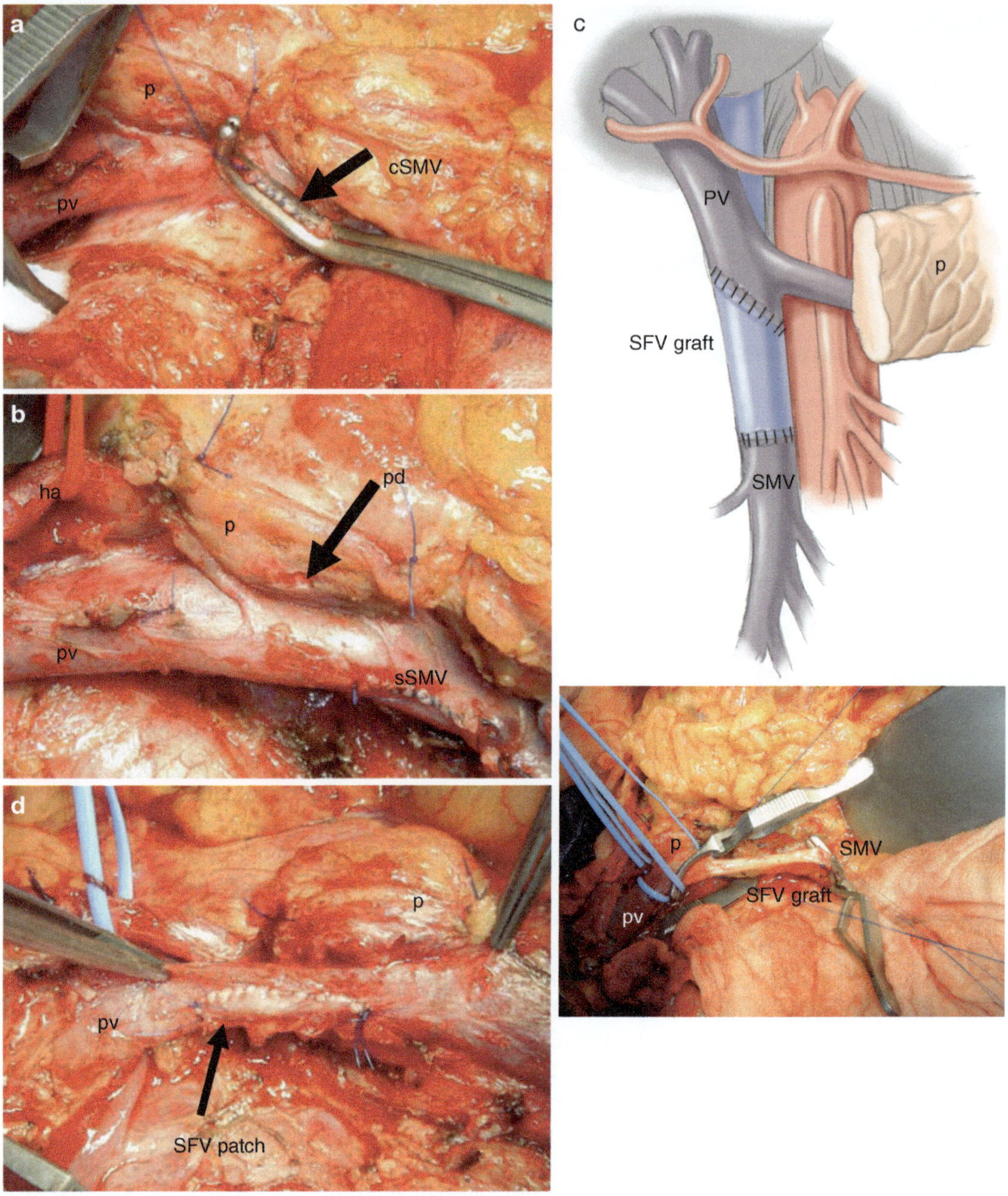

Fig. 1.8 (**a–d**) Portal vein reconstruction. The lateral wedge resection is the simplest procedure. The vein is clamped out laterally and the venous flow is still existent. The defect is closed over the vascular clamp with a continuous non absorbable 5/0 monofilament suture (Prolene®, Ethicon, Johnson and Johnson, Somerville, USA). The open diameter of the SMV or portal vein should not been reduced significantly (**a**, **b**). The drawing shows a tangential technique for interposition of a superficial femoral vein (*SFV*) segment with the intent to save the junction with the splenic vein (**c**). The reconstruction with a superficial femoral vein patch is also possible (**d**). (*cSMV* laterally clamped SMV, *p* pancreas, *pv* portal vein, *sSMV* sutured SMV, *ha* hepatic artery, *pd* pancreatic duct). (Illustration by Reinhold Henkel, Heidelberg)

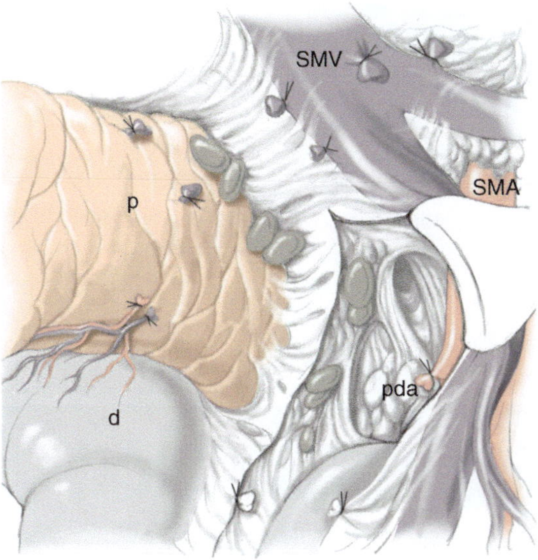

Fig. 1.9 Several small veins from the uncinate process or the pancreatic head which drain directly into the superior mesenteric vein or in the portal vein are ligated. The specimen is only fixed by the retroperitoneal tissue around the SMA. This tissue is divided on the right side of the SMA using sutures. The inferior pancreaticoduodenal artery should be isolated and ligated selectively (*SMV* superior mesenteric vein, *p* pancreas, *d* duodenum, *SMA* superior mesenteric artery, *pda* inferior pancreaticoduodenal artery). (Illustration by Reinhold Henkel, Heidelberg)

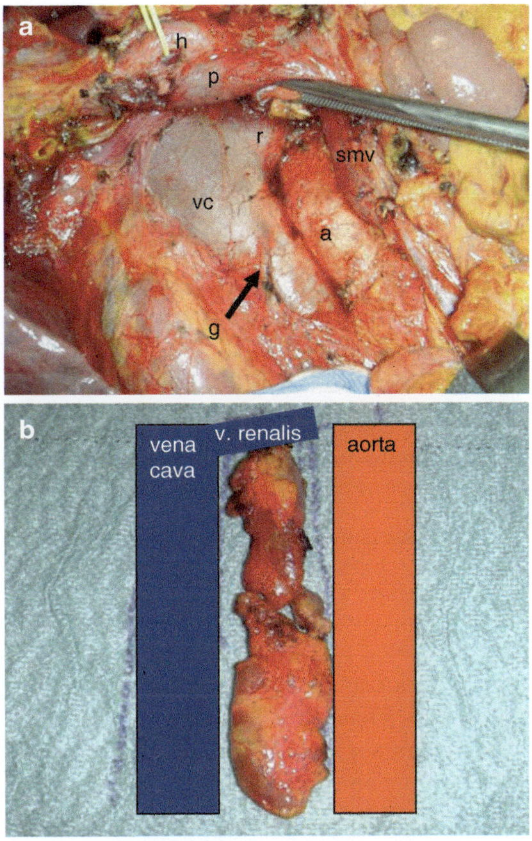

Fig. 1.10 Operation field after resection of the specimen at the retoperitoneal level of the anterior surface of the vena cava (**a**) and after dissection of the lymph nodes in the aortocaval sulcus (**b**) (*h* hepatic artery, *p* portal vein, *smv* superior mesenteric vein, *vc* vena cava, *a* aorta, *r* right renal vein, *g* gonadal vein)

Lymph node metastases are common in periampullary carcinoma and are critically relevant for prognosis. Extended lymphadenectomy is the standard procedure in our opinion. The extent of lymphadenectomy remains a matter of debate. During the pathologic investigation of the margins of the specimen, we complete the lymphadenectomy. The anterior and posterior pancreaticoduodenal lymph nodes are usually located in the specimen. For this reason, it is important to start the Kocher maneuver at the level of the right anterior wall of the inferior vena cava (Fig. 1.2). Usually, the right renal vein is identified at this time. Lymph nodes are removed from the hepatoduodenal ligament (caudal to the former cystic duct junction). Typically, lymph nodes from the cystic duct or from the corner between bile duct and duodenum are removed en bloc with the specimen. Other lymph nodes around the portal vein or hepatic artery are dissected separately (Fig. 1.2). We dissect the hepatic artery from its lymphatic tissue up to the level of the celiac trunk (level of the left gastric artery). We prefer to use bipolar cautery for this procedure. The lymph nodes on the right side of the SMA have been resected with the specimen. We avoid routine dissection of lymph nodes on the anterior and left side of the SMA because of the high morbidity (diarrhea, malnutrition). Other lymph nodes that appear to be malignant, besides the fourth portion of the duodenum and the ligament of Treitz, are also removed with the specimen. Lymph nodes in the aortocaval groove are removed separately (Fig. 1.10).

Reconstruction: The transected jejunum is pulled through a vascular window in the transverse mesocolon and into the subhepatic space. We prefer this pathway for the jejunal limb rather

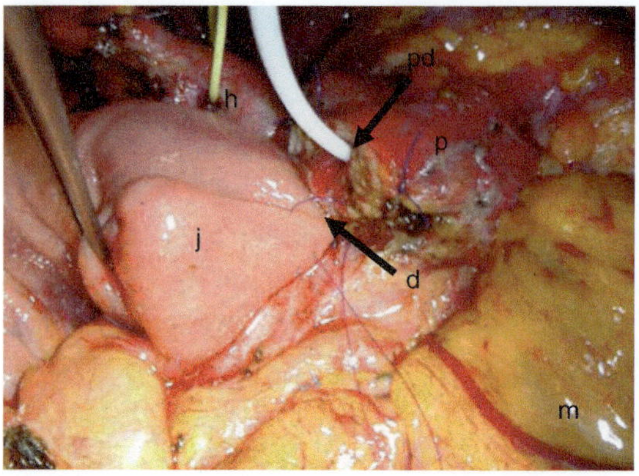

Fig. 1.11 Performing the outer posterior row using a low absorbable monofilament single sutures (PDS® 4/0 Ethicon, Johnson and Johnson, Somerville, USA), end-to-side anastomosis, pancreatic duct intubated with a flexible Simon–Weidner probe (*j* jejunal loop, *p* pancreas, *pd* pancreatic duct, *h* hepatic artery, *d* dorsal layer with single sutures, *m* transverse mesocolon)

than posterior to the mesenteric vessels (in the bed of the duodenum) because of the risk of tumor recurrence in the area of the SMA and possible obstruction of the jejunal limb. The closed end of the jejunum is oversewn using a 4/O absorbable suture (Vicryl®, Ethicon). The jejunal limb placed subhepatic has no tension when positioned near the cut edge of the pancreatic remnant. The posterior surface of the pancreatic remnant is mobilized carefully from the venous confluence and the splenic vein using bipolar forceps cautery.

We perform a modified, Cattell-Warren, duct-to-mucosa anastomosis in an end-to-side fashion without stenting. We start with the outer, posterior row using absorbable, 4/0 monofilament interrupted sutures (PDS®, Ethicon) (Figs. 1.11 and 1.12). Depending on the size of the pancreatic duct, we use one or two sutures on each side (posterior, anterior, cranial, and caudal, minimum four sutures, maximum eight sutures). In some cases with a very small pancreatic duct, an anastomosis of the pancreatic duct to the jejunal mucosa with only two sutures still works. The outer anterior row between the pancreas and the jejunal wall is also done using an interrupted suturing technique using PDS® 4/0 (Ethicon) placed 3–5 mm between stitches (Fig. 1.13). The sutures between the pancreatic tissue and the jejunal limb are sometimes difficult to place

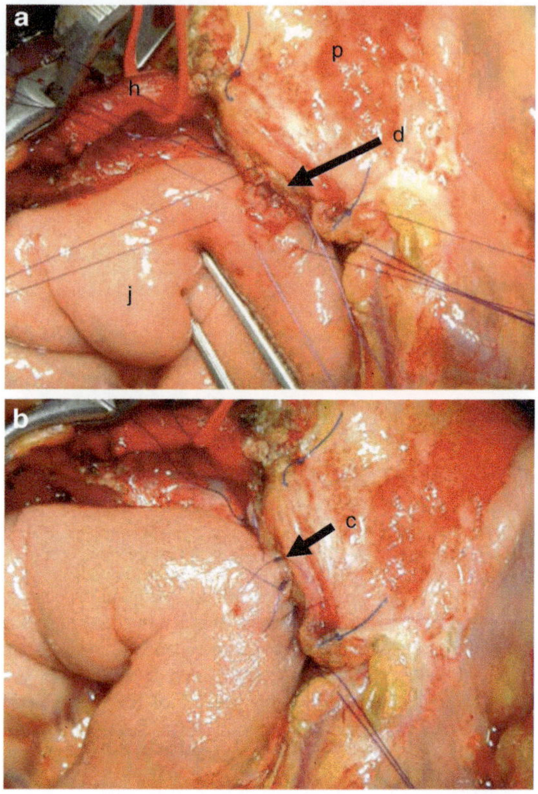

Fig. 1.12 (**a**, **b**) The pancreatic duct is fixed to a small incision in the corresponding jejunal limb using low-absorbable monofilament single sutures (PDS® 5/0, Ethicon, Johnson and Johnson, Somerville, USA). Depending on the size of the pancreatic duct we use 1 or 2 sutures on each side (posterior, anterior, cranial and caudal) (*j* jejunal loop, *p* pancreas, *h*- hepatic artery, *d* not sutured 5/0 PDS sutures – duct-to-mucosa anastomosis with five single interrupted sutures, *c* completed duct-to-mucosa anastomosis)

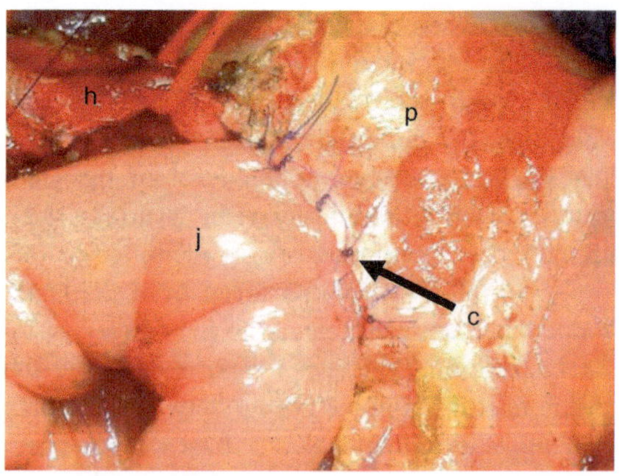

Fig. 1.13 Completed outer anterior row of the pancreaticojejunostomy, using PDS® 4/0 (Ethicon, Johnson and Johnson, Somerville, USA) in an interrupted single suture technique (*j* jejunal loop, *p* pancreas, *h* hepatic artery, *c* completed anterior row)

especially in nonchronic pancreatitis patients because of the softness of the pancreatic tissue. The amount of pancreatic tissue we include in the suture depends on the texture of the pancreas. In a very soft pancreas, the amount of needed pancreatic tissue is greater than in patients with a more fibrotic pancreas like in chronic pancreatitis. Sometimes, it is very helpful to use a U stitch technique to incorporate more tissue in the stitch. The technique of tying the knots itself is important, too. It is crucial to avoid any sawing movements with the suture. The suture should be tied very gently with mild compression of the two tissues with a distance of 3–5 mm between sutures.

Next, the end-to-side hepaticojejunostomy is performed 8–10 cm distal to the pancreatic anastomosis. This point is chosen to avoid kinking of the jejunal limb. The antimesenteric jejunum is opened using electrocautery. The jejunal enterotomy should be a little smaller than the lumen of the hepatic duct, because it will be dilated during manipulation. The posterior part of the anastomosis is performed with a single layer of continuous absorbable monofilament suture (PDS® 5/0, Ethicon) (Fig. 1.14), while the anterior part of the anastomosis is performed with a single layer of the same suture material. To allow better visualization, the sutures are not tied until all have been placed. When the lumen of the hepatic duct is very small, an anastomosis should be performed as described by Goetze-Guetgemann (Fig. 1.15). We do not routinely use t-tubes or stenting jejunal tubes. The jejunum is then fixed with two, single, absorbable sutures (Vicryl® 4/0, Ethicon) to the transverse mesocolon. The defect at the ligament of Treitz is obliterated to avoid hernias. Next, the attention is directed at restoring gastrointestinal continuity. We first inspect the postpyloric duodenum to assure sufficient vascular perfusion of the proximal duodenum. Sometimes the vascular inflow or outflow is compromised and the postpyloric area takes on a purplish, ischemic hue; because we know that is ischemia of the duodenal cuff results in impaired gastric emptying in the postoperative course, we prefer a distal resection of the stomach and reconstruction as described by Kausch-Whipple. If the blood perfusion to the postpyloric duodenum is sufficient, an antecolic, end-to-side duodenojejunostomy is performed in a double layer continuous technique with an absorbable suture (Vicryl® 4/0, Ethicon) (Figure 1.16).

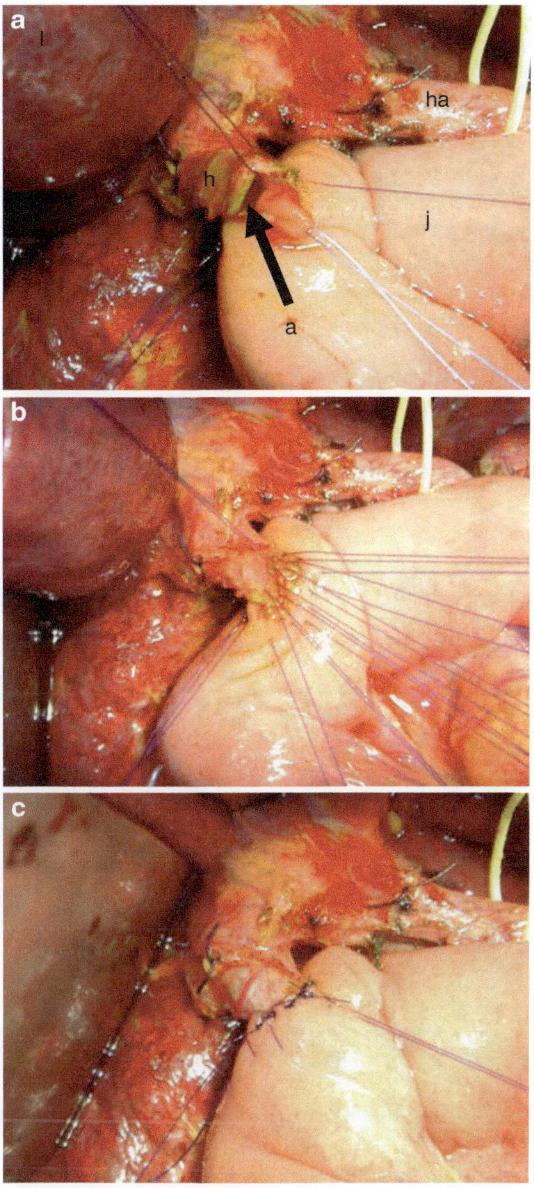

Fig. 1.14 A end-to-side hepaticojejunostomy is performed using a single-layer continuous absorbable monofilament suture (PDS® 5/0, Ethicon, Johnson and Johnson, Somerville, USA) in the back and a single layer interrupted absorbable monofilament suture (PDS® 5/0) in the front. (**a**) Continuous posterior row completed (*j* jejunal loop, *h* hepatic duct, *ha* hepatic artery, *l* liver, *a* anastomosis), (**b**) anterior row not yet sutured, (**c**) anastomosis completed

The biliary anastomosis and the posterior part of the pancreaticojejunostomy is drained by

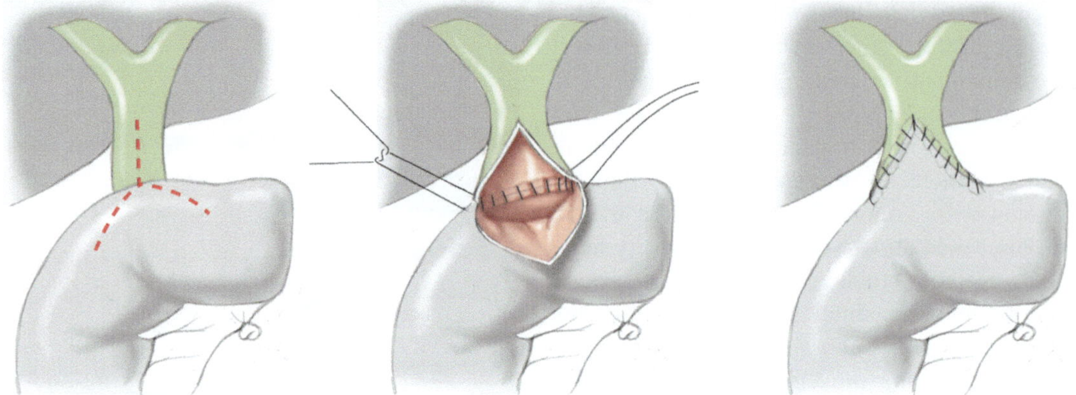

Fig. 1.15 In the case of a small lumen on the hepatic duct an anastomosis is performed as described by Goetze–Guetgemann to avoid stenosis. (Illustration by Reinhold Henkel, Heidelberg)

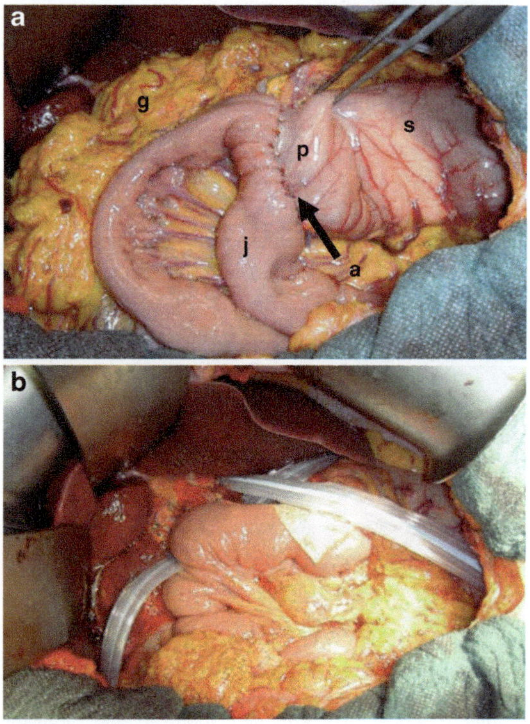

Fig. 1.16 (**a**, **b**) An antecolic end-to-side duodenojejunostomy is performed in a double layer continuous technique with a absorbable suture (Vicryl® 4/0, Ethicon, Johnson and Johnson, Somerville, USA). Multiple perforated easy flow drainage tubes are placed behind and in front of the pancreatic anastomosis. The pancreatic anastomosis is saved using a TachoSil® surgical patch (Nycomed Pharma, Unterschleissheim, Germany) (*s* stomach, *p* pylorus, *j* jejunal loop, *a* anastomosis, *g* the greater omentum is placed in front of the pancreatic anastomosis for a covering effect)

a 12 mm, multi-perforated, closed-suction drain (Easy Flow Drainage, P.J. Dahlhausen & Co. GmbH, Cologne, Germany) which is placed in the right subhepatic space and brought out through a stab wound in the right lateral abdomen. The anterior surface of the pancreatic anastomosis is also drained by a similar 12 mm drain which is placed anterior to the pancreaticojejunostomy and brought out through a stab wound in the left lateral abdomen (Fig. 1.16). The abdominal wound is closed in layers with two continuous layers of an absorbable, monofilament suture (PDS® 2, Ethicon).

1.1.3 Additional Medication and Procedures

- All patients undergoing an elective pancreatic operation are given perioperative antibiotic prophylaxis with a cephalosporin (Cefuroxin® 1.5 g, Fresenius KABI, Bad Homburg, Germany) and metronidazole (Metronidazol® 0.5 g, Fresenius KABI, Bad Homburg, Germany) 30 min preoperatively. The antibiotic is redosed if the operation lasts longer than 4 h. Only in patients with preoperative cholangitis is antibiotic therapy prolonged postoperatively.
- We use octreotide (100 μg subcutaneously; Sandostatin®, Novartis Pharma, Nuernberg,

Germany) for prophylaxis against the potential complications after pancreatic surgery beginning 2 h preoperatively and every 8 h postoperatively for 7 days.

- At the time of operation, we place a double lumen, gastric/jejunal tube (Nasojejunal Feeding tube with Gastric Drainage Tube® 18 FR, Novartis Pharma, Osthofen, Germany) with the end of the tube positioned 5–8 cm distal to the duodenojejunostomy. The distal lumen is used for enteral nutrition starting 4 h postoperatively and continuing at a rate of 10 ml/h until the 5th postoperative day when the tube is removed and oral intake is begun. Sips of water or tea are offered after the first postoperative day.
- All patients receive prophylaxis against deep vein thrombosis with low molecular weight heparin (0.3 ml Certoparin-Natrium, Mono-Embolex®, Novartis Pharma, Nuremberg, Germany) once daily, starting on the evening before operation and given until discharge.
- Prophylaxis against stress gastritis and anastomotic ulceration is given using a once daily dose of 40 mg pantoprazole intravenously (Pantozol®, Atlanta Pharma, Constance, Germany).
- If technically possible, all patients are treated with an epidural catheter for postoperative pain management.
- Postoperative ICU admission with invasive monitoring and laboratory analysis is routine.
- The perianastomotic intraperitoneal drains are removed when the volume of output is less than 50 ml/day (not before the fifth postoperative day). Drain output is not measured routinely for amylase. We only measure the amylase activity in the drain fluid when the output is high or the color is typical for a pancreatic fistula; in this situation, the drain is maintained in place until the amylase activity and the output volume are normalized. In the case of a persistent pancreatic fistula without clinically worrisome symptoms, the drain is removed gradually every day (2–3 cm/day). Usually any persistent fistula is drained into a dermal drain bag and will close by itself over time; for persistent drainage, we obtain an abdominal CT to exclude an undrained peripancreatic fluid collection. When clinical symptoms (fever, pain, leukocytosis) suggest a pancreatic fistula, abdominal CT will show an insufficiently drained, peripancreatic fluid collection; in this situation, the drains are maintained and usually require repositioning, placement of an additional pigtail catheter(s) or, rarely, reoperation. It may be necessary to stop oral nutrition and start octreotide therapy if the output is high. Antibiotics are often required as well, depending on the clinical symptoms and systemic response. Discharge with drains in situ is possible in these patients after clinical stabilization and resumption of oral nutrition.

1.1.4 Results

The results of this study are contained in Table 1.3.

1.2 Carcinoma of the Body and Tail of the Pancreas

1.2.1 Relevant Basic Information, Indications and Contraindications

About 30 % of pancreatic carcinomas are carcinomas of the body or tail of the pancreatic gland. These neoplasms often harbor a silent course because, in contrast to proximal pancreatic cancers which cause objective, obstructive symptoms of the bile duct or duodenum, cancers of the body/tail region do not lead to obstructive symptoms. Weight loss and pain are characteristic of this diagnosis but are often vague and insidious. CT, ERCP, and/or MRI/MRCP lead to the diagnosis of the carcinoma of the pancreatic body and tail. A pancreatic duct cut-off is the most common abnormality observed during ERCP. CT or MRI demonstrate the primary tumor in relation to the surrounding vascular structures or organs and can demonstrate liver metastases or lymph node metastases (Table 1.4). Endoscopic ultrasonography can offer additional information about local infiltration and involvement of surrounding structures as well as confirming or supplementing the findings on CT or MRI/MRCP. Besides ductal adenocarcinoma of the body and tail of the pancreas, endocrine,

Table 1.3 Patients with periampullary carcinoma and resection (2006, 2007)

Parameter	Number	%
Patients	68	100
Hospital mortality	2	2.9
Hospital stay (median, days)	24 (8–84)	
Relaparotomy	5	7
Death without local complications	0	0
Whipple procedure	11	16
Longmire-Traverso procedure	57	84
Tumor stage (UICC)		
Ia	1	1.5
Ib	6	8.8
IIa	18	26.5
IIb	40	58.8
III	2	2.9
IV	1	1.5
R0 resection rate	50	73.5
R1 resection rate	15	22
R2 resection rate	3	4.5
Postoperative local morbidity		
Postoperative bleeding[a]	2	2.9
Delayed gastric emptying[b]	3	4.4
Pancreatic fistula[c]	15	22
Biliary fistula[d]	1	1.5
Wound infection	14	20.6
Other (i.e. abscess, pleural effusion)	21	30.9
Postoperative systemic morbidity		
Systemic complications[e]	6	8.8

[a]Need for relaparotomy

[b]Nasogastric intubation ≥10 days, need for reinsertion of a nasogastric tube because of vomiting, or the inability to tolerate a solid diet after the 14th postoperative day. Other definitions: Inability to eat after 10 postoperative days; intolerance to oral intake and need for nasogastric decompression after the seventh postoperative day

[c]Drain output of any measurable volume of fluid on or after postoperative day 3 with an amylase activity greater than 3 times the serum amylase activity. Other definitions: Persistent drainage of more than 30 ml amylase-rich fluid (>5,000 units) per day for more than 10 days; drainage of more than 30 ml of amylase-rich fluid (at least 3 times the upper normal limit of serum amylase activity) per 24 h after the 5th postoperative day

[d]Bilirubin-rich fluid was drained for more than 5 days

[e]Cardiopulmonary, renal, sepsis, neural, other

neuroendocrine neoplasms, the spectrum of cystic pancreatic neoplasms, and other less common neoplasms (metastases, sarcomas, etc.) can be located in this area. Involvement of the more distal splenic vein or artery is usually no problem for resection, but tumor involvement of the celiac trunk, the superior mesenteric artery, or the superior mesenteric vein almost always indicates unresectability. Partial resection of the superior mesenteric vein or portal vein with a patch repair using tissue from the superficial femoral vein is possible in selected cases if R0 resection seems otherwise possible. Long-term survival after extended resections is described in the literature. Overall, however, the prognosis is influenced strongly by the nodal status. Statistically, node-positive patients may not benefit from such extended resections; however, only resection provides a chance of cure. Distant metastases (liver or peritoneum) are contraindications to resection. In patients noted to be unresectable preoperatively, tissue diagnosis by percutaneous fine needle aspiration biopsy is indicated. Only about 10 % of all pancreatic adenocarcinomas of the body or tail can be resected. In the case of unclear preoperative diagnostic staging, exploration is indicated to confirm unresectability.

1.2.2 Surgical Technique

Distal pancreatectomy with splenectomy is the standard technique for cancer of the pancreatic body and tail (Table 1.5). We prefer an antegrade approach because this technique provides excellent visualization of the operating field and allows easy control of the splenic artery and vein early in the phase of the procedure.

Antegrade distal pancreatectomy with splenectomy is begun with a bilateral, subcostal incision with extension more to the left side of the abdomen. We regularly use a self-retaining retraction system for the costal margin in all pancreatic resections (Fig. 1.1). The liver and the peritoneal cavity are first inspected and palpated to exclude metastases. The lesser omentum is opened for the initial exploration of the lesser sac. After dividing the gastrocolic ligament, the view into the lesser sac is now wide open allowing access to the anterior surface of the entire body and tail of the gland. Using this operating plan, it is necessary to save the right gastroepiploic artery for the blood supply of the

Table 1.4 Diagnostic in patients with suspicion of a carcinoma of the body or pancreatic tail

Diagnostic method	Questions
Clinic	Pain, weight loss, palpable abdominal mass
Laboratory	Evaluation Standard parameters
Standard chest X-ray	Pulmonary lesions, metastases
Ultrasound	Pancreatic tumor, ascites, liver metastases
CT (high quality multiphase contrast-enhanced, thin-section helical CT), Angio-CT	Size and location of the tumor, relationship to the mesenteric and portal vein and hepatic and superior mesenteric artery, liver or lymph node metastases, peritoneal metastases
ERCP	Strictures and obstruction of pancreatic duct
Endoscopic ultrasonography	Size and location of the tumor, relationship to the mesenteric and portal vein and celiac trunk, local lymph node metastases
MRT + MRCP + Angio-MRI	*All in one procedure, Size and location of the tumor, relationship to the mesenteric and portal vein and hepatic and superior mesenteric artery, liver or lymph node metastases, peritoneal metastases, strictures and obstruction of pancreatic or bide duct*
Diagnostic laparoscopy (in combination with the resection procedure – in one step)	*Small liver metastases (which not seen with CT or MRI), peritoneal metastases*
Preoperative biopsy	*Histological confirmation of the tumor, only important for nonresectable patients*

Italic = optional tests for specification of the diagnosis

Table 1.5 Steps of a standard procedure (distal pancreatic resection for cancer)

Resection	
1	Exploration
2	Biopsy of liver or peritoneal metastases if necessary
3	Division of the of the gastrocolic ligament (save the right gastroepiploic artery for the blood supply of the greater omentum if you use this technique)
4	Freed any lienocolic and gastrocolic attachments and divide the short gastric vessels (mobilization of the left colon flexure)
5	The common hepatic artery, the celiac trunk and the origin of the splenic artery are visualized to confirm respectability
6	Identification of the portal vein on the superior border of the pancreas
7	Exposure of the SMV at the inferior border of the pancreas
8	Mobilize carefully the confluence of the superior mesenteric vein, the portal vein and the splenic vein from caudal
9	The splenic artery is divided at the origin o the celiac trunk
10	Division of the pancreas using a stapler, separate ligature of the splenic vein
11	Mobilize the pancreas from medial and caudal to the retroperitoneum in a antegrade way. After passing the SMA go posterior. The anterior surface of the left adrenal gland, the adrenal vein and left renal vein marked the posterior plan of dissection
12	Frozen section of the pancreatic margin on the specimen
13	Complete Lymphadenectomy
14	Drainage and closure of the abdominal wound

greater omentum. An alternative approach involves gaining access to the lesser sac by dissecting the greater omentum off the transverse colon and retracting the omentum rostrally. Any lienocolic and gastrocolic attachments in the left upper abdomen are transected between clamps or with the harmonic scalpel. Use of the harmonic scalpel saves time in this situation and the short gastric vessels can be divided with the harmonic scalpel as well (gastrosplenic ligament).

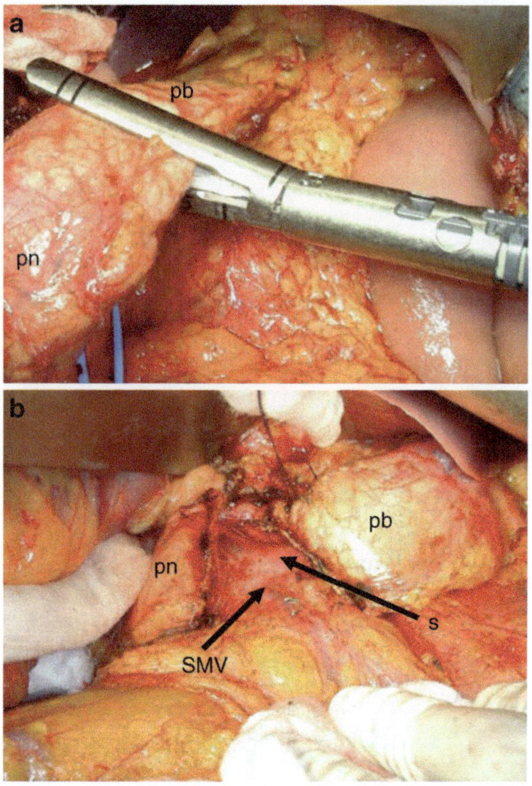

Fig. 1.17 (**a**, **b**) The neck of the pancreas is divided using a stapler (ETS Flex® 45 mm, white magazine, Ethicon, Johnson and Johnson, Somerville, USA). After dividing the pancreatic neck the venous confluence is clearly seen (*pn* pancreatic neck, *pb* pancreatic body, *SMV* superior mesenteric vein, *s* splenic vein)

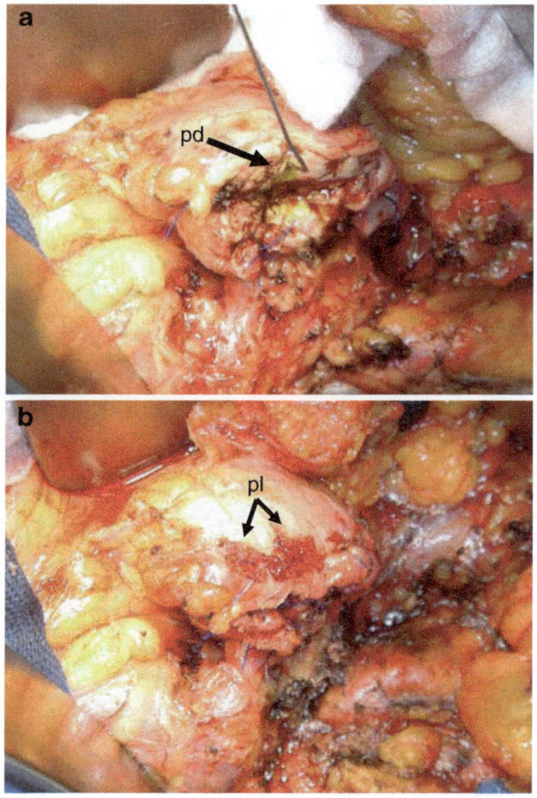

Fig. 1.18 (**a**) A larger pancreas can be closed using a fish mouth incision with selectively ligation of the pancreatic duct. (**b**) To avoid sawing, the use of absorbable undyed pledgets is possible (Ethisorb®, pledget undyed, absorbable, Ethicon, Johnson and Johnson, Somerville, USA) (*pd* with metal probe marked pancreatic duct, *pl* pledgets)

The common hepatic artery, the celiac trunk, and the origin of the splenic artery are visualized and isolated to confirm resectability in this area. Lymph nodes in this area are dissected using bipolar forceps. The suprapancreatic portal vein is exposed by retracting the gastroduodenal artery. Likewise, the SMV is mobilized infrapancreatically. At this point is very important to confirm that the confluence of the superior mesenteric vein and the portal vein is not invaded by tumor. Using a blunt clamp, the pancreatic tissue can be mobilized carefully from the anterior surface of the confluence of the superior mesenteric vein and the splenic vein to the portal vein. If this mobilization is possible and the celiac artery, SMA, and common hepatic artery are uninvolved, resectability is confirmed.

The splenic artery is first divided at the origin of the celiac trunk. The neck of the pancreas is divided using a stapler (Ethicon, Johnson & Johnson, Somerville, USA, ETS Flex® 45 mm, white magazine) (Fig. 1.17). The proximal pancreatic stump is sealed using a small TachoSil® patch (Nycomed Pharma, Unterschleissheim, Germany) (Fig. 1.18). There is usually no need for additional sutures to reinforce the closure of the pancreatic duct. When using this stapling procedure, it is important that the pancreatic duct in the head has no stenosis and a free outflow of the pancreatic secretion into the duodenum is exists (MRCP or ERCP confirmation preoperatively is preferred). Intubation or ductography of the pancreatic duct is not possible after stapling dissection of the pancreas. A narrowing of the pancreatic duct will usually lead to a pancreatic fistula. In the case of stenosis of the remnant proximal pancreatic duct, a Roux-en-Y pancreaticojejunostomy should be performed to prevent a pancreatic stump fistula.

After dividing the pancreatic neck, the venous confluence is seen clearly (Fig. 1.17). The splenic vein is divided between ligatures at the confluence with the SMV, avoiding leaving a redundant segment of splenic vein that would thrombose and potentially propagate into the portal vein to cause portal vein/SMV thrombosis postoperatively. When the neck of the pancreas is thick (>1.5–2 cm), transection/occlusion with a stapler is not reliable; in this situation, we transect the pancreas with a fishmouth-type incision and specifically and selectively ligate the pancreatic duct in the stump (Fig. 1.18). Sutures are also placed to close the anterior and posterior aspects of the pancreatic stump over the ductal closure; to avoid these sutures cutting or sawing through the usually soft, normal pancreatic parenchyma, the use of absorbable pledgets is possible (Ethisorb®, pledget undyed, absorbable, Ethicon, Johnson & Johnson, Somerville, USA).

The posterior surface of the body of the pancreas is next mobilized anteriorly from the retroperitoneum. This plane of dissection is at first anterior to the SMA. Fat and fibrous tissue is divided using bipolar forceps. The plan of dissection then goes posteriorly on the left side of the SMA down to the aorta. The lymph nodes anterior and on the left side of the aorta are taken in this step. The operative plan now shifts to the left side, and the pancreas is mobilized from the retroperitoneum. The anterior surface of the left adrenal gland, the adrenal vein, and the left renal vein mark the posterior plane of dissection (Fig. 1.19). During this maneuver, the inferior mesenteric vein is ligated. Using this technique, the superior part of Gerota's fascia of the kidney is taken with the specimen (Fig 1.19). This dissection is more aggressive than the classic technique of "retrograde" distal pancreatectomy. Our belief is that carcinoma of the body or tail has the same tumor biology as pancreatic head carcinoma. The frequency of retroperitoneal infiltration or lymph node metastases is high, unfortunately,

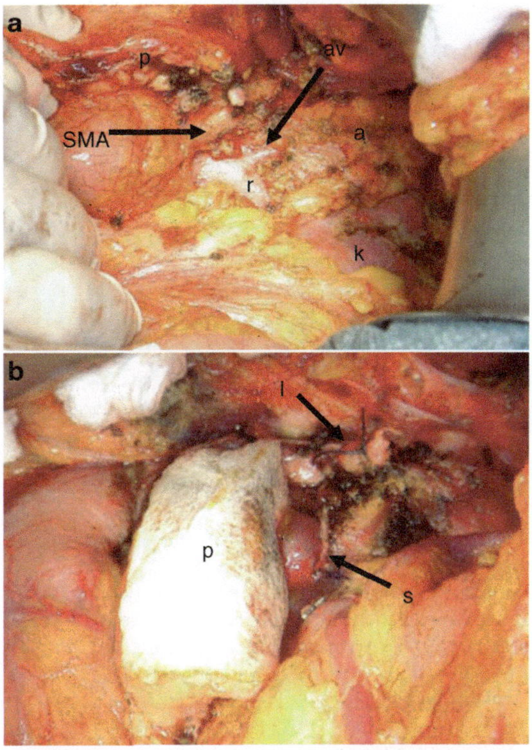

Fig. 1.19 (**a**) The anterior surface of the left adrenal gland, the adrenal vein and left renal vein marked the posterior plan of dissection. The upper part of the Gerota's fascia of the kidney is taken with the specimen. (**b**) The pancreatic stump is additionally saved using a small TachoSil® surgical patch (Nycomed Pharma, Unterschleissheim, Germany) (*k* left kidney, *r* renal vein, *a* adrenal gland, *av* adrenal vein, *SMA* superior mesenteric artery, *p* pancreatic stump, *s* sutured splenic vein, *l* ligated splenic artery)

in both types of carcinoma. Therefore, we have also adopted the use of an aggressive approach of resection in pancreatic body or tail carcinomas which involves resection of retroperitoneal, retropancreatic tissue including several lymphatic vessels and including several lymph node stations (Fig. 1.20). Involvement of the colon, stomach, or adrenal gland needs resection of these structures en bloc with the pancreatic tumor. Special attention is given to the posterior resection margin (adrenal gland, kidney) and the resection margin in the area of the pancreatic neck over the SMV/PV. After dividing the lienorenal ligament, the specimen is completely mobilized. The left lateral aspect of the resection is sometimes

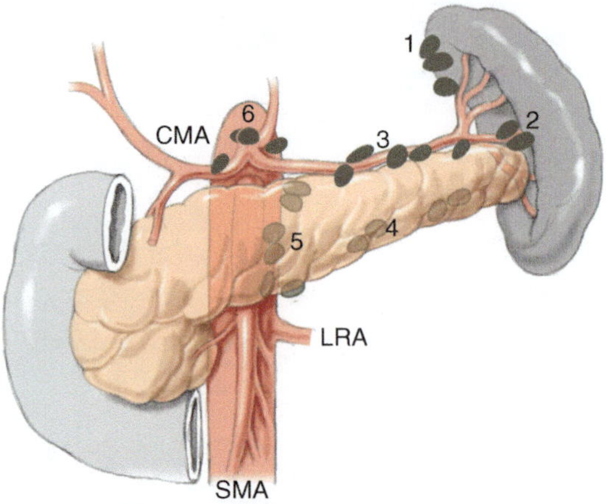

Fig. 1.20 Relevant lymph node stations for carcinomas of the body or tail of the pancreas. Gray drawn nodes are located behind the pancreas (*1* gastrosplenic lymph nodes, *2* splenic lymph nodes, *3* suprapancreatic lymph nodes, *4* infrapancreatic lymph nodes, *5* mesenteric lymph nodes, *6* celiac lymph nodes, *CHA* common hepatic artery, *LRA* left renal artery, *SMA* superior mesenteric artery) (Modified from O'Morchoe (1997)). (Illustration by Reinhold Henkel, Heidelberg)

difficult. In these cases, the spleen is lifted anteriorly to allow the distal part of the pancreas to be dissected.

The pancreatic margin on the specimen is investigated by frozen section to confirm a tumor-free margin. A 12 mm multiply perforated, closed suction drain (Easy Flow Drainage 12 mm®, P. J. Dahlhausen & Co. GmbH) is placed near the pancreatic stump and brought out through a stab wound in the left lateral abdomen. The pancreatic stump is then covered with the greater omentum, which is placed into the lesser sac superior to the transverse colon and posterior to the stomach. The abdominal wound is closed in two layers with continuous absorbable monofilament suture (PDS® 2, Ethicon).

1.2.3 Additional Medication and Procedures

- All patients undergoing an elective pancreatic operation are given perioperative antibiotic prophylaxis with a cephalosporin (Cefuroxin® 1.5 g, Fresenius KABI, Bad Homburg, Germany) and metronidazole (Metronidazol® 0.5 g, Fresenius KABI, Bad Homburg, Germany) 30 min preoperatively. The antibiotic is redosed if the operation lasts longer than 4 h. Only in patients with preoperative cholangitis is antibiotic therapy prolonged postoperatively.
- We use octreotide (100 μg subcutaneously; Sandostatin®, Novartis Pharma, Nuremberg, Germany) for prophylaxis against the potential complications after pancreatic surgery beginning 2 h preoperatively and 8 h postoperatively for 7 days.
- All patients are given sips of tea or water on the first postoperative day. Oral nutrition is started with yogurt and liquid nutrition on the third postoperative day.
- Prophylaxis against stress gastritis and anastomotic ulceration is given using a once daily dose of 40 mg pantoprazole intravenously (Pantozol®, Atlanta Pharma, Constance, Germany).
- If technically possible, all patients are treated with an epidural catheter for postoperative pain management.
- Postoperative ICU admission with invasive monitoring and laboratory analysis is routine.
- The perianastomotic intraperitoneal drains are removed when the volume of output is less than 50 ml/day (not before the fifth postoperative day). Drain output is not measured routinely for amylase. We only measure the amylase activity in the drain fluid when the output is high or the color is typical for a pancreatic fistula; in this situation, the drain is maintained in place until the amylase activity and the output volume are normalized. In the case of a persistent pancreatic fistula without clinically worrisome symptoms, the drain is removed gradually every day (2–3 cm/day). Usually any persistent fistula is drained into a dermal drain bag and will close by itself over time; for persistent drainage, we obtain an abdominal CT to exclude an undrained

Table 1.6 Patients with a carcinoma of the body or tail of the pancreas (2006, 2007)

Parameter	Number	%
Patients	20	100
Hospital mortality	1	5
Hospital stay (median, days)	20 (9–34)	–
Relaparotomy	1	5
Death without local complications	0	0
Tumor stage (UICC)		
Ia	0	0
Ib	3	15
IIa	5	25
IIb	12	60
III	0	0
IV	0	0
R0 resection rate	17	85
R1 resection rate	1	5
R2 resection rate	2	10
Postoperative local morbidity		
Postoperative bleeding[a]	2	10
Pancreatic fistula[b]	3	15
Wound infection	1	5
Other (i.e. abscess, pleural effusion)	8	40
Postoperative systemic morbidity		
Systemic complications[c]	1	5

[a]Need for relaparotomy
[b]Drain output of any measurable volume on or after three postoperative days with an amylase activity greater than three times the serum amylase activity. Other definitions: Persistent drainage of more than 30 ml of amylase-rich fluid (>5,000 units) per day for more than 10 days; drainage of more than 30 ml of amylase-rich fluid (at least three times the upper normal limit of serum amylase activity) per 24 h after the fifth postoperative day
[c]Cardiopulmonary, renal, sepsis, neural, other

peripancreatic fluid collection. When clinical symptoms (fever, pain, leukocytosis) suggest a pancreatic fistula, abdominal CT will show an insufficiently drained, peripancreatic fluid collection; in this situation, the drains are maintained and usually require repositioning, placement of an additional pigtail catheter(s) or, rarely, reoperation. It may be necessary to stop oral nutrition and start octreotide therapy if the output is high. Antibiotics are often required as well, depending on the clinical symptoms and systemic response. Discharge with drains in situ is possible in these patients after clinical stabilization and resumption of oral nutrition.

1.2.4 Results

The results of this study are contained in Table 1.6.

Reference

O'Morchoe CCC (1997) Lymphatic system of the pancreas. Microsc Res Tech 37:456–477

Commentary

2

Claudio Bassi, Giovanni Butturini,
and Roberto Salvia

When we examine Table 1.2, we subscribe to the same surgical steps as suggested by Mantke and Lippert. Similarly, in pancreatic head resection for periampullary cancer, we follow the same sequence of maneuvers but with few different "strategic choices" and "details." For example, Mantke and Lippert prefer a subcostal incision; we use a midline incision, because this incision is quicker to both make and close; in addition, for the majority of patients, the midline incision offers an equally good view of the entire peritoneal cavity. Certainly, whenever the uncinate process and the plane posterior to the head of the gland is "deep" and difficult to access, the surgeon's left hand is going to suffer intermittent, transient ischemia attacks when using a midline approach, but, at least in our experience, the use of the harmonic scalpel technology during this operative step has been able to reduce this specific disadvantage to the surgeon in the obese patient.

We also prefer pylorus-preserving resections. We start with a very wide "extended" Kocher maneuver; at this stage, we prefer to identify the origin of the SMA and the area between SMA and celiac trunk origin, because often this is the site of metastatic lymph nodes leading to a non-therapeutic R2 resection if not completely dissected.

To isolate the retropancreatic mesenteric/portal vein, we usually prefer to dissect the portal vein at the rostral margin of the pancreas and simultaneously to remove the nodes along the common hepatic artery. By doing so, you can get a sense of the direction of the superior mesenteric vein, a helpful hint often not easy to recognize in obese patients. Also, and most importantly, if an injury to the mesenteric/portal venous confluence should occur (and we know that sometimes this type of injury does happen!), the rostral control of the mesenteric-spleno-portal system is facilitated.

We specifically do not use bipolar cautery but rather use the harmonic scalpel extensively with the last generation forceps (FOCUS) which for us has become our "third hand." It is possible to secure most of the vessels with this device using suture ligation only for gastroduodenal, gastroepiploic, and sometimes the pancreatoduodenal arteries during the dissection of the uncinate process. In particular, the anatomic dissection of the retroportal plane is facilitated and speeded markedly using the harmonic scalpel, starting from the anterior aspect of the SMA with gentle traction on the specimen after transection of the neck of the pancreas with a regular scalpel as guided by the left hand of the surgeon.

When resection of the portal or mesenteric vein is necessary, we administer 5,000 IU of heparin in order to minimize the risk of vein thrombosis. In our experience, a primary veno-venous anastomosis is almost always possible and preferable after a complete vein resection. Sometimes, it is necessary to disconnect and ligate the splenic

C. Bassi, M.D., FRCS (✉) • G. Butturini, M.D., Ph.D.
R. Salvia, M.D., Ph.D.
Surgical Department, University of Verona,
Verona, Italy
e-mail: claudio.bassi@univr.it

R. Mantke et al. (eds.), *International Practices in Pancreatic Surgery*,
DOI 10.1007/978-3-540-74506-8_2, © Springer-Verlag Berlin Heidelberg 2013

vein at its junction with the SMV. The in situ pancreatic remnant and spleen maintain adequate venous drainage through the short gastric vessels; we have never had a splenic infarction or other complication with this technique.

Regarding common bile duct, after transection, we do not clamp the duct to avoid microdamage to the duct wall and accept free flow of the bile as controlled with a warm gauze. When the patient has had a previous biliary stent with the expectant bacterobilia, we irrigate the bile duct extensively.

We do not perform the so-called "extended lymphadenectomy" for the simple reason that several randomized, controlled trials have shown clearly that there is no survival advantage; as described by Mantke and Lippert, we also remove the lymph nodes around the common bile duct up to the cystic duct, the hepatic artery, anterior and posterior pyloric nodes, and the nodes along the superior mesenteric artery together with the specimen. We do not remove the lymph nodes in the aortocaval groove routinely but, when enlarged, we do remove them to ensure accurate pathologic staging. With this procedure, one must be very careful to avoid injury to the cysterna chyli, which is close to the left renal vein.

2.1 Reconstruction

Our preferred technique of pancreatic-enteric drainage is a single layer, intussuscepting, end-to-side pancreatojejunostomy using absorbable 4/0 monofilament interrupted sutures (PDS®, Ethicon). We carefully avoid occlusion of the Wirsung duct with the suture, believing that it is better to leave the transected duct "open" without potential damage of its delicate and thin walls by a direct mucosa-to-mucosa anastomosis. We also believe strongly that with a hard or very firm pancreas, every technique is a good option, but for the very soft pancreatic stump, pancreatogastrostomy is a good alternative and appears to decrease the rate of grade B and C pancreatic fistulas; for this latter technique, an anterior gastrostomy allows the surgeon to pull the pancreatic stump into the gastric lumen prior to performing single layer, end-to-side pancreatogastrostomy using absorbable 4-0 monofilament interrupted sutures (PDS®, Ethicon). The trick to these intussuscepting anastomoses is to mobilize the pancreatic stump for at least 5 cm anterior to the splenomesenteric venous confluence.

An end-to-side hepaticojejunostomy is then performed at least 15 cm distal to the pancreaticojejunostomy. We have never yet experienced kinking of the jejunal limb with this technique. Usually, a single-layer suture using 4-0 monofilament interrupted sutures (PDS®, Ethicon) is performed for both the posterior and the anterior wall; for a particularly small duct, a running suture should be avoided to decrease the risk of ischemia and subsequent late stenosis. For the small size duct, we use interrupted 5-0 monofilament sutures (PDS®, Ethicon) without any other particular trick except to not use too many stitches; some bile leak in the first 48 h is preferable to the long-term morbidity of an anastomotic stenosis! Finally, to restore gastrointestinal continuity, we perform a single-layer duodenojejunostomy using 3-0 absorbable interrupted sutures (Vicryl®, Ethicon) in an antecolic fashion.

At the end of the procedure, a smooth, non-suction, passive 2-mm drain is placed from the right flank posterior to the biliary anastomosis and near the rostral edge of the pancreatojejunostomy; a second drain is placed from the left flank and positioned at the caudal edge of the pancreatojejunostomy.

2.2 Postoperative "Fast Track" Management

All patients have a nasogastric tube placed perioperatively, but it is removed the next day. We test the drain fluid for amylase level. If the amylase level is less than 5,000 U/L, we remove the drain on postoperative day 3, because the risk of a pancreatic fistula is very low, while the risk of a drain-related complication (superinfection, erosion of local structures) is possible. Patients are allowed to drink tea and water on day 1 and to start eating on day 3 when the octreotide is stopped. Yes, we use prophylactic octreotide perioperatively to decrease the risk of pancreatic anastomotic leak based on several of our previous studies.

2.3 Distal Pancreatectomy and Splenectomy for Ductal Pancreatic Carcinoma

Most patients are approached via a midline incision just as for a pancreatic head resection. As with pancreatoduodenectomy, the harmonic scalpel has become the third hand of the surgeon which facilitates the management of the short gastric vessels, the retroperitoneal dissection of the pancreas, and the lymphadenectomy. After a wide opening of the gastrocolic ligament, we prefer to perform a Kocher maneuver to allow control of the portomesenteric axis and of the superior mesenteric artery. Lymphadenectomy along the common hepatic artery and celiac trunk is accomplished. The resectability of the tumor can now be verified with the careful mobilization of the pancreatic isthmus maintaining view of the splenoportomesenteric confluence. After division of the splenic artery at its origin, we usually transect the pancreas with a scalpel, but acknowledge that a stapler can also be sued. Although there are studies on the advisability and efficacy of stapling the pancreatic stump, none have shown a convincing advantage of the use of a stapler. A recent report from Mayo Clinic suggested an advantage of the harmonic scalpel when transecting the pancreas during distal pancreatectomy; although we have tried this technique in few patients with good results and our interest is now in that direction, we are also conscious of minimizing the overall cost of the procedures by avoiding staplers or other biologic supports for which there is no sufficient evidence currently to justify their routine use. Finally, we use a similar drain as for pancreatoduodenectomy and manage this drain as described above. Patients are not managed postoperatively in the ICU and are subjected to a "fast track" approach.

An important difference in our technique from that of the authors is related to the lymphadenectomy. We do not remove the lymph nodes along the aorta or the tissue of Gerota fascia. We do not believe that any data support that such an extended lymphadenectomy prolongs survival and, on the contrary, we fear that these procedures could lead to postoperative morbidity, such as chylous fistula or infected intraabdominal collections. We also note the long median hospital stay (20 days) reported by the authors (Table 1.6) when compared with the relatively low rate of pancreatic fistula (15 %), and we wonder why the hospital stay is so prolonged.

Commentary

3

Thilo Hackert, Jens Werner, and Markus W. Büchler

3.1 Relevant Basic Information, Indication and Contraindication

Diagnosis of pancreatic cancer is usually made by high-resolution, thin sliced, contrast-enhanced, multiphase Computed tomography (CT) as the standard tool. We use magnetic resonance imaging (MRI) only in situations when CT cannot be performed (e.g. due to contrast medium allergy/renal failure). Our initial approach is, thus, comparable to the standard procedure in Magdeburg. Evaluation of the pancreatic tumor by CT can be done with a high local resolution that allows very accurate imaging of soft tissue and vascular structures, as well as the presence/absence of liver metastases. To improve quality, the CT protocol includes the so-called "hydro-technique" (Grenacher and Klauss 2009) which involves oral water intake (one liter or more) and the intravenous administration of buscopan (10 mg) prior to the examination to achieve maximum distension of the stomach and duodenum, thereby achieving a negative contrast inside the lumen. In addition, the patient is placed in an oblique, 30°, right-sided down position (Fig. 3.1).

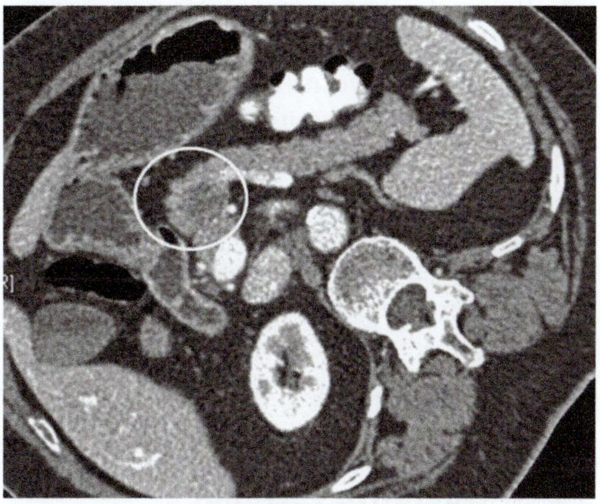

Fig. 3.1 High-resolution CT scan, hydro technique with 30° right-sided position of the patient showing a hypodense tumor in the pancreatic head (*white circle*)

Criteria for resectability are the absence of metastases (liver/peritoneal) and no evident involvement of the central arterial vessels (celiac trunk, superior mesenteric artery). In the latter case, neoadjuvant treatment is initiated with the aim of downstaging the disease for a potential secondary resection. Portal and mesenteric vein involvement are not necessarily regarded as a contraindication, regardless of the extent of tumor infiltration.

Further diagnostic procedures, such as endoscopic ultrasonography and ERCP, are not mandatory. We do not favor stent placement in the bile duct unless the serum bilirubin levels exceed 300 µmol/l, which is usually associated with impairment of liver function and especially coagulation (van der Gaag et al. 2010). In contrast, when the operation has to be postponed because

T. Hackert • J. Werner
Department of Surgery, University of Heidelberg, Im Neuenheimer Feld 110, 69120 Heidelberg, Germany

M.W. Büchler, M.D. (✉)
Professor of Surgery, Chair, Department of Surgery, University of Heidelberg, 69120 Heidelberg, Germany
e-mail: markus_buechler@med.uni-heidelberg.de

R. Mantke et al. (eds.), *International Practices in Pancreatic Surgery*,
DOI 10.1007/978-3-540-74506-8_3,

of cholangitis, neoadjuvant treatment, or need for more medical evaluation and treatment, cholestasis should be relieved before the operation. In these situations, a stent is inserted by endoscopic techniques or transhepatically, and the operation is delayed until the serum bilirubin decreases to <150 μmol/l. Most other patients are operated as soon as possible.

Preoperative tissue diagnosis by endoscopic or percutaneous five needle aspiration is only required in patients who are scheduled for neoadjuvant or palliative treatment, or if the nature of the tumor remains unclear (e.g. no increase in serum CA 19-9 level or unclear radiologic findings).

Concerning patient age, we have no routine cutoff, although 80 years represents a relative age after which a more critical reflection of the patient's condition, symptoms, and perioperative risk profile are considered (Makary et al. 2006). Biologic age and co-morbidities of the patient become the major factors that determine the decision for operative exploration or alternative palliative treatment in case of contraindications that are not directly tumor-related.

3.2 Operative Technique

Our standard approach to pancreatic head neoplasms is the pylorus-preserving partial pancreatoduodenectomy. We perform >90 % of all head resections with preservation of the pylorus; a classic pancreatoduodenectomy procedure with antrectomy is limited to patients with tumor spread toward the pylorus, suspicious lymph nodes in this area, or a history of peptic ulcers. The incision is not standardized. A midline laparotomy is preferred in non-obese patients, because this incision provides a more comfortable exposure during the phase of pancreaticojejunostomy; however, in obese patients, a transverse incision offers better exposure during the resection.

Regarding the resection itself, two approaches have been developed and are used increasingly in our clinical routine. The "standard" resection can be facilitated by the "uncinate-first approach" (Hackert et al. 2010), which involves the retrograde resection of the pancreatic head. The rationale for this approach is to begin the resection at

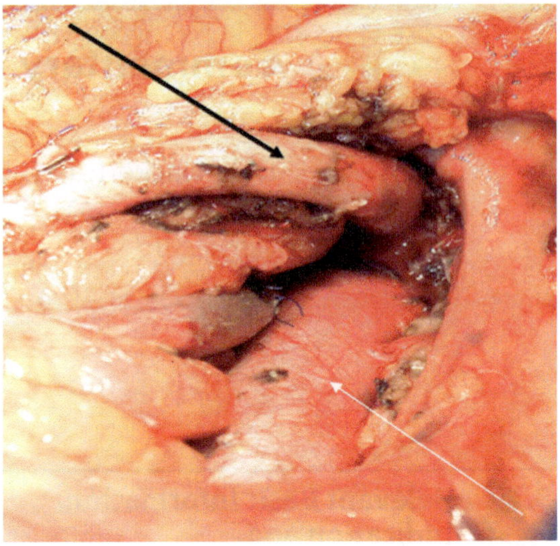

Fig. 3.2 "Artery-first approach" with exposition of the superior mesenteric artery from the left side (*black arrow*: superior mesenteric artery; *white arrow*: aorta)

the first jejunal loop with transposition of the specimen to the right aspect of the celiac axis. The resection is then carried out caudo-cranially under optimal vision of the superior mesenteric vein and artery to allow clear margins and excellent control of potential bleeding. From our experience, this is a very convenient and safe procedure.

The second newer technique is the "artery-first approach" (Weitz et al. 2010). The essential step during this procedure is dissection of the superior mesenteric artery beginning from the left side of the mesenteric axis. The artery is exposed down to its origin so that tumor adherence can be excluded safely and before any other definitive steps of the resection have taken place (Fig. 3.2). This approach is especially appropriate in patients in whom arterial involvement remains unclear in the preoperative evaluation.

Transection of the neck of the pancreas anterior to the portal vein can be performed before completing the dissection along the portal vein or may be done as the last step of the procedure. We prefer to place sutures at the superior and inferior pancreatic margin on both sides of the transection line. This maneuver offers control of bleeding from the vessels in these regions and can be used to lift up the pancreatic remnant during the further mobilization of the body of the gland. We do not use electrocautery for control of bleeding on the

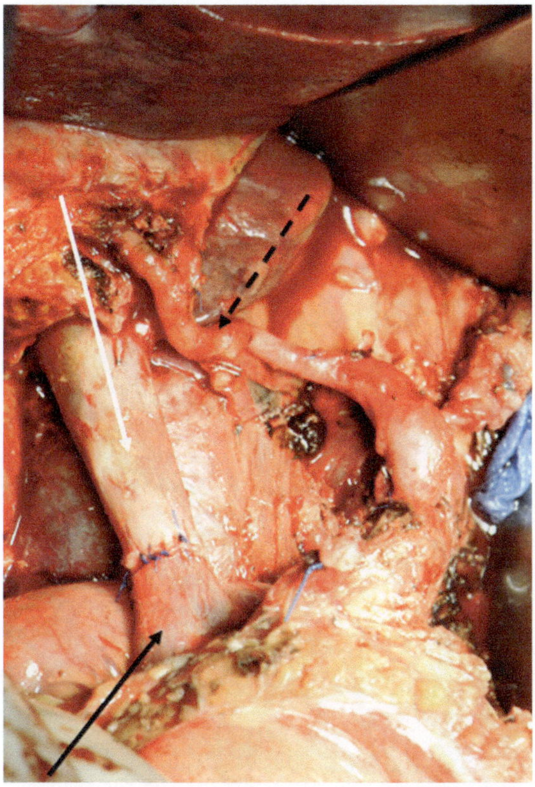

Fig. 3.3 Portal vein reconstruction during total pancreatectomy. End-to-end anastomosis between superior mesenteric vein (*black arrow*) and portal vein (*white arrow*), *broken black arrow*: proper hepatic artery

cut surface of the remnant; instead, atraumatic, non-resorbable sutures are the standard for this step of the operation.

When there is involvement of the superior mesenteric or portal vein, we prefer a reconstruction by direct suture of the vein, either as mentioned in the Magdeburg approach by a lateral venorrhaphy, or when necessary, by an end-to-end anastomosis. For both techniques, non-resorbable suture material (e.g. 5-0 polypropylene) is used with intraoperative assessment of blood flow after the reconstruction (Fig. 3.3). From our experience, a venous or synthetic graft is rarely necessary. To gain enough mobility of the distal superior mesenteric vein for a tension-free anastomosis, it is essential to mobilize the root of the mesentery completely. This technique is accomplished by dividing the attachment of the mesentery of the ileum and right colon from the retroperitoneal plane up to the base of the small bowel mesentery with antero-rostral elevation of the small bowel. After complete mobilization, portal vein defects of 4–5 cm can usually be bridged without any tension.

Our standard lymphadenectomy during partial pancreatoduodenectomy includes the lymph nodes in the hepatoduodenal ligament (group 12), and those nodes along the common hepatic artery (group 8), portal vein (group 12), and the cranial portion of superior mesenteric vein (group 4–6), as well as right-sided lymph nodes of the celiac trunk (group 9) and the right side of the superior mesenteric artery (group 3) (Adler et al. 2007; Japan Pancreas Society 2003).

The impact of extended lymph node dissection (i.e. paraaortic nodes in the aortocaval groove, left-side of the celiac trunk, and the left side of the superior mesenteric artery) has been well investigated in four, randomized, controlled trials between 1998 and 2005 examining survival (Pedrazzoli et al. 1998; Yeo et al. 1999; Farnell et al. 2005; Nimura et al. 2004). Although there were differences in the studies with regard to the number of resected lymph nodes (20 vs. up to 40), three of the studies showed no survival advantage, either in N0 nor in N1 patients who underwent a standard or extended resections. Only Pedrazzoli et al. (1998) found a survival benefit of 7 months in the subgroup analysis for N1 patients who underwent extended resection. Moreover, all groups except for Pedrazzoli et al. observed a markedly increased morbidity and decreased quality of life in the postoperative follow-up related to diarrhea, nutritional difficulties, etc. A metaanalysis published in 2007 (Michalski et al. 2007) analyzed these studies – including an overall number of 297 vs. 311 patients – with regard to their scientific quality and results. No benefit for such an extended lymphadenectomy could be determined concerning either local tumor control or survival. Furthermore, an increased rate of perioperative complications and a decreased quality of life were demonstrated. Therefore, with regard to these studies and consequently based on a level 1 evidence, the concept of ultra-radical lymphadenectomy should be abandoned, and a defined standardized lymph node dissection should be performed during partial pancreatoduodenectomy (Fig. 3.4).

We maintain that the most important operative step in preventing severe postoperative complications is the pancreaticojejunostomy. We prefer to perform the anastomosis end-to-side in a two-layer fashion suturing the pancreatic duct separately (Figs. 3.5, 3.6, and 3.7). Three atraumatic, resorbable sutures are placed at the anterior and posterior aspect of the pancreatic duct at the beginning. These sutures are later integrated in the inner suture row. The outer row is performed with interrupted, 5-0 PDS sutures between the pancreatic capsula and the seromuscular layer of the jejunum. After incision in the jejunal wall, the second back row is performed with interrupted sutures which incorporates the previously placed posterior ductal stitches. The anterior wall of the anastomosis is sutured in a similar fashion with two layers of interrupted stitches. We do not use intraductal stents in the pancreatic duct because of concerns that they tend to obstruct the outflow in small diameter ducts. Using our technique, rates of Grade Band C leaks occur in about 3 % (Büchler et al. 2003; Wente et al. 2006). Bile duct reconstruction is standardized by a one-layer, end-to-side technique using resorbable monofilament sutures approximately 10–15 cm distal to the pancreatic anastomosis to minimize the risk of bile reflux toward the pancreas. An end-to-side duodenojejunostomy completes the reconstruction. Recent studies have shown that an antecolic reconstruction is more favorable in terms of preventing delayed gastric emptying (Hartel et al. 2005). Two closed suction drains (12 mm, EasyFlow®) are used routinely and positioned near the pancreatic anastomosis and in the subhepatic space from the right side of the abdomen. Drain removal, which can usually be done

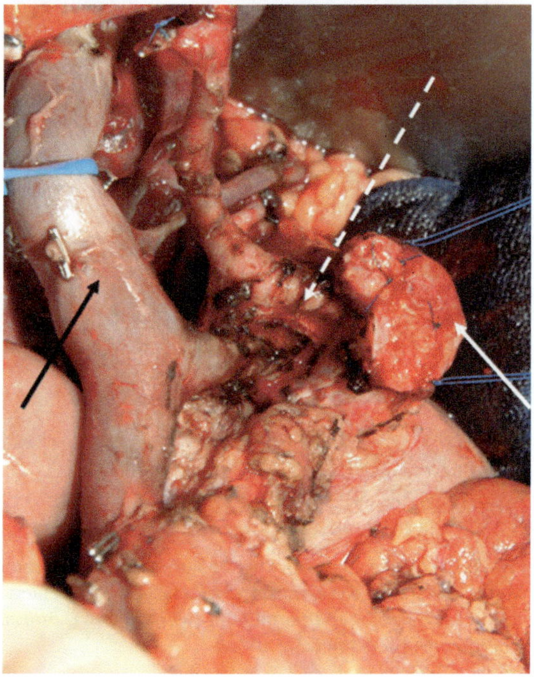

Fig. 3.4 Situs after partial duodeno-pancreatectomy with standardized lymphadenectomy. Dissection has been performed along the portal vein (*black arrow*) and right side of the celiac axis (*broken white arrow*), *white arrow*: pancreatic remnant

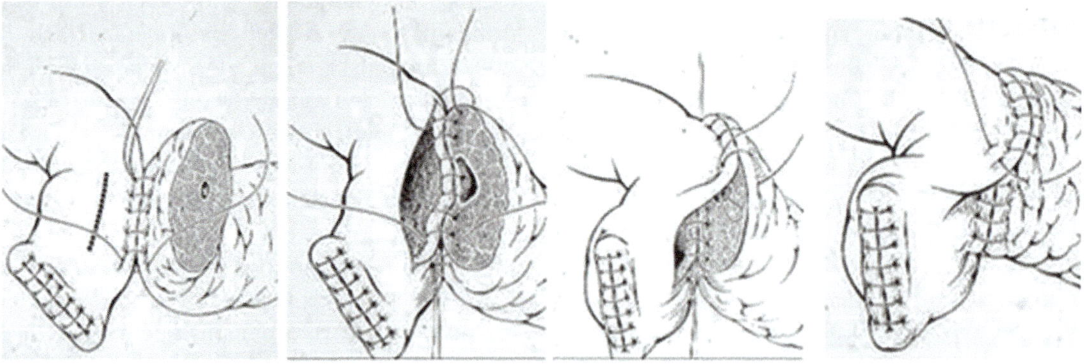

Fig. 3.5 Scheme of the anastomosis technique showing the two layer suture of the posterior wall (*two left pictures*) and the anterior wall (*two right pictures*)

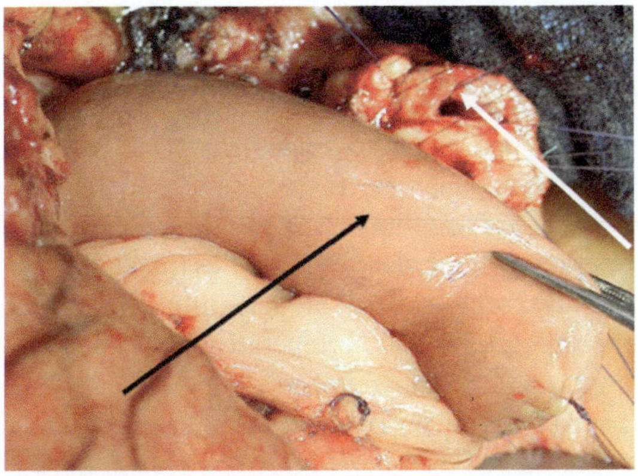

Fig. 3.6 Intraoperative situs during pancreatico-jejunostomy. Prepared duct sutures (*white arrow*) and jejunal loop (*black arrow*)

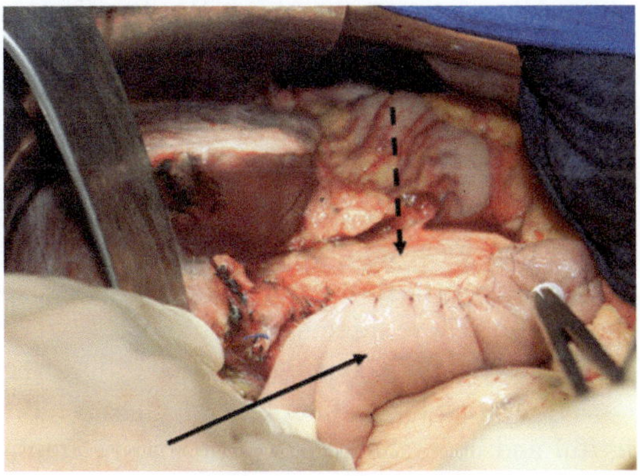

Fig. 3.7 Intraoperative situs of the completed end-to-side pancreatico-jejunostomy. *Black arrow*: jejunal loop, *broken black arrow*: pancreatic remnant

48 h postoperatively, should be preceded by analysis of pancreatic enzyme levels in the drain fluid (Bassi et al. 2010).

The perioperative management includes perioperative, prophylactic antibiotics using mezlocillin (or ciprofloxacin in case of penicillin allergy) and metronidazole beginning before the operation, and repeated just once after 4 h. We do not use prophylactic, perioperative octreotide as a routine procedure unless the pancreas has a soft tissue texture intraoperatively. In these cases, octreotide is administered during the operation and continued for 5 days at a dosage of 200 μg 3 times/day. Because of good evidence from a recent metaanalysis (Gurusamy et al. 2010) that routine perioperative octreotide prophylaxis does not prevent pancreatic leakage, we believe that the use of octreotide should be restricted to individual situations and only if the surgeon classifies the pancreatic anastomosis as "high risk" due to soft tissue and a small diameter pancreatic duct.

A nasogastric tube is inserted at the beginning of the operation under general anesthesia and removed at the end of the operation. Oral intake of fluids is allowed beginning on the first postoperative day with progression to a more regular diet by about the fifth postoperative day.

For neoplasms of the body and tail of the pancreas, similar diagnostic measures are used as described above for pancreatic head neoplasms. We do not use diagnostic laparoscopy routinely and only when there is strong suspicion of tumor spread to the peritoneal cavity when there is a markedly increased serum CA 19-9 level without visible extrapancreatic spread or ascites on the CT. If there are no contraindications, distal pancreatectomy is performed by an open approach via a median or transverse laparotomy, depending on individual patient anatomy.

Distal pancreatectomy for oncologic indications always includes splenectomy to achieve a radical resection and a sufficient lymphadenectomy. After dissection of the superior mesenteric and portal mesenteric vein, the neck of the pancreas is transected. We prefer sharp transaction of the pancreatic neck for several reasons. First, the results of the recently completed DISPACT study (Diener et al. 2011) did not show any advantage of closure of the stump of the pancreatic remnant with a mechanical stapler, and second, the use of staplers may be contraindicated in thick or fibrotic glands. After dissection, bleeding is controlled by individual, non-resorbable atraumatic sutures (e.g. 5-0 Novafil). The pancreatic duct is cannulated, and if there is free passage toward the duodenum, the duct is closed selectively with a Z-shaped suture. The cut surface is then oversewn systematically using U- or Z-shaped sutures of slowly absorbable monofilament (e.g. 5-0 PDS). We do not use any synthetic patches for sealing of the pancreas. If possible, the falciform ligament is mobilized and transposed through the lesser omentum to serve as an autogenous tissue

Results from Heidelberg 01/2006–12/2008

Parameter	Number	%
Patients	537	100
Pylorus-preserving pancreatoduodenectomy	287	53.4
Classic pancreatoduodenectomy (including antrectomy)	40	7.4
Total pancreatectomy	82	15.3
Distal pancreatectomy	128	23.9
30-day mortality	15	2.8
Hospital stay (median, IQR)	12 (10–17)	
Tumor stage (UICC)		
0	24	4.5
I	13	2.4
II	438	81.6
III	45	8.4
IV	17	3.1
R0	194	36.1
R1[a]	327	60.9
R2	16	3.0
Morbidity		
Postoperative bleeding	34	6.3
Pancreatic fistula (grades B and C)	23	4.2
DGE	125	23.9
Wound infection	16	3.0

[a]According to Esposito et al. (2008)

patch and fixed with resorbable sutures on the posterior and anterior aspect of the cut surface of the pancreatic stump.

The lymphadenectomy during distal pancreatectomy includes the lymph nodes in the hepatoduodenal ligament, the celiac trunk, and the left side of the superior mesenteric artery. In addition, all fat and soft tissue on the anterior aspect of Gerota's fascia is removed en bloc with the specimen and the spleen. Usually 25–30 lymph nodes are included in the specimen for histopathologic evaluation. During the lymph node dissection of the hepatoduodenal ligament, a cholecystectomy is performed routinely.

At the end of the operation, two closed suction drains (12 mm, EasyFlow®) are placed routinely near the pancreatic stump and in the subdiaphragmatic space from the left side of the abdomen. Drain removal is preceded by analysis of pancreatic enzyme levels in the drain fluid and can usually be performed 72–96 h postoperatively.

The perioperative management of patients after distal pancreatectomy is similar to that after partial pancreatoduodenectomy in terms of perioperative, prophylactic antibiotics (mezlocillin or ciprofloxacin in case of penicillin allergy and metronidazole) and perioperative octreotide prophylaxis if the pancreas has a soft texture intraoperatively. The nasogastric tube inserted at the beginning of the operation is removed at the end of the operation. Oral intake of the patients is allowed on the first postoperative day with fluid, and the diet is advanced quickly.

For histopathologic evaluation of the pancreatic cancer specimen, the revised R1 classification is used in Heidelberg (Esposito et al. 2008). This staging includes an R1 classification whenever tumor cells are close to (<1 mm) or infiltrate the resection margin, which leads to a substantially greater proportion of R1 resections in our patient cohort due to a large number of specimens in which tumor cells do not infiltrate but are close to the margin. These resections would be classified as R0 resections in other institutions; however, we believe that the new R1 classification is more useful and accurate regarding prognostic implications and have implemented this standardized definition since 2005.

References

Adler G, Seufferlein T, Bischoff SC et al (2007) S3-Guidelines "exocrine pancreatic cancer" 2007. Z Gastroenterol 45:487–523

Bassi C, Molinari E, Malleo G, Crippa S, Butturini G, Salvia R, Talamini G, Pederzoli P (2010) Early versus late drain removal after standard pancreatic resections: results of a prospective randomized trial. Ann Surg 252(2):207–214

Büchler MW, Wagner M, Schmied BM et al (2003) Changes in morbidity after pancreatic resection: toward the end of completion pancreatectomy. Arch Surg 138(12):1310–1314, discussion 1315

Diener MK, Seiler CM, Rossion I et al (2011) Efficacy of stapler versus hand-sewn closure after distal pancreatectomy (DISPACT): a randomised, controlled multicentre trial. Lancet. 2011 Apr 30;377(9776): 1514–22.

Esposito I, Kleeff J, Bergmann F, Reiser C, Herpel E, Friess H, Schirmacher P, Büchler MW (2008) Most pancreatic cancer resections are R1 resections. Ann Surg Oncol 15(6):1651–1660

Farnell MB, Pearson RK, Sarr MG, DiMagno EP, Burgart LJ, Dahl TR, Foster N, Sargent DJ, Pancreas Cancer Working Group (2005) A prospective randomized trial comparing standard pancreatoduodenectomy with pancreatoduodenectomy with extended lymphadenectomy in resectable pancreatic head adenocarcinoma. Surgery 138(4):618–628

Grenacher L, Klauss M (2009) Computed tomography of pancreatic tumors. Radiologe 49(2):107–123, Review

Gurusamy KS, Koti R, Fusai G, Davidson BR (2010). Somatostatin analogues for pancreatic surgery. Cochrane Database Syst Rev. (2):CD008370. Review

Hackert T, Werner J, Weitz J, Schmidt J, Büchler MW (2010) Uncinate process first – a novel approach for pancreatic head resection. Langenbecks Arch Surg 395(8):1161–1164, Epub 2010 Jun 27

Hartel M, Wente MN, Hinz U, Kleeff J, Wagner M, Müller MW, Friess H, Büchler MW (2005) Effect of antecolic reconstruction on delayed gastric emptying after the pylorus-preserving Whipple procedure. Arch Surg 140(11):1094–1099

Japan Pancreas Society (2003) Classification of pancreatic carcinoma, 2nd edn. Kanehara, Tokyo

Makary MA, Winter JM, Cameron JL, Campbell KA, Chang D, Cunningham SC, Riall TS, Yeo CJ (2006) Pancreaticoduodenectomy in the very elderly. J Gastrointest Surg 10(3):347–356

Michalski CW, Kleeff J, Wente MN, Diener MK, Büchler MW, Friess H (2007) Systematic review and meta-analysis of standard and extended lymphadenectomy in pancreaticoduodenectomy for pancreatic cancer. Br J Surg 94(3):265–273

Nimura Y, Nagino M, Kato H, Miyagawa S, Yamaguchi A, Kinoshita T et al (2004) Regional versus extended lymph node dissection in radical pancreaticoduodenectomy for pancreatic cancer: a multicenter, randomized controlled trial. HPB (Oxford) 6(Suppl 1):2

Pedrazzoli S, DiCarlo V, Dionigi R, Mosca F, Pederzoli P, Pasquali C, Klöppel G, Dhaene K, Michelassi F (1998) Standard versus extended lymphadenectomy associated with pancreatoduodenectomy in the surgical treatment of adenocarcinoma of the head of the pancreas: a multicenter, prospective, randomized study. Lymphadenectomy Study Group. Ann Surg 228(4): 508–517

van der Gaag NA, Rauws EA, van Eijck CH, Bruno MJ, van der Harst E, Kubben FJ, Gerritsen JJ, Greve JW, Gerhards MF, de Hingh IH, Klinkenbijl JH, Nio CY, de Castro SM, Busch OR, van Gulik TM, Bossuyt PM, Gouma DJ (2010) Preoperative biliary drainage for cancer of the head of the pancreas. N Engl J Med 362(2):129–137

Weitz J, Rahbari N, Koch M, Buchler MW (2010) The "artery first" approach for resection of pancreatic head cancer. J Am Coll Surg 210:e1–e4

Wente MN, Shrikhande SV, Kleeff J et al (2006) Management of early hemorrhage from pancreatic anastomoses after pancreaticoduodenectomy. Dig Surg 23(4):203–208, Epub 2006 Jul 26

Yeo CJ, Cameron JL, Sohn TA, Coleman J, Sauter PK, Hruban RH, Pitt HA, Lillemoe KD (1999) Pancreaticoduodenectomy with or without extended retroperitoneal lymphadenectomy for periampullary adenocarcinoma: comparison of morbidity and mortality and short-term outcome. Ann Surg 229(5):613–622, discussion 622–624

4 Commentary

Philippe Bachellier, E. Rosso, and D. Jaeck

4.1 Comments

The chapter entitled "Surgery of pancreatic carcinoma" by Mantke and Lippert reflects their personal experience; their recommendations are supported by the reputation of their institution, the literature, and the excellent results reported. In our department, the standard pancreatic resection is performed in a similar way to that described by the authors; however, some differences should be underlined:

1. We perform mainly the classic Kausch-Whipple procedure for pancreatic cancer instead of the pylorus-preserving pancreatoduodenectomy (PD). In our experience, the partial gastrectomy allows a better extended lymphadenectomy and also decreases the rate of delayed gastric emptying.
2. The "superior mesenteric artery (SMA) first approach" is performed systematically.
3. The lymphadenectomy is "extended", including the lymph nodes of the hepatic pedicle, the celiac trunk up to its origin on the aorta, the root of the mesentery, and the interaortocaval area.
4. Pancreatic reconstruction is achieved by a double-layer, invaginated, pancreatogastrostomy which, in our hands, has decreased the rate of pancreatic fistula as well as the re-laparotomy rate after pancreatoduodenectomy.

4.2 Standard Pancreatoduodenectomy

A high-quality, multiphase, contrast-enhanced, thin-section, helical-CT including angio-CT constitutes the main preoperative, radiologic investigation adopted in order to choose the therapeutic strategy for patients with pancreatic cancer, particularly, in case of vascular involvement.

We have developed a "vascular" approach for pancreatic resection for cancer. Indeed, the plane of dissection during PD is the tunica adventitia of the SMA, which is identified at its origin on the aorta at the beginning of the operation (the "artery first" approach) (Fig. 4.1). For a small tumor in the head of the pancreas without portal vein involvement, only the right border of the SMA is skeletonized from its origin on the aorta to the root of the mesentery, including a right splanchnicectomy (Fig. 4.2a).

The duodenum is mobilized with a Kocher maneuver starting from the inferior edge of the foramen of Winslow and continuing downward along the posterior plane to the Treitz fascia and includes all the tissue covering the inferior vena cava and the left renal vein. The right colon and the root of the mesentery are mobilized allow-

P. Bachellier, M.D., Ph.D. (✉) • E. Rosso, M.D. •
D. Jaeck, M.D., Ph.D., FRCS
Service de Chirurgie Générale, Pancréatique, Hépatique et Transplantation, Hopital de Hautepierre, avenue Molière, 67098 Strasbourg, France
e-mail: philippe.bachellier@chru-strasbourg.fr

R. Mantke et al. (eds.), *International Practices in Pancreatic Surgery*,
DOI 10.1007/978-3-540-74506-8_4, © Springer-Verlag Berlin Heidelberg 2013

ing excellent exposure of the aortocaval area. At this time, the right colon and the small intestine are lifted anteriorly and are kept so retracted by the first assistant by placing his two hands, one on each side of the SMA. The origin of the SMA is exposed where the left renal vein crosses the aorta (Fig. 4.1). Dissection of the SMA continues along the plane of the adventitia up to the junction of the third and fourth parts of the duodenum. In the presence of a replaced right hepatic artery arising from the SMA, its origin is identified easily at this time of the dissection. Once proximal control of the SMA is obtained, distal control is secured by identifying the SMA below the transverse colon along the left border of the superior mesenteric vein (SMV) (Fig. 4.3). The Treitz ligament is divided, then the lymphovascular tissue of the anterior side of the root of the mesentery is divided between thin ligatures, plane-by-plane, until the SMV is identified and controlled by a vessel loop. The SMA is now identified and encircled with a vessel loop. In case of malignant invasion of the mesentericoportal axis, the root of the transverse mesocolon is divided preserving the Riolan arcade. Therefore, the middle colic artery is ligated proximally and divided at its origin on the SMA distally, proximal to the anastomotic arcades between the right and left colic arteries.

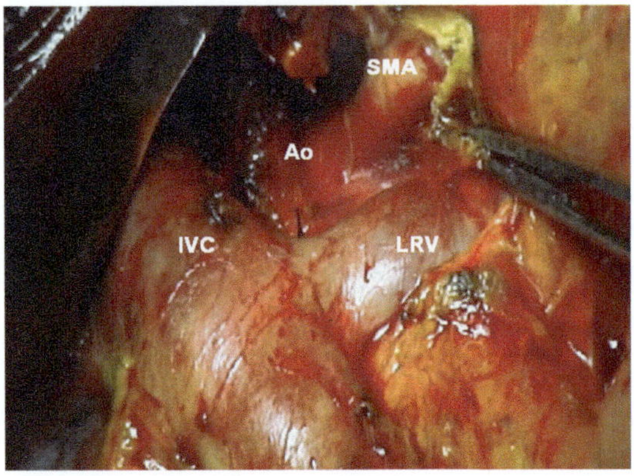

Fig. 4.1 Intraoperative views of "the artery first approach". The origin of the SMA is exposed at the point where the left renal vein crosses the aorta. *IVC* inferior vena cava, *LRV* left renal vein, *Ao* aorta, *SMA* superior mesenteric artery

Attention is then directed toward the hepatic pedicle. The bile duct, portal vein, right and left branches of the hepatic artery, hepatic artery, origin of the splenic artery, left gastric artery, and celiac trunk are skeletonized in order to remove not only the lymph nodes but all the nervous and lymphatic tissue as well (Fig. 4.2b). The right gastric artery is ligated and divided at its origin.

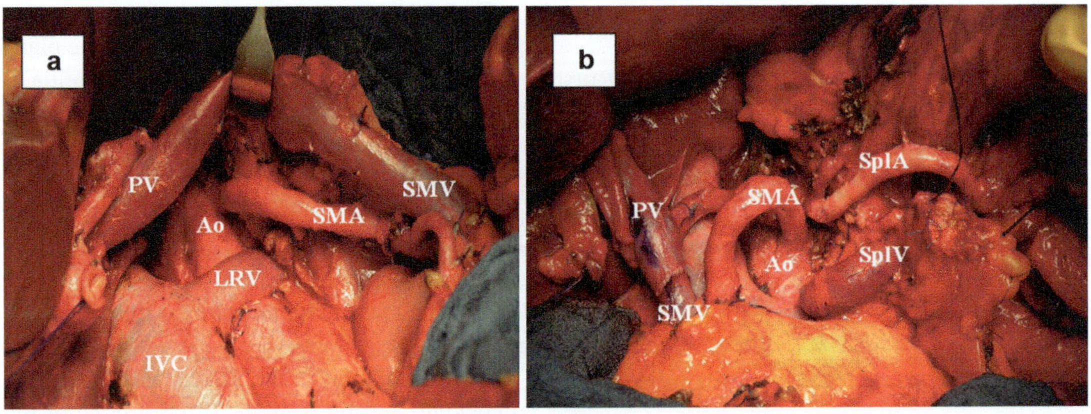

Fig. 4.2 Intraoperative view of: (**a**) pancreatoduodenectomy without portal vein resection. The right border of the SMA is skeletonized from its origin from the aorta to the root of the mesentery including a right splanchnicectomy. (**b**) Pancreatoduodenectomy with portal vein resection. *SMV* superior mesenteric vein. The SMA is skeletonized on both sides from its origin on the aorta to the root of the mesentery including a bilateral splanchnicectomy. *SMA* superior mesenteric artery, *PV* portal vein, *Ao* aorta, *IVC* inferior vena cava, *LRV* left renal vein, *SplA* splenic artery, *SplV* splenic vein

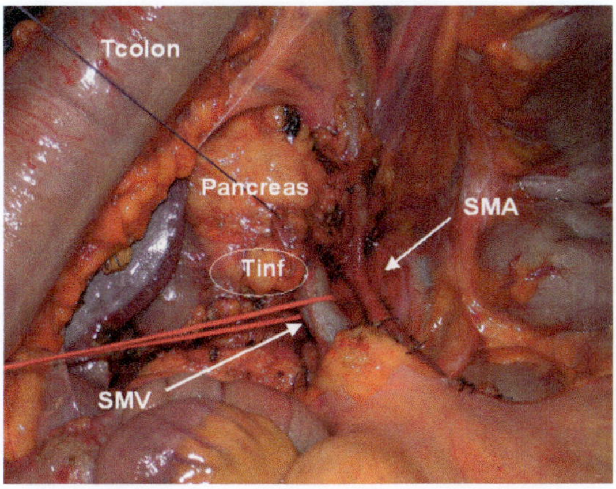

Fig. 4.3 Intraoperative view of the SMV and SMA dissected in the root of the mesentery below the transverse colon and at a distance from the tumour. *SMA* superior mesenteric artery, *SMV* superior mesenteric vein, *Tinf* tumor infiltration, *Tcolon* transverse colon

The gastroduodenal artery is dissected, and a trial of clamping is performed before ligation of the gastroduodenal artery to determine if a clinically-relevant celiac trunk stenosis is present. When the pulse in the hepatic artery disappears during the trial of clamping, the arcuate ligament is sectioned. If the hepatic artery remains pulseless, stenosis of the celiac trunk should be suspected and treated accordingly (jump graft to hepatic artery or endarterectomy). The above mentioned conditions should be identified on the pre-operative CT; indeed, most cases of celiac artery stenosis can be treated pre-operatively by interventional radiology (dilation, stent, etc.). When the clamping test is negative, the gastroduodenal artery is double-ligated and divided.

The stomach is first transected using a linear stapler, and the pancreas is divided with a surgical knife with a frozen section performed. The proximal jejunum is transected using a linear stapler after which its mesentery is divided up to the first jejunal branch which is divided. This maneuver reaches the distal part of the SMA at the point where it was tagged at the beginning of the operation. The inferior pancreatoduodenal artery is identified, double-ligated, and divided. At this stage of the operation, the dissection is tailored accordingly to the need (or not) of a portal vein resection.

The proximal jejunum is passed behind the mesenteric root to the right side. The inferior pancreatoduodenal veins and all the small tributaries to the PV are ligated individually and divided. The PV is retracted with an eyelid retractor to the left side. The right and posterior side of the SMA is dissected toward the aorta removing all the neurolymphatic tissue covering the SMA and the origin of the celiac trunk (Fig. 4.2a). Special attention should be paid during this step to preserve a replaced right hepatic artery arising from the SMA. The final step is the division of the bile duct immediately below the biliary duct confluence. A sample of bile is obtained for bacteriologic examination.

4.3 Extended Pancreatoduodenectomy

Tumor invasion of the mesentericoportal (MP) axis is a frequent event in pancreatic cancer and should not be considered a contraindication to a curative resection. The operative strategy, however, should be tailored and adapted according to the extent of the venous invasion as shown by the pre-operative CT. In case of radiologic contact between the tumor and the mesentericoportal axis without narrowing of the vein (Nakao type A) or unilateral narrowing of the mesentericoportal axis (Nakao type B), venous resection can be planned preoperatively and performed. In contrast, for borderline resect able or locally advanced pancreatic cancer with bilateral narrowing (Nakao type C) or venous occlusion (Nakao type D) of the mesentericoportal axis, the resection is contraindicated initially. Preoperative chemotherapy should be administered to these patients for about 3 months, then resection can be re-evaluated in case of disease stability or response. Similarly, radiologic involvement of the hepatic artery or of the superior mesenteric artery does not constitute an absolute contraindication to pancreatic resection provided: (1) the tumor has not progressed after neoadjuvant chemotherapy, and (2) the resection can be performed safely

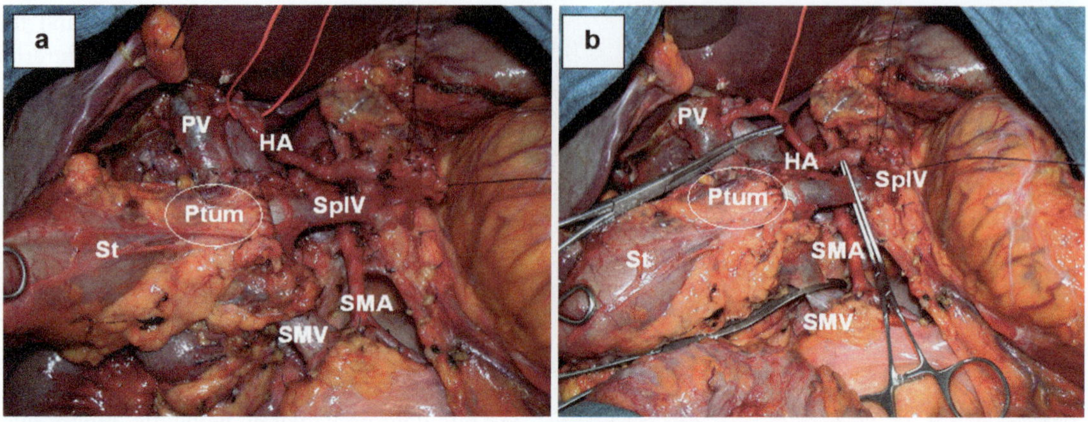

Fig. 4.4 Intraoperative views of the final step of a pancreatoduodenectomy with portal vein resection (**a**) before and (**b**) after the positioning of vascular clamps. The specimen is attached only to the venous vascular axis and it is freed completely from the retro-portal attachments. *SMA* superior mesenteric artery, *SMV* superior mesenteric vein, *SplV* splenic vein, *HA* Hepatic artery, *PTum* pancreatic tumour, *St* stomach

with curative intent. In fact, only a minority of patients with a radiologic arterial involvement present true histologic invasion of the artery. Pre-operative radiotherapy is not performed due to the risk of damage to the vascular wall which constitutes a major obstacle in case of subsequent resection with venous or arterial resection and reconstruction.

4.4 Portal Vein Resection

During PD with venous resection, the main technical objectives to achieve a safe venous resection are:

1. to resect completely the retroportal lamina before performing the vascular resection in order to minimize the venous clamping time (Fig. 4.4).
2. to perform systematically a segmental venous resection. In the majority of the cases, there is no need for an interposition venous graft. Indeed, extensive mobilization of the mesenteric root as well as the complete lymphadenectomy of the area between the celiac trunk and the SMA, allows a tension-free anastomosis for up to 7 cm of venous resection.

The first part of the operation is performed as for a standard PD. After division of the proximal jejunum, the anterior and the left sides of the SMA are skeletonized up to the aorta. The right colon and the small bowel are retracted anteriorly as above. The proximal jejunum is pulled behind the mesenteric root. The posterior and right side of the SMA is skeletonized up to the aorta, thereby performing a bilateral splanchnicectomy. The common hepatic duct is divided immediately below the hepatic hilum. At this point of the dissection, the specimen is attached exclusively by the mesentericoportal axis. The venous axis is clamped above and below the zone of invasion, and then divided. A direct, end-to-end venous anastomosis is performed using 6/0 non-absorbable suture (Fig. 4.4). In case of resection of the venous trifurcation (spleno-mesenterico-portal axis), we usually reimplant the splenic vein to avoid left-sided portal hypertension. If the length of the splenic vein resection does not exceed 3 cm, the splenic vein is sutured to the SMV in a double lumen fashion and re-implanted on the PV. If the length of the splenic vein resection exceeds 3 cm, two options can be considered:

1. If the inferior mesenteric vein is still draining the splenic vein, re-implantation of the splenic vein is not necessary.
2. If the inferior mesenteric vein has been resected, then two vascular anastomoses have to be performed, the first between the PV and the SMV and the second between the splenic vein and the inferior mesenteric vein (Fig. 4.5).

A special approach is required for patients with type C (bilateral narrowing) venous

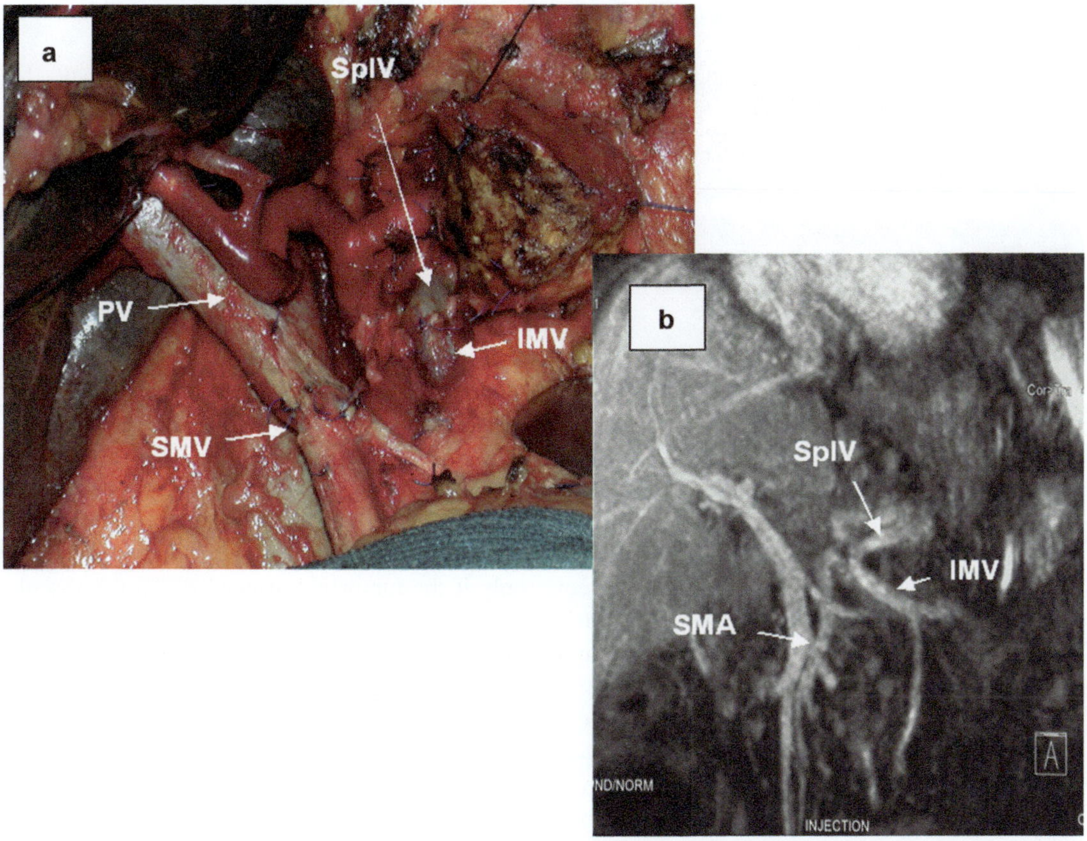

Fig. 4.5 Intraoperative view (**a**) and post-operative MRI (**b**) after pancreatoduodenectomy with resection of the spleno-mesenterico-portal axis. Two vascular anastomoses are shown, the first between the *PV* and the *SMV* and the second between the *SplV* and the *IMV*; in order to avoid left-sided portal hypertension. *PV* portal vein, *SMV* superior mesenteric vein, *IMV* inferior mesenteric vein, *SMA* superior mesenteric artery

involvement and with type D (venous occlusion) with the presence of collateral circulation persisting after neo-adjuvant chemotherapy. In such cases, the dissection around the pancreas determinates a gradual interruption of the collateral venous circulation for the liver and the gut, causing prolonged hepatic venous ischemia and a gut congestion. Therefore, in order to avoid the above mentioned potentially lethal intra-operative complications, a temporary mesenterico-portal shunt (TMPS) is performed using a prosthesis of 20 cm ePTFE (FEP*Ringed Gore-Tex®, WL Gore and Associates) (diameter 14–20 mm) which is inserted between the distal stump of the PV and the proximal stump of the SMV by two, end-to-end anastomoses with 5/0 non-absorbable monofilament running sutures. The anastomosis between the SMV and the distal side of the prosthesis is performed first, to preserve as much as possible portal flow to the liver from the bowel through the splenic vein. Subsequently, the hilar PV is clamped and divided. The venous stumps on the specimen side are sutured. Finally the anastomosis between the hilar PV and the proximal side of the prosthesis is achieved. The distal clamp is removed from the SMV to purge the prosthesis. Then, the proximal clamp is removed from the PV: the temporary shunt is now operational. The PD is completed as above, and the specimen is removed en-bloc with the involved tract of the PV/SMV. After clamping the PV and the SMV, the Gore-Tex® shunt is removed and a direct, end-to-end anastomosis between the PV and

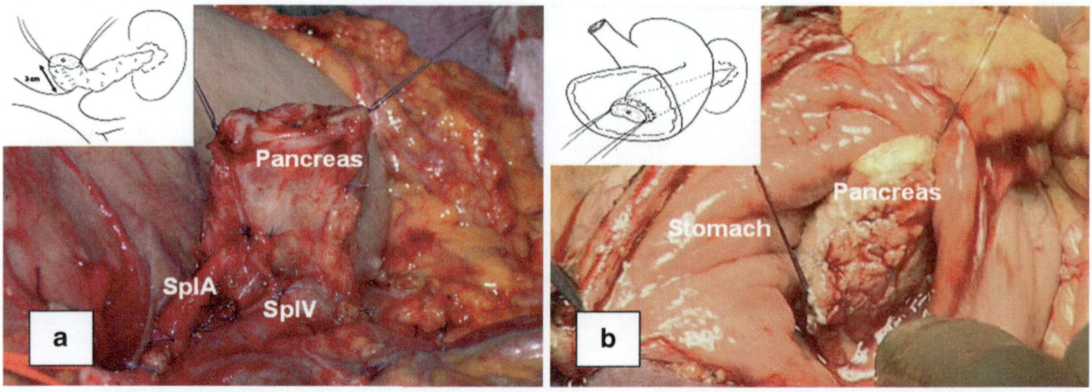

Fig. 4.6 Intraoperative views of a pancreaticogastrostomy. (**a**) The pancreatic stump is dissected for about 3 cm from the *SplV*. (**b**) The pancreatic stump is telescoped in the stomach. *SplV* splenic vein, *SplA* splenic artery

SMV is performed with a 6/0 non-absorbable monofilament running suture. Finally a direct end-to-end anastomosis without graft interposition is performed between the splenic vein and the inferior mesenteric vein.

4.5 Arterial Resection

Pancreatic resection for persistent arterial invasion after neoadjuvant chemotherapy is considered only if a single artery is invaded, otherwise the tumor is considered unresectable with curative intent. The arterial resection is performed en-bloc with the pancreatic specimen to avoid the risk of tumor seeding and/or arterial damage. For arterial reconstruction requiring a graft interposition, an autologous vein (e.g. saphenous vein) is used preferentially. A synthetic interposition graft (Gore-Tex®) is avoided whenever possible. Vascular anastomoses are performed with 7/0–8/0 non-adsorbable monofilament running sutures using microsurgical instruments magnification. In patients requiring an associated portal vein resection, venous resection is performed after arterial resection/reconstruction and is conducted with portal vein occlusion but with preservation of the arterial hepatic flow. The most common presentations are: (1) invasion of a right hepatic artery originating from the SMA, (2) invasion of the common hepatic artery at the origin of the gastroduodenal artery, (3) invasion of the SMA, and (4) invasion on the CT. In the case of SMA or CT invasion, the resection is performed only if the tumor is "suspended" on the vascular axis. In the case of invasion of the aorta, resection in contraindicated. It should be emphasized that arterial reconstruction should be performed by surgeons with experience in both pancreatic and vascular surgery.

4.6 Reconstruction, Additional Medication, and Procedures

We use exclusively a double-layer, invaginated pancreatogastrostomy for pancreatic reconstruction (Fig. 4.6). In patients with a prior total gastrectomy, we adopt an invaginated, suture-free pancreatojejunostomy. Two abdominal drains are inserted routinely. Amylase activity in the drainage fluid is measured daily for the first 7 days. In case of pancreatic fistula, the drain is maintained in place until the complete healing of the pancreatic fistula. A postoperative abdominal CT is performed routinely prior to discharge.

4.7 Distal Pancreatectomy Without Portal Vein Invasion

After division of the gastrocolic ligament, the inferior border of the pancreas is dissected and the portal vein is freed from the posterior side of the pancreas. Lymphadenectomy with skeletonization of the hepatic artery, left gastric artery, and celiac trunk is performed. The splenic artery is double ligated and divided. The neck of the pancreas is transected using a Cavitron Ultrasonic Surgical Aspirator (CUSA®, Cavitron Lasersonics, Division of Cavitron Corp). The main pancreatic duct is identified and selectively suture-ligated. In case of a soft pancreatic parenchyma, the pancreatic stump is closed with a few non-adsorbable, invaginating sutures. The splenic vein is divided between ligatures. The SMA is identified and skeletonized on its left side up to its origin from the aorta (Fig. 4.3a). All the lymphovascular tissue on the left side of the celiac trunk and on the left side of the aorta is removed. Then we proceed in the same way as described by Mantke and Lippert.

4.8 Distal Pancreatectomy with Portal Vein Resection

In case of portal vein invasion after division of the neck of the pancreas, we proceed as described above for pancreatoduodenectomy with portal vein resection. The SMV is identified and encircled below the root of the transverse mesocolon. The middle colic artery is divided preserving the arcade of Riolan. The SMA is dissected on the left border of the SMV and skeletonized bilaterally up to its origin from the aorta removing entirely the retroportal lamina. The distal pancreas and the spleen are mobilized completely. The specimen is now attached only to the spleno-mesenterico-portal axis. The vascular axis is clamped above and below the zone of invasion, and a direct end-to-end anastomosis is performed using 6/0 non-absorbable suture. A note of caution should be mentioned; on the left side, vascular resections are more difficult to perform due to the reduced possibility of mobilization of the mesenteric root. Therefore, mobilization of the PV and of the SMV above and below the zone of invasion should be extensive. In case of persistent tension, we use the left renal vein as an interposition graft.

4.9 Arterial Resection (Appleby Procedure)

In case of invasion of the celiac trunk, an Appleby procedure may be considered as a curative resection. The common hepatic artery proximal to the gastroduodenal artery is dissected early during the operation. A clamping test of the common hepatic artery is then performed. If the pulse of the proper hepatic artery is still present and effective hepatic arterial flow is confirmed by the intra-operative Doppler sonography, then the common hepatic artery is divided below the origin of the gastroduodenal artery. The first part of the duodenum is divided with a linear stapler, the stomach is mobilized, and the distal esophagus is sectioned. Finally, the distal pancreas and the spleen are mobilized, and the celiac trunk is divided at its origin on the aorta. During the skeletonization of the SMA, meticulous attention should be paid to avoid injury of the pancreatoduodenal arteries (inferior and superior) on the right side of the SMA. If the pulse of the common hepatic artery is reduced, during the clamping test, then the procedure should be modified. The celiac trunk and the common hepatic artery should be divided only after the complete mobilization of the stomach and of the distal pancreas and after having obtained a saphenous graft. After removing the specimen, the common hepatic artery should be revascularized by reimplanting it into the aorta or into the right renal artery using the saphenous graft.

Commentary

5

Michael G.T. Raraty and John P. Neoptolemos

In general, our approach to surgery for pancreatic carcinoma is very similar to that described by the authors; however, there are a number of differences in the details of our management.

5.1 Staging

We prefer a high-quality, multi-phase contrast-enhanced CT as the principal modality for radiologic staging of pancreatic carcinoma. Our radiologic criteria for resection are as described but in addition, we utilize staging laparoscopy plus laparoscopic ultrasonography (L/LUS) much more frequently. Laparoscopic assessment for pancreatic cancer can be useful in selected patients by demonstrating small volume peritoneal or hepatic disease and may also be utilized in assessment of venous involvement. We have found, however, that in patients with low serum levels of the tumour marker Ca19-9, the rate of positive L/LUS is very low, and therefore we use L/LUS selectively based on Ca19-9 values. If the pre-operative Ca19-9 is greater than 150 kU/l in the absence of jaundice, or >300 kU/l in the presence of jaundice (bilirubin > 35 μmol/l), we recommend L/LUS preoperatively, as long as there are no other contra-indications to laparoscopy. In the presence of a markedly increased serum Ca19-9, L/LUS identifies radiologically undetected evidence of unresectability in approximately 20 % of patients.

In addition, we have recently commenced a trial of the role of PET-CT in the pre-operative staging of pancreatic cancer. It is possible that PET-CT will detect evidence of small volume metastatic disease that would otherwise not be detected pre-operatively.

5.2 Carcinoma of the Pancreatic Head/Periampullary Region

5.2.1 Operative Technique

Our preferred option for lesions within the head of the pancreas is the pylorus-preserving pancreatoduodenectomy as described. Initial mobilization consists of wide Kocher manoeuvre of the duodenum and opening of the lesser sac. Rather than dividing the gastro-colic omentum, however, we prefer to separate this from the transverse colon along the anatomic plane. Mobilization of the hepatic flexure of the colon is usually necessary in order to obtain adequate access to the duodenum.

The superior mesenteric vein and inferior border of the pancreas are then exposed, allowing early assessment of the degree of venous involvement, followed by exposure of the portal vein at the superior border of the pancreas above the pancreatic neck as described.

M.G.T. Raraty • J.P. Neoptolemos (✉)
Division of Surgery and Oncology,
University of Liverpool, Liverpool, UK
e-mail: j.p.neoptolemos@liverpool.ac.uk

R. Mantke et al. (eds.), *International Practices in Pancreatic Surgery*,
DOI 10.1007/978-3-540-74506-8_5, © Springer-Verlag Berlin Heidelberg 2013

After exposure of the gastroduodenal artery cephalad to the neck of the pancreas, patency of the common hepatic artery is checked by temporary occlusion of the gastroduodenal artery with a small vascular clamp or bulldog clip to ensure that the liver is not reliant on retrograde flow through the gastro-duodenal artery secondary to celiac artery compression. If, after occlusion, there remains flow through the hepatic artery, then we divide the gastroduodenal artery.

The proximal duodenum is transected with a linear stapling device and the gallbladder separated from the liver. The cystic artery is divided, but the cystic duct is ligated in continuity so that it remains connected to the resection specimen. The common hepatic duct is transected just cephalad to the cystic duct insertion; however, contrary to the practice of the authors, we prefer not to clamp the stump as this could potentially lead to ischaemic damage to the common hepatic duct stump. Instead, we merely place a swab over the cut end. Leakage of a small amount of bile is thus contained and does not cause any clinically important problems.

The first jejunal loop is then transected with a linear stapler and mobilized as described, and we would agree that use of the harmonic scalpel for this manoeuvre speeds the process. After mobilization, the distal duodenum and proximal jejunum are passed behind the superior mesenteric vessels to the right side of the patient and the pancreatic neck can then be divided between stay sutures. Our preference is to use diathermy to perform this division, and we have not encountered any problems in terms of pathologic assessment using this technique. Any tumour cells within 1 mm of the resection margin are deemed to represent a positive resection margin.

After transection of the pancreatic neck, the retro-pancreatic tissues are divided as close to the superior mesenteric artery as possible by serial ligation and division of the numerous small vessels in this area. If the tumour is particularly adherent to the vein, a limited vein resection may be performed; we have found bovine collagen vein patches to be useful for reconstruction in this situation.

We do not send samples routinely for frozen section analysis; however, if the surgeon is suspicious of the presence of residual tumour tissue, then further specimens may be sent for frozen section and a further resection considered. This approach is particularly pertinent for mucinous cystic lesions or main-duct IPMN, where there may be high-grade dysplasia within the residual pancreatic duct such that a further pancreatic resection may be entertained.

The pancreatic anastomosis is performed using either the Cattell-Warren technique, as described, or the Blumgart technique, using four 3-0 PDS, mattress sutures through the pancreatic body approximately 1 cm away from the cut margin and taking the jejunum both anteriorly and posteriorly to buttress the sutures. The pancreatic duct is treated in the same way as for the Cattell-Warren technique using 4-0 PDS. In both techniques, we utilise a fine-bore, paediatric feeding tube as a pancreatic duct stent. This stent is cut to a length of approximately 10 cm and placed across the pancreatic anastomosis to discourage stricture formation.

The hepaticojejunostomy is performed using a single layer of interrupted, 4-0 PDS. The duodenojejunostomy is constructed in an antecolic position with 3-0 monocryl or 3-0 PDS, again as a single layer of interrupted sutures. Interrupted sutures are preferred to a continuous layer because of the risk of ischaemia with the latter (Fig. 5.1).

In the event that a pylorus-preserving procedure is not possible due to proximity of the tumour to the pylorus and proximal duodenum, then reconstruction of the gastro-jejunostomy is performed using a Roux-en-Y loop in order to reduce bile reflux into the stomach (Fig. 5.2).

We place two simple, corrugated, "passive" drains adjacent to the anastomosis. We prefer not to use suction drains in proximity to bowel due to the risk of injury to the bowel wall.

5.2.2 Additional Medication and Procedures

All patients receive antibiotic prophylaxis with cefuroxime and metronidazole and octreotide, 100 μg subcutaneously, 3 times a day for 7 days, commencing on the evening before surgery.

All patients are admitted routinely to a postoperative critical care unit for the first night post-

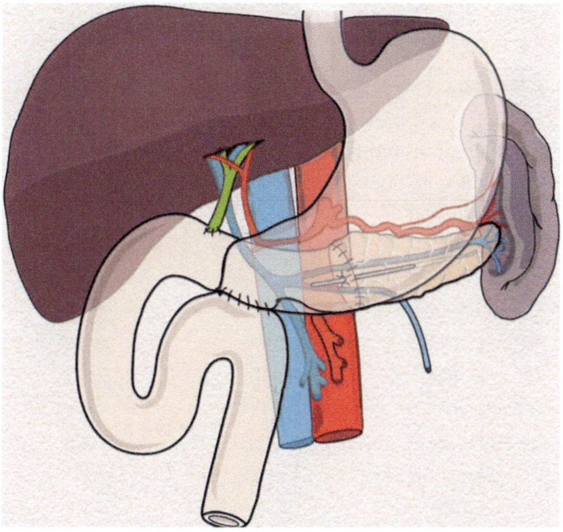

Fig. 5.1 Reconstruction after standard, duodenum-preserving pancreatoduodenectomy. Retrocolic pancreatojejunostomy with 4-0 PDS, hepaticojejunostomy with 4-0 PDS and antecolic duodenojejunostomy with 3-0 PDS or monocryl (Copyright University of Liverpool (2003)

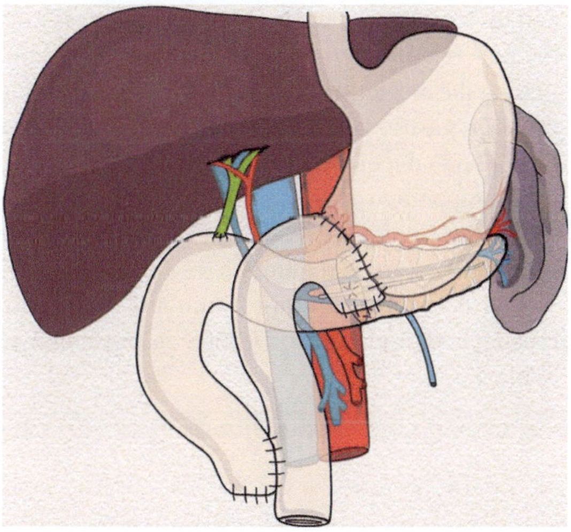

Fig. 5.2 Roux-en-Y reconstruction following a classic Kausch-Whipple pancreatoduodenectomy with removal of the pylorus. Retrocolic pancreatojejunostomy with 4-0 PDS, and hepaticojejunostomy with 4-0 PDS and antecolic gastrojejunostomy with 3-0 PDS or monocryl, and jejunojejunostomy with linear stapler plus 3-0 PDS or monocryl. *Note* the separate Roux limb for the gastrojejunostomy (Copyright University of Liverpool (2003)

operatively, but transferred to the Pancreatic Enhanced Recovery Unit the following day, where they remain until fit for discharge on day 7-10.

Table 5.1 Patients with carcinoma of the pancreatic head/periampullary region undergoing pancreatic resection 2007–2008

Parameter	Number	%
Patients	151	100
In-hospital mortality	3	2
Hospital stay – days (median, range)	17.5	(4–84)
Reoperation	5	3
Classic Kausch-Whipple	20	13
Pylorus-preserving pancreatoduodenectomy	118	78
Total pancreatectomy	9	6
Pancreas-preserving duodenectomy	3	2
Tumour stage (UICC)	112	
Ia	3	3
Ib	3	3
IIa	17	15
IIb	63	63.4
III	12	11
IV	6	5
R0 resection	84	56
R1 resection	64	42
R2 resection	3	2
Vascular resection	11	7
Complications	85	56
Bleeding	3	2
Delayed gastric emptying	10	7
Pancreatic fistula	10	7
Biliary fistula	2	1
Wound infection	41	27
Collection requiring drainage	9	6

A nasogastric tube is routinely left in situ postoperatively but is not used routinely for supplemental feeding; instead we encourage early introduction of fluids – sips of water may be taken as soon as the patient has recovered sufficiently from the anaesthetic – and oral intake is increased gradually over the next few days until the patient is taking solids by day 4. Early mobilization is encouraged.

The drains are shortened gradually, commencing on day 3 provided the output is not excessive, and there is no clinical suspicion of an anastomotic leak.

Our data for resections of tumours of the pancreatic head 2007/2008 is presented in Table 5.1.

5.3 Carcinoma of the Body/Tail of Pancreas

5.3.1 Operative Technique

Our approach to the pancreatic body/tail is very similar to that described by the main authors. Initial exposure of the pancreas proceeds as for a pancreatoduodenectomy with separation of the greater omentum from the transverse colon, although for a left-sided resection, this separation is continued all the way across to the splenic flexure.

The duodenum is Kocherized in the same way as we would for a pancreatic head resection in order to allow control of the superior mesenteric and portal veins if necessary. This manoeuvre is particularly important if the pancreas is to be transected formally across the neck. For more distal lesions, it sometimes possible to transect the pancreas further to the left, however, adequate access for control of the veins is still essential before dissection of the pancreas commences.

After mobilisation of the pancreatic neck in a manner similar to that employed for a pancreatic head resection (although preserving the gastroduodenal artery and right gastroepiploic vessels) the splenic artery is ligated and divided and the pancreatic neck divided. Transection of the pancreas may be performed using a stapling device as described, or using diathermy as we described above for the pancreatic head resection. In the latter case, the stump must be oversewn with 4-0 PDS, taking care to identify and close the pancreatic duct separately. The splenic vein is then ligated and divided behind the body of the pancreas, and the pancreatic body mobilised as described, continuing the dissection around the spleen and taking the short gastric vessels with the harmonic scalpel or ligatures depending on circumstances.

Postoperative care is similar to that for pancreatoduodenectomy, although often only a single corrugated drain is required.

Our data for resections of tumours of the pancreatic body/tail for 2007/2008 is presented in Table 5.2.

Table 5.2 Patients with carcinoma of the body/tail of pancreas undergoing pancreatic resection 2007–2008

Parameter	Number	%
Patients	23	100
In-hospital mortality	0	0
Hospital stay – days (median, range)	19.5	(8–57)
Reoperation	0	0
Left pancreatectomy	20	87
Total pancreatectomy	3	13
R0 resection	20	87
R1 resection	3	13
R2 resection	0	0
Vascular resection	1	4
Complications	14	61
Bleeding	1	4
Pancreatic fistula	1	4
Wound infection	1	4
Collection requiring drainage	6	26

6 Commentary

Tadahiro Takada, Keita Wada, and Keiji Sano

6.1 Carcinoma of the Pancreatic Head/Periampullary Adenocarcinoma

6.1.1 Relevant Basic Information, Indications and Contraindications

Diagnosis and staging is a crucial step to provide appropriate treatment for individual patients with pancreatic adenocarcinoma. Our gold standard modality for diagnosis and staging is multiphase "pancreas protocol," thin-slice, multi-detector CT (MDCT) including chest scans. Recently introduced multi-detector technology allows high scanning speed with thin collimation, which decreases the time needed to cover a volume of interest for imaging during clearly defined perfusion phases. If the findings on MDCT are equivocal, endoscopic ultrasonography (EUS) with or without fine needle aspiration (FNA) is indicated. ERCP, MRI/MRCP, and PET-CT are indicated only for selected patients.

MDCT provides high diagnostic accuracy for assessing resectability and unresectability based on the relationship between the primary tumor and the major vessels, including the hepatic artery (HA), superior mesenteric artery (SMA), and superior mesenteric and portal vein (SMV & PV). In our practice, vascular involvement itself does not necessarily mean unresectability. If vascular involvement is limited to a short segment and allows for reconstruction, those cases are still candidates for operative resection (as of 2010, we prefer neoadjuvant therapy before surgery rather than a "surgery-first" approach). In addition to vascular involvement, nodal status is also important for determining indications for operative intervention. Distant lymph node metastasis including the paraaortic lymph nodes which means systemic disease and is a contraindication for operation. If the diagnosis of distant lymph node metastasis by MDCT is equivocal, we prefer to proceed with a PET-CT and/or open biopsy. The indication for operative exploration for each patient should be determined by a comprehensive workup that includes physiologic and nutritional status.

6.1.2 Operative Technique

6.1.2.1 Resection

Our standard operative procedure for adenocarcinoma of the head of the pancreas and periampullary region is the pylorus-preserving pancreatoduodenectomy (Traverso-Longmire procedure), if it is possible to preserve the pylorus. We use an upper midline incision from the xiphoid down to the umbilicus, or sometimes we extend the incision to the right (J-shape incision) when the patient is obese and/or exposure is difficult. Any distant

T. Takada, M.D., FACS, FRCS (HON) (✉)
K. Wada, M.D. • K. Sano, M.D.
Department of Surgery, Teikyo University, School of Medicine, 2-11-1 Kaga, Itabashi-ku, Tokyo 173-8605, Japan
e-mail: t-takada@jhpbs.jp

R. Mantke et al. (eds.), *International Practices in Pancreatic Surgery*,
DOI 10.1007/978-3-540-74506-8_6, © Springer-Verlag Berlin Heidelberg 2013

metastasis, including liver metastases and peritoneal seeding, is a contraindication for resection. We routinely sample lymph nodes in the aortocaval groove following the Kocher maneuver (before proceeding with resection). If any positive lymph nodes are seen in this area, operation is concluded.

We prefer that the greater omentum be detached from the transverse colon rather than being divided between ligatures to preserve omentum vascularity. We agree with Drs. Mantke and Lippert's perspective that the well-vascularized omentum helps to control postoperative complications of the pancreatic anastomosis. We sometimes use the segmental omentum (omentum flap) to cover the pancreatic anastomosis to prevent serious complications.

After mobilizing the transverse mesocolon caudally from the pancreatic head and dividing the right gastroepiploic vein and artery, the nerve-plexus-covered SMV and SMA are taped separately at the inferior border of the pancreas. In cases involving SMV from which the middle colic veins drain, this tape should be placed more caudally, below the transverse mesocolon. The transverse mesocolon with middle colic artery and vein is often divided for better exposure in this area. Ischemic change in the transverse mesocolon is seen only rarely provided the marginal vessels are preserved. These tapes prove helpful in subsequent portal vein resection and plexus resection along the SMA (Fig. 6.1).

For pancreatic head adenocarcinoma without findings of vascular involvement, a retropancreatic tunnel is made under the pancreas from the SMV to the portal vein in the groove for the portal vein where the pancreas is divided. In contrast, however, in cases with vascular resection, the pancreas is divided at the level of the SMV, which provides better exposure in the area where the SMV-PV is involved. This also allows us to secure the root of the SMA and celiac artery for proximal vascular control when hepatic artery and/or SMA resection is performed (Fig. 6.2).

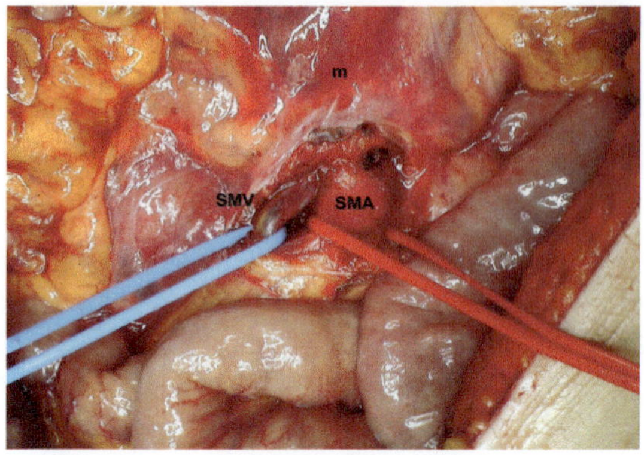

Fig. 6.1 The superior mesenteric artery and vein are identified below the transverse mesocolon. The superior mesenteric artery is secured with the surrounding plexus. (*SMA* superior mesenteric artery, *SMV* superior mesenteric vein, *m* transverse mesocolon)

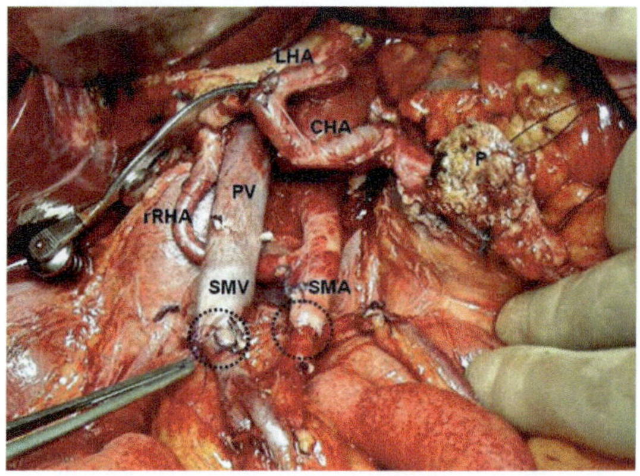

Fig. 6.2 Radical pancreatoduodenectomy with resection and reconstruction of the superior mesenteric artery and vein (*SMA* superior mesenteric artery, *SMV* superior mesenteric vein, *PV* portal vein, *CHA* common hepatic artery, *LHA* left hepatic artery, *rRHA* replaced right hepatic artery, *P* pancreas). A *block dotted circle* represents the size of vascular reconstruction of *SMA* and *SMV*

The extent of lymphadenectomy for pancreatic head adenocarcinoma in our practice is similar to Drs. Mantke and Lippert's description. We do not perform routine extended lymphadenectomies based on the results of several randomized, controlled trials (Yeo et al. 1999, 2002; Nguyen et al. 2003; Nimura et al. 2004; Farnell et al. 2005). The paraaortic lymph node is only sampled for staging, and the lymph node on the left side of the SMA is not resected routinely unless positive lymph nodes are observed in this region.

In addition to lymphadenectomy, the extent of resection of the neurolymphatic plexus along the SMA is crucial for achieving an R0 resection for pancreatic head adenocarcinoma, especially in

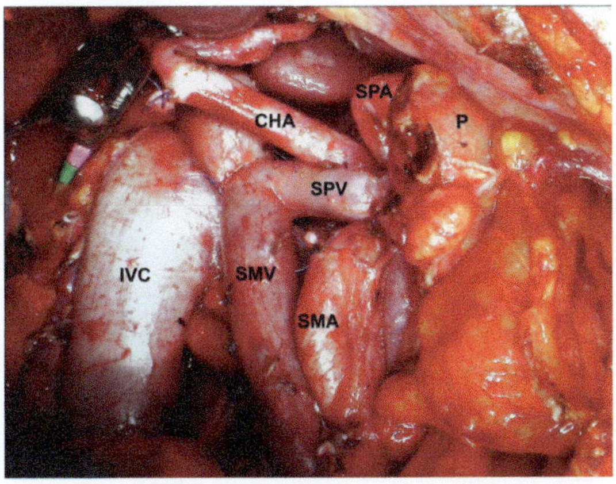

Fig. 6.3 Radical pancreatoduodenectomy. About one-half to two-thirds circle of the plexus around the superior mesenteric artery is resected (*SMA* superior mesenteric artery, *SMV* superior mesenteric vein, *CHA* common hepatic artery, *SPA* splenic artery, *SPV* splenic vein, *IVC* inferior vena cava, *P* pancreas)

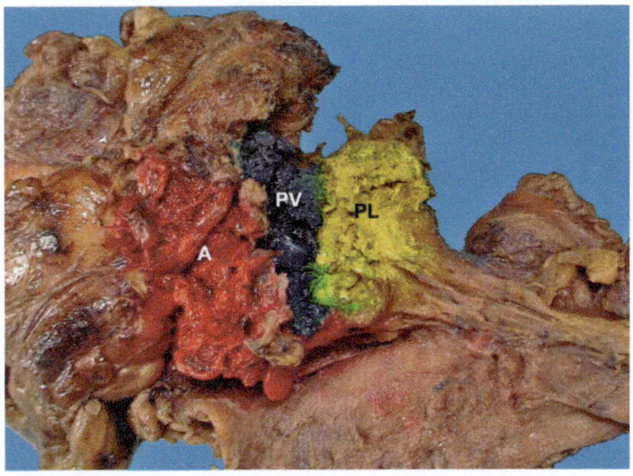

Fig. 6.4 All surgical margins are inked in separate colors (*PL* uncinate-SMA margin, *PV* PV groove, *A* anterior margin)

cases where the main tumor is located in the uncinate process. Although we do not undertake routine resection of the nerve plexus along the SMA, it is indicated if an R0 resection is deemed. For plexus resection, the anterior surface of the SMA with the plexus is divided longitudinally, exposing the adventitia of the SMA itself. The dissection is extended toward the root of the SMA, where it is cancer-free. At this point, the inferior pancreaticoduodenal artery (IPDA) is ligated and divided at its origin, usually prior to portal vein resection or dissection of the uncinate process from the SMV and PV. Ligating the IPDA first helps to decrease bleeding by preventing congestion of the specimen. Next, rightward traction is applied to the cut margin of the plexus, which is then resected longitudinally from the right side to the posterior side (about one-half to two-thirds circle of the plexus is resected) (Fig. 6.3). The margin in this region is inked separately on the specimen as the SMA plexus margin (Fig. 6.4). Postoperative diarrhea may be happened but it can usually be managed successfully by medication and resolves in 6–12 months.

For portal vein resection, our procedure is almost identical to that described by Drs. Mantke and Lippert. We prefer an external iliac vein graft because of its size. The junction of the splenic vein is not always preserved after using test clamps to ensure the prevention of splenic congestion.

6.1.2.2 Reconstruction

Our reconstruction procedure is similar to that described by Drs. Mantke and Lippert. The jejunal limb is brought up through a window in the transverse mesocolon. Anastomosis of the end of the pancreas to the side of the jejunal stump is accomplished using a duct-to-mucosa anastomosis for the inner layer and transfixing sutures for the outer layer. We use 5-0, absorbable, monofilament, interrupted sutures with an RB-2 needle (PDS™ II, Ethicon, Johnson and Johnson, Somerville, NJ, USA) for duct-to-mucosa suture without a stent. We usually place 6 to 8 sutures using a Castroviejo needle holder aided by surgical loupes (2.5X). A Castroviejo needle holder under magnification is easy to handle for fine sutures. Transfixing outer sutures are made between the full thickness of the pancreas and the wider seromuscular layer of the jejunum using 3-0, nonabsorbable, monofilament, interrupted sutures (Prolene™, Ethicon). We usually place four sutures in the outer layer, two for the cranial and two for the caudal positions to the inner anastomosis. The ligatures should be tied gently and not too tightly.

For the end-to-side hepaticojejunostomy, we use 5-0, absorbable, monofilament, interrupted sutures (PDS™ II, Ethicon) without a stent. For the antecolic, end-to-side duodenojejunostomy, we use a double continuous technique with 4-0 absorbable sutures (PDS™ II, Ethicon).

6.1.2.3 Drainage

We routinely place two closed-suction drains (Silicone Flat Drains™, BARD, Covington, GA, USA) for pancreatic and biliary anastomosis. One drains the biliary anastomosis and posterior pancreatic anastomosis, and the other drains the anterior and cranial pancreatic anastomosis (around the stump of the gastroduodenal artery).

6.1.3 Additional Treatment and Postoperative Care

- Antibiotic prophylaxis is used with a second-generation cephalosporin. The initial dose is given in the operating room prior to skin incision and is continued until postoperative day (POD) #3.
- Octreotide is not used.
- A nasogastric tube is placed intraoperatively and is removed on POD #1–2. Clear water is resumed on the day following nasogastric tube removal, and a liquid diet is started on POD #5–6.
- Enteral feeding is used selectively and only for patients with malnutrition.
- A proton pump inhibitor is used routinely for prevention of peptic ulcer.
- Drain volume and amylase content are measured daily. If the drain amylase activity is less than three times that of the serum on POD #3, the drains are removed by POD #7 regardless of the volume. In contrast, if the drain amylase activity is greater than three times that of the serum on POD #3, the drain is maintained until the amylase activity is normalized or the pancreatic fistula is well localized. If clinical symptoms (fever, leukocytosis) are observed, we obtain a CT to exclude an undrained peripancreatic fluid collection. Drain exchange or percutaneous drainage is indicated if necessary. Antibiotics are also administrated if infection is evident.

6.1.4 Results

Our results are summarized in Table 6.1.

Table 6.1 Outcomes after resection for pancreatic head adenocarcinoma at Teikyo University Hospital (2006/2007)

Parameter	Number	%
Patients	40	
Hospital mortality	1	3
Hospital stay (median, range) (in days)	28 (7–75)	
Relaparotomy	2	5
Death without local complications	0	0
Classic pancreatoduodenectomy	14	35
PPPD	26	65
Portal vein resection	25	63
HA resection	2	5
SMA resection	1	3
Tumor stage (UICC)		
Ia	1	3
Ib	0	0
IIa	12	30
IIb	23	56
III	1	3
IV	3	8
R0 resection	33	83
R1 resection	6	15
R2 resection	1	2
Postoperative local morbidity		
Postoperative bleeding[a]	2	5
Delayed gastric emptying[b]	3	8
Pancreatic fistula[c]	5	13
Bile leak[d]	1	3
Wound infection	2	5
Other	8	20
Postoperative systemic morbidity		
Systemic complications	3	8

[a]Any bleeding requiring intervention
[b]By ISGPS definition
[c]By ISGPF definition
[d]Any bilirubin-rich drainage on or after POD #3

6.2 Carcinoma of the Body and Tail of the Pancreas

6.2.1 Relevant Basic Information, Indications and Contraindications

Preoperative resectability is assessed from the MDCT results, which image the relationship between the tumor and the adjacent vessels, including the splenic, common hepatic, celiac, superior mesenteric artery, and splenic and portal veins.

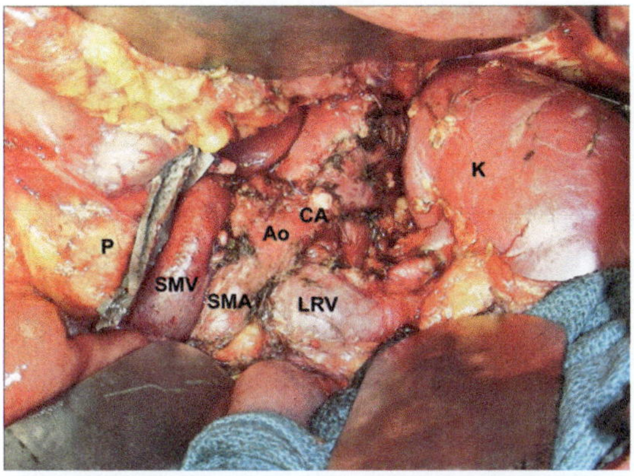

Fig. 6.5 Radical distal pancreatectomy with celiac artery resection (DP-CAR) (*SMA* superior mesenteric artery, *SMV* superior mesenteric vein, *Ao* aorta, *CA* celiac artery, *LRV* left renal vein, *P* pancreas, *K* kidney)

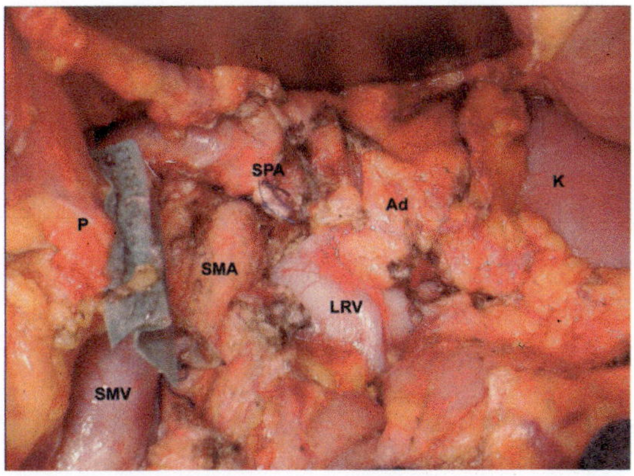

Fig. 6.6 Radical distal pancreatectomy. The left adrenal gland is preserved (*SMA* superior mesenteric artery, *SMV* superior mesenteric vein, *SPA* splenic artery, *LRV* left renal vein, *P* pancreas, *Ad* adrenal gland, *K* kidney)

We pay special attention to the extent of invasion into the retroperitoneal soft tissue and left adrenal gland, because the retroperitoneal margin is the area where is most likely to be involved with cancer cells (R1 resection). In our practice, cases with vascular involvement including the celiac artery, hepatic artery, and portal vein are still considered potential operative candidates. In selected cases, a radical resection is possible with distal pancreatectomy combined with celiac artery resection with or without portal vein resection as described by Hirano et al. (as of 2010, we prefer neoadjuvant therapy before resection rather than a "surgery-first" approach) (Hirano et al. 2007) (Fig. 6.5). In addition to vascular involvement, nodal status is also important for determining resectability. Distant lymph node metastasis including the paraaortic lymph nodes means systemic disease and is a contraindication for resection. If the diagnosis of distant lymph node metastasis by MDCT is equivocal, we prefer to proceed with PET-CT and/or open biopsy. Operative indication for each patient should be determined by a comprehensive workup, including physiologic and nutritional status.

6.2.2 Operative Technique

6.2.2.1 Resection

Our standard procedure for carcinoma of the body and tail of the pancreas is antegrade distal pancreatectomy with splenectomy, which is almost identical to the description by Drs. Mantke and Lippert. The antegrade approach (divide pancreas first) has advantages over the conventional approach (mobilize spleen first) in terms of better exposure of the root of the celiac artery and SMA, and securing the retroperitoneal margin as described by Strasburg et al. (Strasberg et al. 2007) (Fig. 6.6).

We divide the pancreas using a stapler with Neoveil® bioabsorbable staple-line reinforcement material (Gunze, Kyoto, Japan) or Duet TRS™ (Covidien, Mansfield, MA, USA), if applicable. When the stapler is used, it is closed very slowly to prevent breakdown of the pancreatic parenchyma. If the pancreatic parenchyma is thick, we use Doyen intestinal forceps to make the parenchyma thinner before stapling. If the parenchyma is either too thick or too fragile, we divide the pancreas by means of electrocautery with or without a fishmouth closure.

6.2.2.2 Drainage

A closed-suction drain (Silicone Flat Drains™, BARD, Covington, GA, USA) is placed near the pancreatic stump.

6.2.3 Additional Treatment and Postoperative Care

- Antibiotic prophylaxis is used with a second-generation cephalosporin. The initial dose is given in the operating room prior to skin incision, and is continued until postoperative day (POD) #3.

Table 6.2 Outcomes after resection for pancreatic body/tail adenocarcinoma at Teikyo University Hospital (2006/2007)

Parameter	Number	%
Patients	16	
Hospital mortality	0	0
Hospital stay (median, range) (in days)	21 (12–54)	
Relaparotomy	0	0
Death without local complications	0	0
Portal vein resection	4	25
Celiac artery resection	4	25
Tumor stage (UICC)		
Ia	0	0
Ib	0	0
IIa	5	31
IIb	3	19
III	3	19
IV	5	31
R0 resection	10	63
R1 resection	4	25
R2 resection	2	12
Postoperative local morbidity		
Postoperative bleeding[a]	0	0
Delayed gastric emptying[b]	4	25
Pancreatic fistula[c]	3	19
Wound infection	2	12
Other	2	12
Postoperative systemic morbidity		
Systemic complications	0	0

[a]Any bleeding requiring intervention
[b]By ISGPS definition
[c]By ISGPF definition

- Octreotide is not used.
- A nasogastric tube is placed intraoperatively and removed on POD #1. Clear water is resumed on the day following nasogastric tube removal, and a liquid diet is started on POD #3.
- Drain volume and amylase activity are measured daily. If the drain amylase activity is less than three times that of the serum on POD #3, the drains are removed by POD #7 regardless of the volume. If the drain amylase activity is greater than three times that of the serum on POD #3, the drain is maintained until the amylase value is normalized or pancreatic fistula is well localized. If clinical symptoms (fever, leukocytosis) are observed, we obtain a CT to exclude an undrained peripancreatic fluid collection. Drain exchange or percutaneous drainage is indicated if necessary. Antibiotics are also administrated if infection is evident.

6.2.4 Results

Our results are summarized in Table 6.2.

References

Farnell MB, Pearson RK, Sarr MG, DiMagno EP, Burgart LJ, Dahl TR, Foster N, Sargent DJ, Pancreas Cancer Working Group (2005) A prospective randomized trial comparing standard pancreatoduodenectomy with pancreatoduodenectomy with extended lymphadenectomy in resectable pancreatic head adenocarcinoma. Surgery 138:618–630

Hirano S, Kondo S, Hara T et al (2007) Distal pancreatectomy with en bloc celiac axis resection for locally advanced pancreatic body cancer: long-term results. Ann Surg 246:46–51

Nguyen TC, Sohn TA, Cameron JL, Lillemoe KD, Campbell KA, Coleman JA, Sauter PK, Abrams RA, Hruban RH, Yeo CJ (2003) Standard vs. radical pancreaticoduodenectomy for periampullary adenocarcinoma: a prospective, randomized trial evaluating quality of life in pancreaticoduodenectomy survivors. J Gastrointest Surg 7:1–11

Nimura Y, Nagino M, Kato H, Miyagawa S, Yamaguchi A, Kinoshita T, Takao S, Takada T, Miyazaki K, Ishiyama S, Shimada H, Kawarada Y, Takeda H, Sagota K, Yasui K (2004) Regional vs. extended lymph node dissection in radical pancreaticoduodenectomy for pancreatic cancer. A multicenter randomized controlled trial. HPB (Off J Int Hepato Pancreato Biliary Assoc) 6(Suppl 1):2 [Abstract]

Strasberg SM, Linehan DC, Hawkins WG (2007) Radical antegrade modular pancreatosplenectomy procedure for adenocarcinoma of the body and tail of the pancreas: ability to obtain negative tangential margins. J Am Coll Surg 204:244–249

Yeo CJ, Cameron JL, Sohn TA, Coleman J, Sauter PK, Hruban RH, Pitt HA, Lillemoe KD (1999) Pancreaticoduodenectomy with or without extended retroperitoneal lymphadenectomy for periampullary adenocarcinoma. Comparison of morbidity and mortality and short-term outcome. Ann Surg 229: 613–624

Yeo CJ, Cameron JL, Lillemoe KD, Sohn TA, Campbell KA, Sauter PK, Coleman J, Abrams RA, Hruban RH (2002) Pancreaticoduodenectomy with or without distal gastrectomy and extended retroperitoneal lymphadenectomy for periampullary adenocarcinoma, part 2. Ann Surg 3:355–368

7 Commentary

Andrew L. Warshaw

7.1 Preoperative Management

Effective, appropriate surgery for pancreatic carcinoma depends on accurate diagnosis and staging for resectability (Fig. 7.1). Although a preoperative tissue diagnosis is not required and may even have adverse consequences (dissemination or seeding along the needle tract, pancreatitis), it is important to discriminate lesions such as autoimmune pancreatitis or lymphoma, for which resection is unnecessary and other treatment is preferred. In these latter examples, a core tissue biopsy will be more diagnostic than fine-needle aspiration cytology.

While fine-slice or spiral contrast-enhanced CT provides excellent information about vascular involvement and good information about metastatic disease, small liver or peritoneal metastases <1 cm are missed frequently. We utilize laparoscopic evaluation and peritoneal cytologic washings for cancers at high risk for metastatic spread: neoplasms larger than 2 cm, borderline resectable lesions because of possible major vascular involvement, and most neoplasms located in the body, tail, or uncinate which may have presented relatively late because of pain in the absence of jaundice.

A.L. Warshaw, M.D.
Department of Surgery, Massachusetts General Hospital, 55 Fruit St., BULF 370, Boston, MA 02114-2696, USA

Department of Surgery, Harvard Medical School, Boston, MA, USA
e-mail: awarshaw@partners.org

We reserve neoadjuvant chemoradiation generally for cases of borderline resectability. Nevertheless, we are conducting currently a trial of preoperative proton beam therapy in conjunction with chemotherapy for resectable adenocarcinoma. Biliary decompression, preferably by endoscopic stent placement, is indicated for treatment of pruritis, serum bilirubin concentrations greater than 10–15 mg/dl, or when definitive operative treatment will not occur promptly.

Although many patients with pancreatic malignancies will have lost considerable body weight, there is no substantial evidence that preoperative nutritional repletion with TPN decreases perioperative complications or mortality. Bowel preparation is unnecessary unless colonic resection is anticipated and even then may not be necessary. Broad-spectrum antibiotics targeting biliary flora are given prior to skin incision and continued for only one dose postoperatively unless there is a specific indication for continuing treatment.

7.2 Pancreatoduodenectomy: General Considerations

This operation should incur a 30-day mortality rate of less than 5 %. It has been our experience that the postoperative hospital duration of stay is significantly greater with the pylorus-preserving operation because of delayed gastric emptying in about one-third of patients. Given that there is neither a nutritional advantage conferred nor any

R. Mantke et al. (eds.), *International Practices in Pancreatic Surgery*,
DOI 10.1007/978-3-540-74506-8_7, © Springer-Verlag Berlin Heidelberg 2013

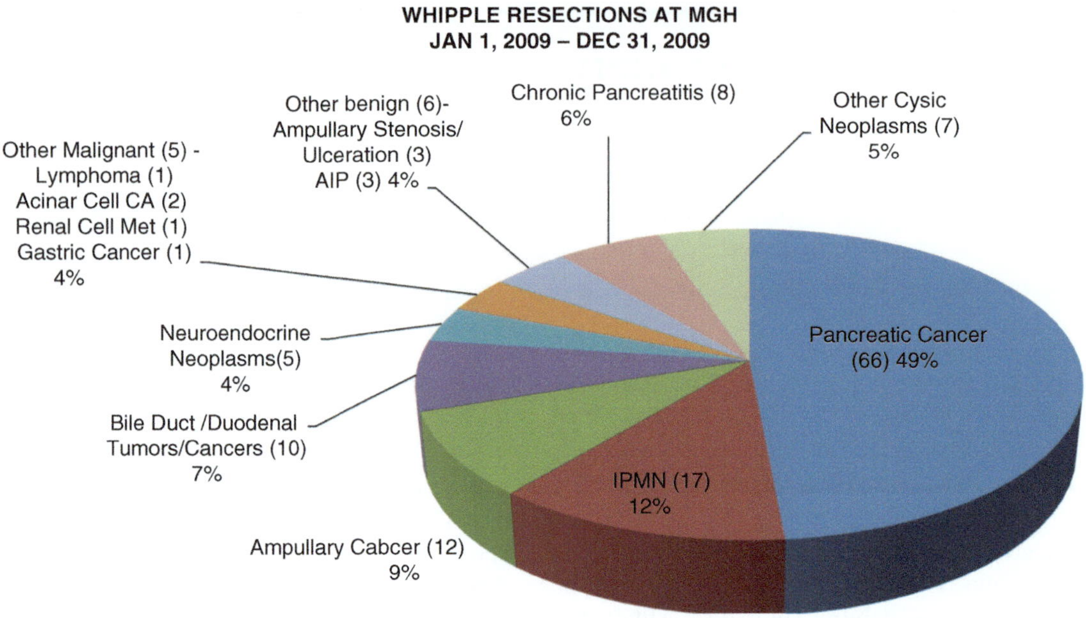

Fig. 7.1 The spectrum of diagnoses leading to a pancreatoduodenectomy at MGH in 2009. Approximately half were for ductal adenocarcinoma and only 10 % were for non-neoplastic conditions

difference in cure rates between the two operations, we have favored the classic pancreatoduodenectomy with antrectomy.

Recent interest has been directed at extending the operation to include tissues outside the standard field of dissection, such as the aorto-caval lymph nodes and the nerve plexuses surrounding the superior mesenteric artery. These extended dissections have shown no benefit in clinical trials in Europe and the United States. In addition, circumferential dissection around the artery leads frequently to debilitating diarrhea and gastrointestinal dysfunction.

Lateral or segmental resection of the portal or superior mesenteric vein may allow completion of the pancreatoduodenectomy but has not convincingly increased the rate of cure even if an R0 resection (negative margin) is accomplished.

7.2.1 Surgical Technique

Step 1: A vertical midline incision provides excellent access. The liver and peritoneal surfaces are examined for unexpected extrapancreatic metastases. Routine biopsy of apparently normal regional lymph nodes is unnecessary, but suspicious lesions and enlarged lymph nodes outside the planned field of resection should be biopsied and examined by frozen section; we abort resection if these nodes are positive for metastatic cancer.

Step 2: The hepatic flexure of the colon is mobilized from its retroperitoneal attachments to access the third and fourth portions of the duodenum. Extensive mobilization of the entire right colon and small bowel mesentery (Cattell-Braasch maneuver) is unnecessary except for lesions involving the fourth portion of the duodenum or for the approach to mobilization and resection of a segment of the superior mesenteric vein. The duodenum and head of the pancreas are separated from the retroperitoneal bed medially past the aorta and distally to the ligament of Treitz. The superior mesenteric artery is palpated posteriorly as it originates from the aorta to establish that the cleft between the artery and uncinate process of the pancreas is not obliterated by tumor. A silk suture placed in the duodenum to mark the junction of the third (D3) and fourth

(D4) portions is particularly helpful for identification of the proximal point of devascularization of the duodenum later when working back from the transected jejunum (Step 7).

Step 3: The gallbladder is removed if still present. The bile duct is dissected free from the adjacent portal structures and divided proximally (hepatic side) to the site of entry of the cystic duct. The proximal bile duct is left unclamped to avoid ischemic trauma to the duct, but the distal bile duct orifice is sutured closed to minimize spillage of tumor cells. The tissues lateral to the portal vein are separated carefully, divided, and ligated with considerable care such that a replaced right hepatic artery off the proximal superior mesenteric artery will be recognized and not ligated.

Step 4: The portal dissection is continued down the anterior aspect of the portal vein. Division of the right gastric artery and gastrojejunal artery greatly facilitates access to the portal vein behind the pancreas. The gastrojejunal artery should be doubly ligated or suture ligated in order to minimize the chance of erosion and bleeding in the event of a pancreatic fistula. Lymph nodes anterior to the proper hepatic artery are taken with the specimen. Although there are no direct anterior branches to the portal vein, there are substantial branches at the upper and lower margins of the pancreas which enter the anteromedial aspect of the portal-mesenteric vein, and these can be injured/avulsed easily during development of the tunnel.

The approach to the mesenteric vein below the neck of the pancreas is facilitated by dividing the gastrocolic omentum outside the gastroepiploic arcade down to the level of the head of the pancreas. Tracing the middle colic vein and gastroepiploic vein down to the superior mesenteric provides rapid and reliable identification.

Step 5: After dividing the descending branch of the left gastric and gastroepiploic vessels at the gastric wall, the stomach is divided across the proximal antrum with a stapler. The lesser curvature portion of the stomach is turned in with nonabsorbable sutures over the staple line, leaving a sufficient portion of the staple line for a 4-cm gastrojejunal anastomosis.

Step 6: The dissection of the tunnel behind the pancreatic neck should be completed by blunt dissection under direct vision. Although traditional descriptions cite this maneuver as critical to proving resectability, it is only relevant to cancers in the neck and body of the pancreas: periampullary tumors are much more likely to involve the lateral and posterior aspects of the portal/mesenteric vein. The final determination of involvement of the vein may not be possible until much later in the operation and only after division of the pancreas during attempted separation of the uncinate process from the right lateral and posterior aspect of the superior mesenteric vein. A soft rubber drain is passed behind the pancreas both for anterior retraction of the pancreatic neck and protection of the portal vein. Sutures are placed at the four quadrants of the transection line to ligate the vascular arcades which run along the cephalad and caudad anterior and posterior margins of the pancreatic parenchyma. The pancreas is divided with electrocautery and additional bleeding points on the cut margins controlled. Suture closure of the pancreatic duct on the side of the specimen may help to decrease potential spillage of tumor cells during subsequent manipulation.

Step 7: The transverse colon and its mesentery are retracted cephalad, and the entire small bowel is eviscerated to facilitate exposure and dissection of the distal duodenum proximal to the ligament of Treitz. The jejunum is divided with a stapler 6–10 cm distal to the ligament of Treitz at a point which will provide sufficient mobility of the distal jejunum to reach easily to the right upper quadrant for the biliary and pancreatic anastomosis. The feeding vessels to the proximal jejunum and distal duodenum are divided at the enteric wall back to the previously placed marker suture at the junction of D3/D4.

Step 8: The final step in removal of the specimen is division of the venous tributaries of the uncinate to the superior mesenteric portal venous confluence and dissection along the lateral margin of the superior mesenteric artery, taking both the arterial branches and the antero-lateral periarterial soft tissues, which include both lymphatics and nerve plexuses that can contain tumor. The space between the pancreas and the mesenteric vessels is exposed by retracting the specimen to the right and the superior mesenteric vein to the left. The safety of this dissection may be increased by passing vessel loops around the portal vein and superior mesenteric vein for retraction. This maneuver is of particular value if there is inflammatory reaction or tumor in the region of the dissection. In the event of laceration of the vein or need for venous resection, an additional vessel loop must be placed around the splenic vein distal (splenic side) to the spleno-portal junction. Traction on the vessel loops and vascular clamps are used for venous control as necessary. Lateral venorrhaphy with a running, fine, nonabsorbable suture may suffice for repair or reconstruction as long as the lumen is not narrowed unacceptably. Segmental resection and reconstruction, either end-to-end or with interposition of a polytetrafluoroethylene (PTFE) graft may be necessary in some cases. As noted previously, extensive mobilization of the right colon and small bowel mesentery may facilitate access to and mobilization of the superior mesenteric vein. Further mobility can be obtained by dividing the splenic vein proximal to the spleno-portal junction.

Traction on the portal/mesenteric venous junction to the left exposes the groove lateral to the superior mesenteric artery. The tissues overlying the artery anteriorly are divided and the dissection is carried carefully down the lateral wall of the artery, and thereafter skeletonizing the medial aspect (Fig. 7.2). Care must be taken to identify and protect a right hepatic artery or a common hepatic artery originating from the superior mesenteric artery. The attachments of the uncinate, including the arterial branches, are then taken sequentially along the lateral margin of the superior mesenteric artery.

After removal of the specimen metal clips are placed at the margins of the resection field to target postoperative radiation therapy.

We place a safety pin in the uncinate margin and a long suture on the posterior soft tissue margin to orient the specimen for the pathologist.

Step 9: The peritoneum at the ligament of Treitz is closed with interrupted nonabsorbable sutures. The end of the jejunum is oversewn with nonabsorbable Lembert sutures over the staple line and brought through the right side of the transverse mesocolon. The pancreaticojejunostomy is performed first. This 2-layer, end-to-side, duct-to-mucosal anastomosis is created using an outer row of interrupted, nonabsorbable, 3-0 sutures that includes most of the cut surface of the pancreas and an inner row of 4-0 interrupted synthetic absorbable sutures, duct-to-mucosa (Fig. 7.3). It is almost always possible, even with a small/normal pancreatic duct, to perform this type of anastomosis. When the duct is very small, we place a #5 pediatric feeding tube into the lumen and place a minimum of 8 sutures circumferentially through the cut edge of the duct. All of the inner layers of duct sutures, anterior and posterior rows, are placed first and arrayed carefully to avoid entanglement (Fig. 7.4). The outer posterior sutures are then laid in between the pancreas posterior to the duct and the seromuscular layer of the bowel. Before tying them, a duct-sized

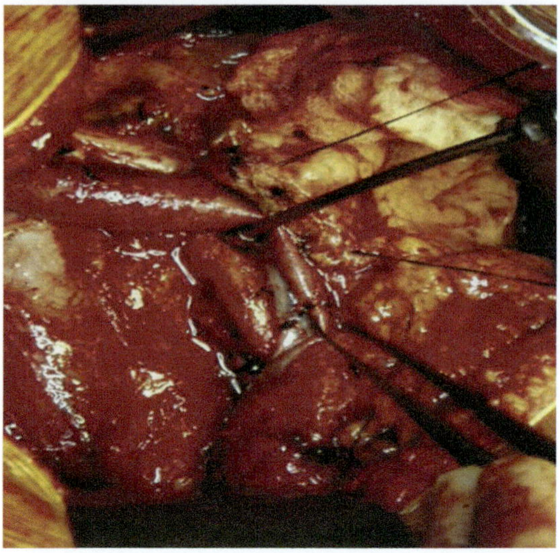

Fig. 7.2 After dividing venous tributaries from the uncinate process to the SMV/portal vein, the vein is retracted to the left with instruments or vessel loops to identify and expose the superior mesenteric artery behind and to the left. The lymphatic, neural, and arterial branches are dissected from the antero-lateral surface of the artery. If it is necessary to retract the vein to the right to expose the artery, division of the splenic vein may also be required for adequate exposure (Warshaw and Thayer 2004, p. 736)

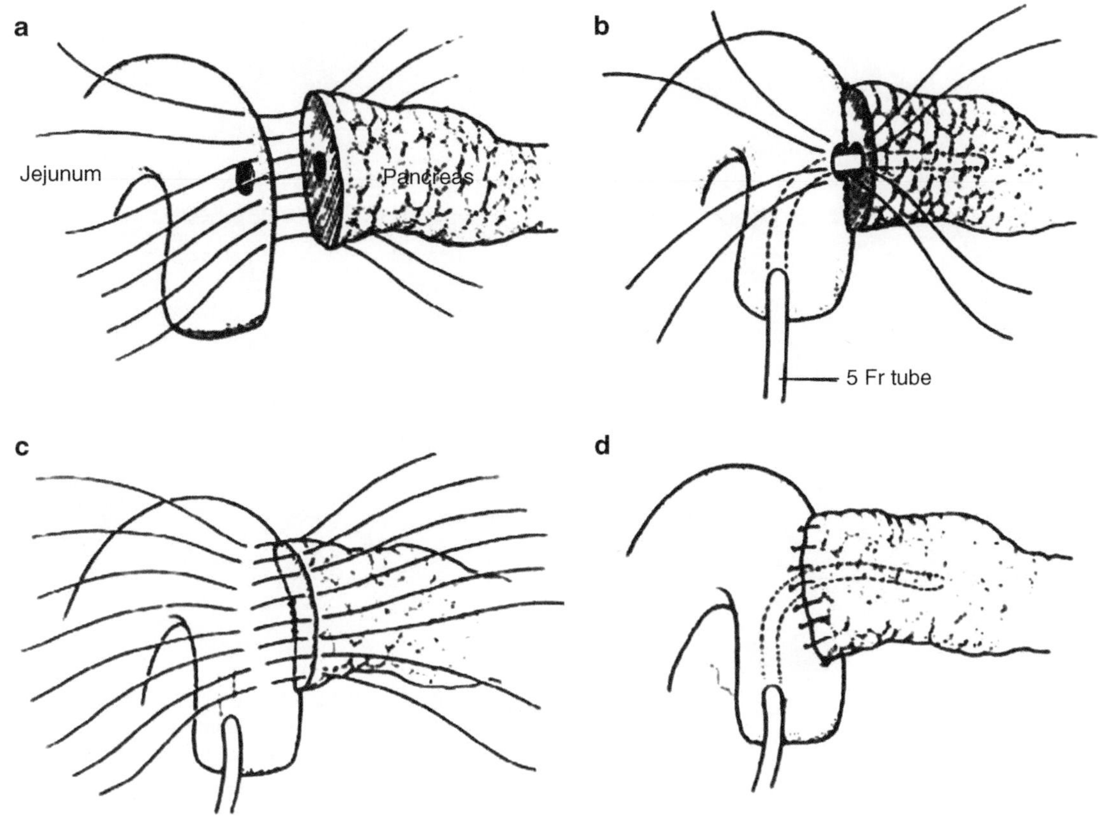

Fig. 7.3 Pancreaticojejunostomy. A 2-layer, end-to-side, duct-to-mucosa pancreaticojejunostomy is preferred (Warshaw and Thayer 2004, p. 737)

incision is made in the jejunum directly opposite the pancreatic duct lumen. The #5 pediatric feeding tube is then brought through the jejunal wall via a #14 needle (Fig. 7.5). The posterior row of sutures is tied and the posterior row of duct sutures is placed through the full thickness of the jejunum. The feeding tube is then placed into the pancreatic duct, and its exit point in the jejunal wall is fixed with a purse-string of chromic catgut and a Witzel tunnel of interrupted silk Lembert sutures. The anterior row of duct sutures is then placed in the full thickness of the jejunal orifice and tied. The anastomosis is completed with an anterior row of silk sutures. It is desirable to have the outer anterior and posterior rows of sutures include 1-cm of the pancreas in order to create a wider surface of apposition. The pancreatic intraductal tube will later be brought through the omentum and out through the right side of the abdominal wall. If there is a very dilated pancreatic duct, this ductal tube is not necessary.

Step 10: Distal to the pancreatic anastomosis, an end-to-side hepaticojejunostomy is made with a single layer of interrupted, closely-spaced, synthetic, absorbable sutures (Fig. 7.6). Unless the bile duct is small or fragile, no transanastomotic drainage tube is necessary. In the event it is needed, a small (#8 pediatric feeding tube) catheter can be left through the anastomosis and brought out distally through the jejunum and through the abdominal wall. If placed preoperatively, a transhepatic drain can be left in place instead of a retrograde tube placed from the jejunum.

Step 11: After fixing the jejunal loop to the transverse mesocolon with interrupted nonabsorbable sutures, gastrointestinal continuity is restored with a retrocolic, Hofmeister-type

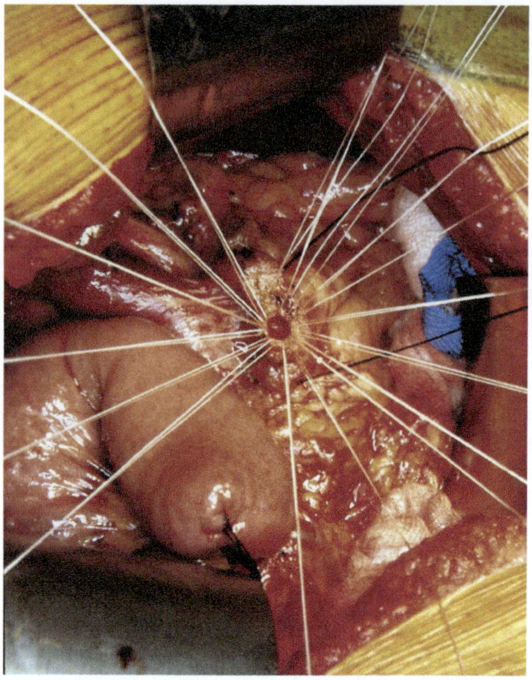

Fig. 7.4 Interrupted synthetic absorbable sutures are place circumferentially through the margins of the pancreatic duct and laid aside until after the posterior row of non-absorbable sutures between the pancreas and jejunum are in place. This sequence allows precise suture placement even in small, normal pancreatic ducts without risk of lacerating injury to a soft gland (Warshaw and Thayer 2004, p. 738)

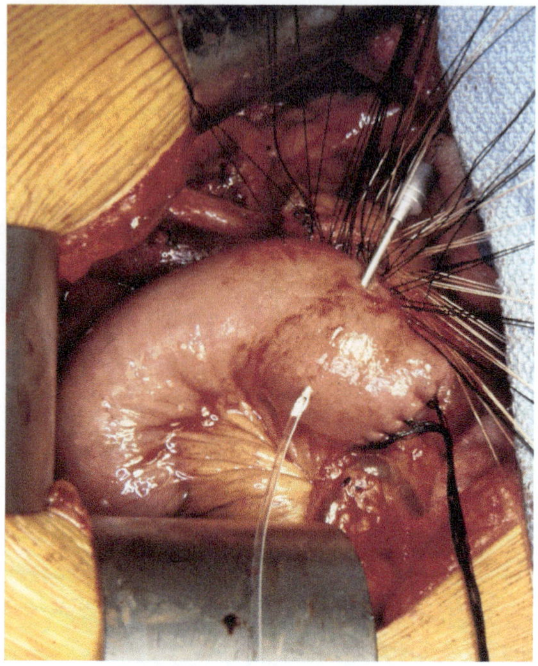

Fig. 7.5 A #5 pediatric feeding tube is introduced into the lumen of the jejunum and then into the pancreatic duct through 14-ga needle and laid aside until the outer and inner posterior rows of sutures have been tied (Warshaw and Thayer 2004, p. 739)

Billroth II gastrojejunostomy. This anastomosis is made with running absorbable sutures for the inner layer and interrupted nonabsorbable sutures for the outer layer. The anastomosis is fixed below the mesocolon with interrupted silk sutures.

Step 12: Omentum is placed over the biliary and pancreatic anastomoses. Soft, closed-suction drains are placed in the right upper quadrant, anterior and posterior to the biliary and pancreatic anastomoses. These drains are brought out through separate incisions in the right side of the abdomen. Neither gastrostomy nor feeding jejunostomy tubes are necessary.

7.2.2 Postoperative Care

The nasogastric tube is discontinued typically on postoperative day 1, and clear liquids are allowed on day 2. The diet is advanced to low-fat, soft solids in frequent small feedings as tolerated. Blood glucose should be monitored and diabetes treated as appropriate. The amylase activity in the drainage is measured on day 5 when the patient is eating. If there is no indication of an anastomotic leak, the suction drains are removed individually on days 5 and 6. Most patients are discharged 7–10 days after the operation (Table 7.1). The pancreatic (and biliary) stents are removed in the clinic, generally at 3 weeks.

Pancreatic fistula is the most common, pancreas-related complication of this operation, occurring in about 15 % of cases, particularly if the pancreas is soft (Table 7.2). The drainage catheters should be left in place long enough to ensure formation of a secure tract and then withdrawn sequentially in segments to allow the tract to close behind as drainage diminishes. In the case of low-volume fistulas (<200 ml/day), patients may eat and be discharged to home.

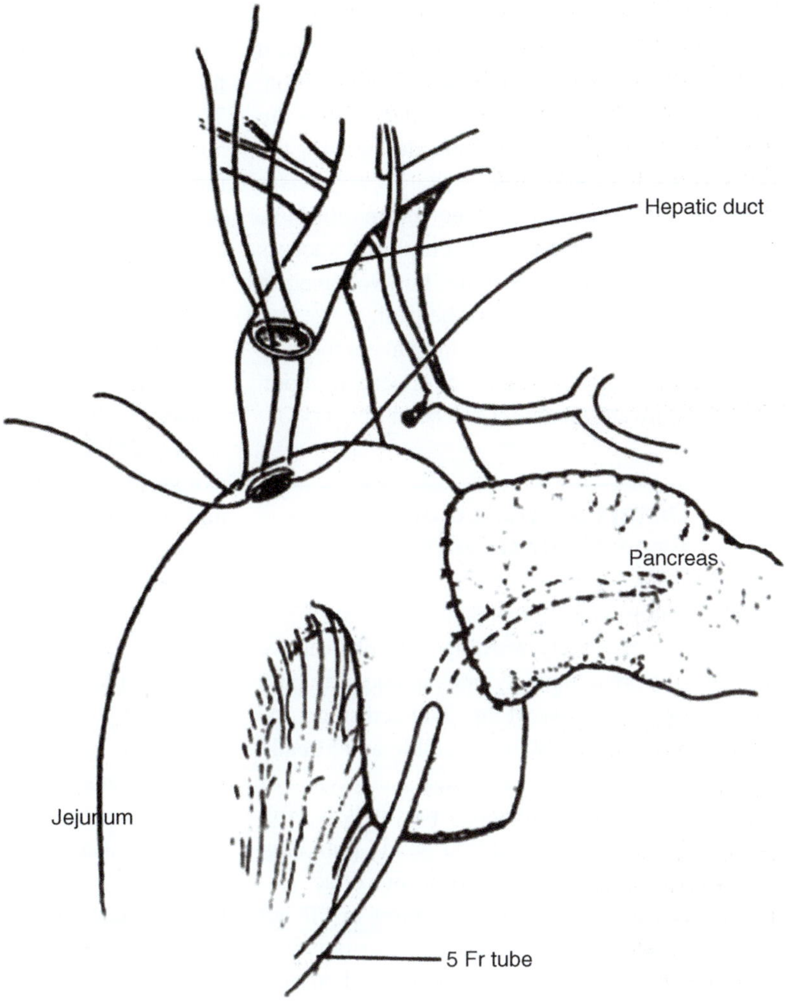

Fig. 7.6 The hepaticojejunostomy made with a single layer of interrupted, closely placed, 3-0 or 4-0 absorbable sutures is constructed several centimeters distal to the pancreaticojejunostomy. It is preferable that all duct sutures be placed first and arranged carefully to avoid entanglement. The posterior row is then sewn and tied prior to completing the anterior row (Warshaw and Thayer 2004, p. 740)

Table 7.1 Pancreatic resections at MGH Jan 1, 2009–Dec 31, 2009

Type of operation	Number	Average duration of stay
Whipple operation	134	9.3
Middle pancreatectomy	14	6.0
Distal pancreatectomy	40	6.6
Lap distal pancreatectomy	17	6.1
Total pancreatectomy	4	12.8
Other	22	8.8
Total	231	8.4

Table 7.2 Complications of pancreatic resections Jan 1, 2009–Dec 31, 2009

Nature of complication	WHIPPLE resection (N=134) (%)	Distal resection (N=57) (%)
Pancreatic fistula	16	25
Biliary fistula	3	N.A.
Delayed gastric emptying	2	N.A.
Abdominal abscess	6	13
Intraabdominal bleeding	2	3
Other	39	40
Death	1	2

High-output fistulas may require a more aggressive approach with fasting, maintenance of fluid and electrolyte balance, and parenteral nutrition. There is no conclusive evidence that fistulas are prevented or that closure is accelerated by the administration of octreotide.

Prokinetic agents such as erythromycin have been used with a modicum of purported success for promoting gastric emptying, but we have not found them to be necessary or helpful.

Most patients will receive adjuvant chemotherapy, with or without irradiation, depending upon what neoadjuvant treatment has been given.

7.3 Distal Pancreatectomy: General Considerations

Because carcinoma of the pancreatic body and tail does not give early warning with obstructive jaundice, the great majority present late with pain and cachexia indicative of an advanced stage, the disease, then, is usually unresectable and already metastatic to liver and peritoneal surfaces. For this reason, we use laparoscopy routinely to augment preoperative evaluation and planning. Invasion involving the mesenteric or celiac vessels or metastases preclude resection in all but 5 % of patients. Nonetheless, a gastrojejunostomy may be necessary if the distal duodenum is obstructed near the ligament of Treitz. While spleen preservation may be desirable for benign tumors, either with or without division of the splenic vessels (Warshaw technique), optimal lymphatic dissection demands a splenectomy for cancers. Lesser pancreatic resections, such as middle resection and enucleation, should be reserved for benign lesions (Table 7.1).

7.3.1 Surgical Technique

Although distal pancreatectomy can be accomplished by either laparoscopic or open technique, our preference for adenocarcinoma has been an open approach, because resection of adjacent retroperitoneal tissues, including those encapsulating the kidney, and involved viscera (stomach, colon) is facilitated. We find either the antegrade (right to left) or retrograde (left to right) method may be appropriate in individual circumstances. The retrograde approach (Steps 3a–5a below) allows for better visualization of the superior mesenteric vessels and mobilization to the right of the tumor for cancer of the pancreatic body especially when the cancer is primarily anterior to the splenic vessels. The antegrade approach (Steps 3b–4b below) may allow more complete dissection of retroperitoneal tissues, including the kidney and adrenal gland, for locally invasive cancers in the pancreatic tail.

Step 1: We utilize an upper midline incision to assess for metastases, adjacent organ invasion, and mesenteric vascular encasement. Gastric varices and enlarged gastroepiploic veins signify splenic vein obstruction but do not necessarily preclude respectability. Ligation of the proximal splenic artery, if accessible, will decrease operative blood loss.

Step 2: The gastrocolic omentum is opened outside the gastroepiploic vessels; the stomach is retracted anteriorly, and the lesser sac is explored for potential invasion of the posterior gastric wall, possibly necessitating a gastric resection. The short gastric vessels are divided and ligated up to the esophagus (the highest short gastric vessels communicate with the tail of the pancreas, not the spleen, and care must be taken to avoid disruption of the cancer).

Step 3a: The posterior peritoneum is opened cephalad and caudad to the pancreas, to the left of the mesenteric/portal vein and to the right of the cancer, and outside the lymphatic arcade along the splenic vessels. A tunnel is developed bluntly behind the pancreas and in front of the portal vein unless there is insufficient space to the right of the neoplasm. A Penrose drain is passed through the tunnel and used to retract the neck of the pancreas anteriorly and to the right.

Step 4a: The pancreas is divided with a sheathed stapler and 4.5 mm staples to minimize crush injury. The splenic artery and vein are divided, ligated, and suture ligated close to the celiac axis and portal vein, respectively. A row of horizontal mattress sutures is placed behind the staple line of the remnant pancreas to provide a bulwark against a pancreatic leak when/if the tissues at the staple line necrose.

Step 5a: The pancreas is mobilized progressively toward the spleen. The inferior mesenteric vein is divided when encountered. Otherwise only small collateral vessels are encountered along the inferior margin of the pancreas. Surrounding tissues, including the transverse mesocolon, Gerota's fascia, and occasionally the kidney itself, are taken with the specimen as necessary to provide a margin outside the cancer. The peritoneal attachments to the spleen are opened, and the lieno-colic ligament is divided, freeing the spleen. The specimen is removed.

Step 3b: When the cancer is located in the neck/body of the pancreas, a retrograde approach allows the dissection of the neoplasm away from the mesenteric vessels under better direct vision and facilitates venous resection and reconstruction if necessary. In this circumstance, the spleen and tail of the pancreas are mobilized as in step 5a, but the dissection and mobilization proceed from left to right.

Step 4b: With the pancreas retracted anteriorly and to the right, the portal/mesenteric vein is exposed, the splenic artery and vein are identified proximally and divided as in step 4a, and a point of pancreatic transaction at least 1 cm to the right of the identifiable tumor margin is chosen. If the pancreas here is too thick to accommodate stapling without undue crushing, the pancreas is transected sharply or with electrocautery and the stump is closed in a "fish-mouth" fashion with interrupted sutures of silk after suture ligation of the pancreatic duct. If possible, a second row of horizontal silk mattress sutures is placed behind the closure as a bulwark against a pancreatic leak.

Step 6: Metal clips are placed circumferentially around the resection margins for postoperative radiation therapy. If possible, omentum is laid against the pancreatic closure. A soft, closed-suction drain is placed in the left upper quadrant adjacent to the pancreatic closure and brought out separately through the abdominal wall.

7.3.2 Postoperative Care

The nasogastric tube is removed on the first postoperative morning. Liquid feedings are begun on the following day, and alimentation is increased as tolerated. Discharge is planned for 5–7 days after operation.

Amylase activity in the drainage is measured on day 4 or 5. The drain is removed on day 5 if the amylase activity is low. Pancreatic leak occurs in up to 25 % of cases, independent of the method of pancreatic closure or the use of octreotide (Table 7.2). In the event of a pancreatic leak, the removal of the drain is managed by sequential segmental extraction as the drainage volume decreases.

Adjuvant chemoradiation is routine.

Reference

Warshaw AL, Thayer SP (2004) Pancreaticoduodenectomy: how I do it. J Gastrointest Surg 8:733–741

Part II

Chronic Pancreatitis Surgery

8 Basic Chapter

Hans-Ulrich Schulz, René Mantke, and Hans Lippert

8.1 Relevant Basic Information, Indications, and Contraindications

Surgical techniques for chronic pancreatitis may be divided into resections and drainage procedures. From a functional point of view, drainage operations in patients with chronic pancreatitis are superior, because less parenchyma is removed. Due to the frequency of local complications in chronic pancreatitis, however, the majority of operations in our hospital are resections. The most frequent indication for resection is pancreatic head enlargement with stenosis of the bile duct, pancreatic duct, and/or duodenum. Resection of the pancreatic body and/or tail is indicated only rarely in chronic pancreatitis. Drainage procedures include enteric drainage of pseudocysts or a dilated pancreatic duct into the jejunum or stomach. We prefer an anastomosis to Roux-en-Y jejunal limb which will protect the pancreatic duct or pseudocyst from entry of intestinal content. Both approaches, resection and drainage, can be combined. Total pancreatectomy for chronic pancreatitis is performed only in very selected patients because of its overriding metabolic sequelae in these often difficult patients, especially if they are alcoholics.

Chronic pancreatitis is not a primary surgical disease. Resection of pancreatic parenchyma may lead to deterioration of exocrine and endocrine function of the gland. The major aims of operative intervention are to relieve pain and to treat the local complications of this chronic inflammatory disease that may develop as sequelae of narrowing, stenosis, or even occlusion of the pancreatic duct and/or focal enlargement of the head of the pancreas with compression of neighboring organs, such as the bile duct, duodenum, portal venous system, stomach, or colon.

General indications for operative intervention include extrinsic compression or inflammatory sclerotic stenosis of the bile duct, pancreatic duct, duodenum, or portal/splenic vein as well as the development of symptomatic pseudocysts. Carcinoma is often part of the differential diagnosis and is best ruled out by resection. Rarely, pancreatic ascites, pancreaticopleural fistula, and bleeding complications lead to operation. Every patient needs an individual treatment plan, which should be developed through an interdisciplinary approach by surgeons, gastroenterologists, and, in special situations, interventional radiologists.

H.-U. Schulz (✉)
Department of Surgery, Otto von Guericke University, Magdeburg, Germany
e-mail: hans-ulrich.schulz@med.ovgu.de

R. Mantke
Professor of Surgery, Chair, Department of Surgery, City Hospital Brandenburg, 14770 Brandenburg, Germany
e-mail: mantke@klinikum-brandenburg.de

H. Lippert, M.D.
Professor of Surgery, Chair, Department of Surgery, Otto von Guericke University of Magdeburg, 39129 Magdeburg, Germany
e-mail: hans.lippert@med.ovgu.de

R. Mantke et al. (eds.), *International Practices in Pancreatic Surgery*,
DOI 10.1007/978-3-540-74506-8_8, © Springer-Verlag Berlin Heidelberg 2013

Table 8.1 Diagnostic preoperative setup in patients with chronic pancreatitis

Diagnostic method	Questions
Clinic	Pain, nausea, weight loss, glucose intolerance, new diabetes, steatorrhea, duodenal stenosis, bile duct stenosis, pancreatic duct stenosis, pseudocyst
Laboratory evaluation	Standard parameters, CA 19-9
Standard chest X-ray	Pulmonary lesions
Ultrasound	Pancreatic tumor, ascites, liver metastases
MRT + MRCP + angio-MRI	All-in-one procedure, exclusion of a malignant tumor, pathology of the mesenteric and portal vein and hepatic and superior mesenteric artery, strictures and obstruction of pancreatic or bile duct
Endoscopic ultrasonography	*Strictures and obstruction of pancreatic or bile duct, exclusion of a malignant tumor, pathology of the mesenteric and portal vein and hepatic and superior mesenteric artery*
Preoperative biopsy	*Unnecessary, in case of tumor suspicion oncological resection is indicated*
In case of all- in- one MRI is not possible:	
CT + ERCP is used	
CT (high-quality multiphase contrast-enhanced, thin-section helical CT), angio-CT	*Exclusion of a malignant tumor, pathology of the mesenteric and portal vein and hepatic and superior mesenteric artery, ascites*
ERCP	*Strictures and obstruction of pancreatic or bide duct, endobiliary stenting, biopsy – cytologic investigations*

Italic = optional tests for specification of the diagnosis

Thrombosis or stenosis (compression) of portal or superior mesenteric veins due to pancreatic head enlargement may lead to severe portal hypertension which, in turn, will become a relative contraindication for aggressive resection because of the high risk for bleeding. When pancreatic head resection is planned, patency of the celiac trunk and superior mesenteric artery should be checked by computed tomography angiography (angio-CT) or magnetic resonance imaging (MRI). When occlusion/stenosis of the celiac trunk or common hepatic artery and the associated variations in arterial supply to the liver is not appreciated, liver ischemia may result. We do not yet perform prophylactic pancreatic resections in patients with hereditary pancreatitis because data supporting such an aggressive procedure is scarce and the sequelae of total pancreatectomy currently outweigh the benefits. In patients with chronic pancreatitis, the often substantial co-morbidity due to chronic alcohol or nicotine abuse should always be taken into consideration. In patients with concomitant liver cirrhosis, cardiomyopathy, pulmonary emphysema, or severe arteriosclerosis, thorough preoperative evaluation is necessary. We will not perform elective pancreatic surgery in patients with severe liver or respiratory insufficiency or in those patients with a left ventricular ejection fraction below 35 %. A thorough preoperative evaluation with correction of abnormalities of electrolytes, nutrition, and coagulation are essential. A strict indication for operative intervention is mandatory to avoid unnecessary risk of complications to the patient.

In general, only patients with a long-standing history of chronic pancreatitis are referred to the surgeon. For this reason, a lot of investigations have usually already been done at this time. To plan an operation, a recent contrast-enhanced, three-phase, thin-layer (1 mm), multidetector computed tomography (MD-CT) or high-quality MRI is required to image the entire pancreatic parenchyma, duct pathology, and vascular anatomy (Table 8.1). In addition, liver (cirrhosis), vessel (thrombosis, stenosis), peritoneal (ascites), and pleural (effusions) pathology should be sought for and excluded or at least acknowledged. 3D reconstruction should allow the recognition of either anatomic vascular abnormalities or functional variant arterial blood supply to the liver related to arteriosclerotic stenosis of the celiac and mesenteric arteries, respectively. Imaging of the pancreatic duct by magnetic resonance cholangiopancreaticography (MRCP) or endoscopic retrograde cholangiopancreaticography (ERCP) is obligatory. Endoscopic ultrasonography (EUS) has lost some of its value with the introduction of MD-CT and high-resolution MRI but offers advantages in patients who present with a conventional helical

CT or MRI performed on a scanner of older generation. There is no specific need for angiography or positron emission tomography (PET). Routine laboratory parameters (blood count, electrolytes, coagulation, renal, liver enzymes, and albumin) serve to evaluate relevant organ functions and allow correction of deficits preoperatively. The tumor marker CA 19-9 is always determined, and a clinically important increase (>200 U/ml) leads us to a more aggressive surgical approach, keeping in mind that jaundice may increase CA 19-9 serum level as well. A conventional chest x-ray is performed only when the thoracic organs were not visualized previously by CT or MRI. Any suggestions of cardiac or pulmonary insufficiency are evaluated by echocardiography and spirometry, respectively.

8.2 Surgical Technique

Two units of packed red blood cells are ordered for each patient on the day of operation. In general, the patient is placed supine on a flexible operation table. The table is adjusted to bring the patient into hollowback hyperextended position and rotated slightly to the right. A curved, right subcostal incision allows for convenient exposure of the pancreas and all other relevant structures. If required, this incision may be extended to the left to improve exposure of the pancreatic tail and spleen. For patients with a prior midline incision or those with a narrow costal margin, a vertical midline incision extending from the xiphoid to just below the umbilicus is equally appropriate. We prefer a Stieber self-retaining retractor to keep the incision open wide and to protect the left lobe of the liver from falling into the operative site. Every operation starts with thorough exploration of the entire peritoneal cavity to detect concomitant pathology of the liver, bowel, and other organs. If indicated, representative tissue specimens are taken for frozen section analysis.

8.2.1 Pancreatic Resection Procedures

Traditionally, pancreatic head resection in chronic pancreatitis follows the same operative rules as in pancreatic cancer, i.e. pancreatoduodenectomy in combination with subtotal resection of the stomach. In contrast, organ-sparing resections have been developed over the past several decades that include pylorus preservation and several techniques for preservation of the duodenum and distal bile duct. The classic Kausch-Whipple (KW) procedure is used typically in patients with chronic pancreatitis who have had a prior gastric resection for ulcer, in rare situations of extensive adhesions between the pancreatic head and the pyloric region, and if the duodenum stump becomes ischemic during an attempted pylorus preservation. Pylorus-preserving pancreatoduodenectomy is indicated in patients who present with suspicion of cancer and those with combined stenoses of the intrapancreatic bile duct, pancreatic duct, and duodenum due to inflammatory pancreatic head enlargement.

The Longmire-Traverso, Frey, and Kausch-Whipple procedures are used frequently in our department in patients with chronic pancreatitis. These methods following this chapter (Table 8.4).

The *classic pancreatoduodenectomy* or Kausch-Whipple procedure begins with mobilization of the hepatic flexure and transverse colon (Table 8.2). The duodenocolic ligament is divided and the superior mesenteric vein identified. An extended Kocher maneuver is then performed so that the common bile duct, the vena cava, and both renal veins become visible (Fig. 8.1). This maneuver allows for palpation of the pancreatic head and uncinate process and evaluation of the retroperitoneal space for pathology, such as enlarged lymph nodes. Next the lesser sac is entered by transection of the right portion of the gastrocolic ligament but with preservation of the gastroepiploic vessels. Use of the harmonic scalpel (SonoSurg®, Olympus, Hamburg, Germany) can be extremely beneficial, because operation time can be reduced. After division of fibrous adhesions between the pancreas and the posterior wall of the stomach, the entire anterior surface of the pancreas is freed up. Care must be taken to avoid injury to the blood vessels and branches of the vagus nerve along the lesser curve of the stomach and the splenic artery at the superior margin of the pancreas.

Table 8.2 Steps of a standard Kausch-Whipple procedure

Resection	
1	Exploration
2	Biopsy of liver or peritoneal metastases if necessary
3	Elevation of the duodenum and pancreatic head (Kocher maneuver)
4	Mobilization of the right colon flexure
5	Division of the duodenocolic ligament
6	Division of the right portion of the gastrocolic ligament
7	Division of adhesions between pancreas and the posterior gastric wall
8	Identification and banding of the gastroduodenal artery and identification of the portal vein on the superior border of the pancreas
9	Exposure of the SMV at the inferior border of the pancreas
10	Division of the gastroduodenal artery
11	Division of the pancreas
12	Resection of the gastric antrum
13	Division of the jejunum distal the ligament of Treitz and delivery of the jejunum and the distal duodenum to the right of the superior mesenteric vessels
14	Freeing the uncinate process and division of the lateral branches of the SMV and SMA
15	Freeing of the gallbladder and transection of the common hepatic bile duct
16	Pancreaticojejunostomy
17	Hepaticojejunostomy
19	Gastrojejunostomy
20	Braun's entero-enterostomy
21	Drainage and closure of the abdominal wound

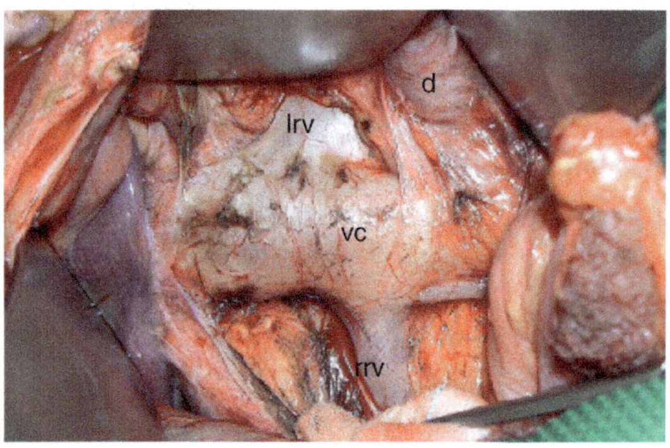

Fig. 8.1 Kocher maneuver. Following mobilization of the duodenum, the inferior vena cava and both renal veins become visible (*vc* vena cava, *rrv* right renal vein, *lrv* left renal vein, *l* liver, *d* duodenum)

Next, the hepatoduodenal ligament is dissected so that the common hepatic artery becomes visible. The origin of the gastroduodenal artery is identified, and the vessel is encircled and retracted to the left. Identification of the portal vein is easy now, because it is situated in the triangle between the common hepatic artery, gastroduodenal artery, and superior margin of the pancreas. Next, starting at the caudal margin of the neck of the pancreas and the superior mesenteric vein, the groove of the portal vein on the dorsal surface of the pancreas is carefully dissected bluntly using an Overholt clamp. In the presence of severe inflammatory adhesions or a large pancreatic head compressing the portal vein, the groove of the portal vein may not be identifiable without causing potentially severe bleeding from the veins. In this situation, the pancreatic parenchyma is transected anterior to the presumed course of the superior mesenteric and portal veins behind the neck of the pancreas. After dissection of the superior mesenteric/portal vein groove from the dorsal pancreatic capsule is completed, a suture of 3/0 diameter (any material possible) is positioned around the neck of the pancreas at the right margin of the superior mesenteric vein and tightly tied. This suture ligation compresses the pancreaticoduodenal arteries and enables the neck of the pancreas to be lifted. Two stay sutures (4/0 monofilament resorbable, e.g. PDS®, Ethicon, Norderstedt, Germany) are placed and tied in the pancreatic neck, one each at the upper and lower margin of the organ (Fig. 8.2). In contrast to other groups, we do not dissect circumferentially and loop the portal and superior mesenteric veins for control of possible bleeding. In our hands, control of bleeding can be achieved easily by bidigital compression of the veins when a wide Kocher maneuver has been performed.

The next step consists of the ligation of the gastroduodenal artery near its origin at the common hepatic artery. The stump of the gastroduodenal artery is secured by a transfixion suture using 4/0 monofilament nonresorbable material (Prolene®, Ethicon). The pancreatic neck then is now lifted by traction of the stay sutures and the pancreatic parenchyma is transected using an

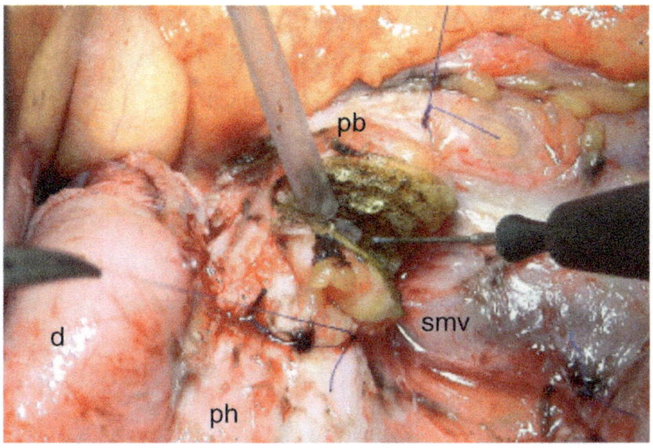

Fig. 8.2 Following the placement of stay sutures, the pancreas is transected in front of the superior mesenteric vein using a cautery needle (*ph* pancreas head, *pb* pancreas body, *smv* superior mesenteric vein, *d* duodenum)

electrocautery needle beginning anteriorly at the right margin of the portal vein, starting at the uncinate edge of the superior mesenteric vein. Details of this transection have been described and illustrated in Chap. 1. Bleeding from small, intrapancreatic vessels is controlled immediately by bipolar coagulation. After transection of the pancreas, the gastric antrum is resected. We never perform the classic 2/3 Billroth resection when resecting a pancreatic head. Transection of the antrum is performed using two firings of a 75-mm, reloadable linear cutter (TLC 75 Proximate®, blue magazine, Ethicon, Norderstedt, Germany). The jejunum is transected about 15 cm distal to the ligament of Treitz also using a TLC 75 Proximate® linear cutter, and the vessels in its mesentery and the mesentery of the fourth portion of the duodenum are transected using a harmonic scalpel. The jejunum is then pulled behind the mesenteric root and into the right subhepatic region. By gently retracting the gastric antrum and the jejunal loop to the right, the superior mesenteric and portal veins become better exposed allowing removal of the pancreatic head from its retroperitoneal surroundings. Resection of the uncinate and head of the pancreas along the right side of the mesentericoportal vessel axis using a harmonic scalpel. Bleeding is controlled by bipolar coagulation and placement of titanium clips (Ligaclip® Multiple Clip Applier MCM-30, Ethicon). After ligation and transection of cystic artery, the gallbladder is mobilized subserously from the liver. In the final step of the resection, the common hepatic duct is transected just proximal to the cystic duct using a cautery needle.

Reconstruction starts by creating a window in the right transverse mesocolon through which the jejunum is pulled through. First, an end-to-side anastomosis between the remnant left pancreas and the jejunal loop is created using the Warren-Cattell technique as described in Chap. 1. The inner duct-to-mucosa layer of the anastomosis is performed using 4–6 (seldom more) single stitches of 5/0 monofilament resorbable sutures (PDS®, Ethicon). For completion of the anastomosis, an outer layer of single stitches of 4/0 monofilament resorbable sutures (PDS®, Ethicon) is carried out with seromuscular sutures in the jejunum and sutures through the capsule and pancreatic parenchyma. We do not perform intraoperative stenting of the pancreatic duct.

The bile duct is then anastomosed to the same jejunal limb about 6–8 cm distal to the pancreatic anastomosis. This biliodigestive anastomosis is created using two running sutures of 5/0 or 4/0 monofilament resorbable material (PDS®, Ethicon). We do not routinely place a Kehr T-tube. When the bile duct lumen is small, reconstruction using the Goetze-Gutgemann technique (for a comparison, see Chap. 1) is advantageous. For this technique, the anterior part of the anastomosis is performed with interrupted stitches instead of a running suture. Monofilament resorbable 5/0 material (PDS®, Ethicon) is used for these cases involving a small bile duct and a small diameter t-tube or transhepatic drain is inserted if deemed necessary by the surgeon.

Next, the stomach stump is anastomosed using an omega-shaped jejunal loop positioned anterior to the transverse colon (antecolic). The distance between biliodigestive and gastric anastomosis is about 60 cm. A Braun anastomosis is created about 10 cm distal to the defect in the transverse mesocolon through which jejunal limb was passed. Both enteric anastomoses are performed using two layers of polyfilamentous resorbable 4/0 (jejunum) or 3/0 (stomach) running sutures (Vicryl®, Ethicon). Figure 8.3 illustrates the reconstruction used. Finally, one silicone drain (Easy Flow Drainage, P. J. Dahlhausen & Co.,

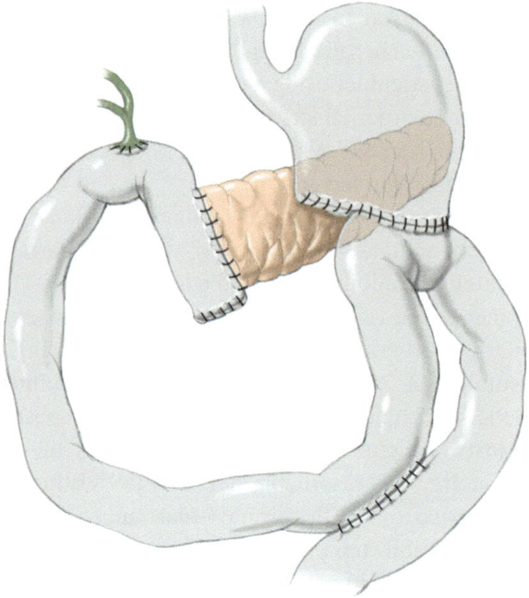

Fig. 8.3 Reconstruction following classical Kausch-Whipple procedure. End-to-side duct-to-mucosa pancreaticojejunostomy using Warren-Cattell's technique is performed followed by end-to-side hepaticojejunostomy. Antecolonic gastrojejunostomy is performed next and reconstruction is completed by side-to-side entero-enterostomy in accordance with Braun

GmbH, Cologne, Germany) is placed into the subhepatic region with its tip in the former epiploic foramen about 2 cm from the pancreatic anastomosis.

Pylorus-preserving pancreatic head resection (PPPHR) is performed in cases where there is a serious concern about pancreatic head carcinoma or when there is a long intrapancreatic stenosis of the bile duct. Longmire's surgical technique for this procedure (Fig. 8.4) was described in Section 1.1.2.

The *Frey procedure* is a combination of a non-anatomic, subtotal resection of the pancreatic head with longitudinal opening (filleting) and drainage of the pancreatic ducts. Pancreatic duct pathology is associated with pancreatic head enlargement in about 30 % of our patients with chronic pancreatitis. Pancreatic head resection alone is inadequate if there is associated pathology of the pancreatic duct (e.g., stones, strictures, retention cysts) in the remnant body or tail of the gland. In contrast, it is unlikely that an enlarged pancreatic head can be drained sufficiently by standard, longitudinal pancreaticojejunostomy

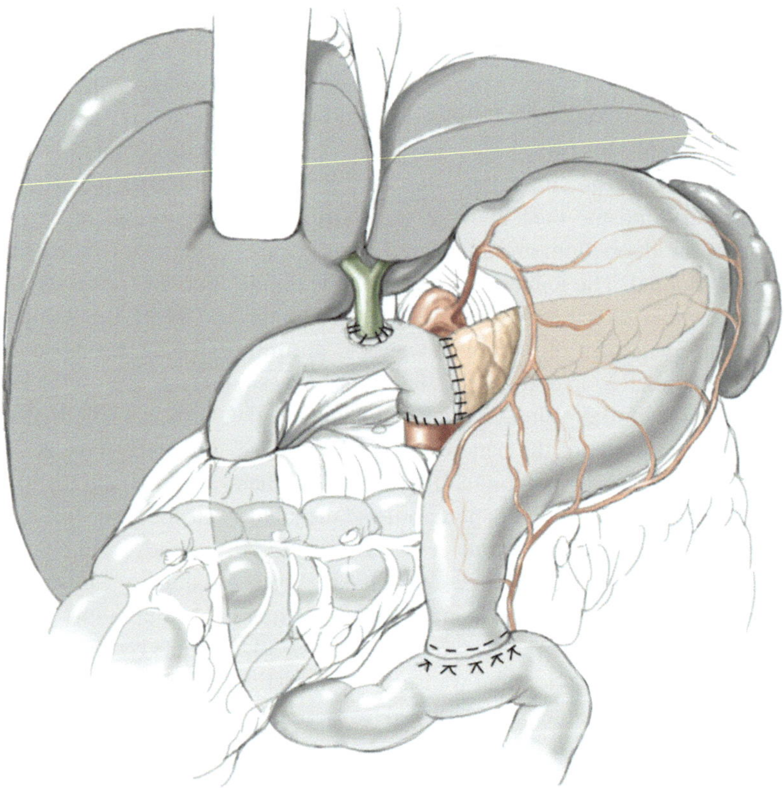

Fig. 8.4 Reconstruction following pylorus-preserving cephalic pancreatoduodenectomy. As in the Kausch-Whipple procedure, the first step consists of end-to-side duct-to-mucosa pancreaticojejunostomy using Warren-Cattell's technique. End-to-side hepaticojejunostomy follows. Antecolonic duodenojejunostomy is performed next. In contrast to the classical Kausch-Whipple operation, no entero-enterostomy is needed

Table 8.3 Steps of the Frey procedure

Resection	
1	Exploration
2	Biopsy of liver or peritoneal metastases if necessary
3	Elevation of the duodenum and pancreatic head (Kocher maneuver)
4	Mobilization of the right and left colon flexure
5	Division of the duodenocolic ligament and gastrocolic ligament
6	Identification and transection of the gastroduodenal artery and identification of the portal vein on the superior border of the pancreas
7	Exposure of the SMV at the inferior border of the pancreas
8	Complete opening of the main pancreatic duct, starting in the body of the pancreas
9	Subtotal resection of the pancreatic head
10	If indicated, drainage of the bile duct into the resection cavity
Reconstruction	
11	Pancreaticojejunostomy using Y-Roux limb
12	Jejunojejunostomy

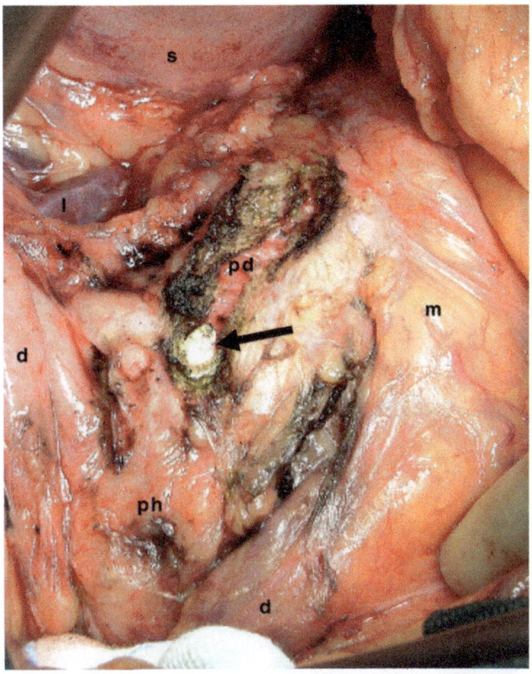

Fig. 8.5 First step of the Frey procedure. The duct of Wirsung is opened in the body of the pancreas using a cautery needle. Note the appearance of a stone within the duct (*arrow*). All stones and strictures must be removed to achieve efficient duct drainage. For this reason, the incision of the duct is carried out as far as possible in both directions to the splenic hilum and to the duodenum (*pd* opened pancreatic duct, *s* stomach, *d* duodenum, *ph* pancreatic head, *l* liver, *m* mesocolon transversum)

(Partington-Rochelle procedure). For these reasons, pancreatic resection and drainage techniques should be entertained and are often combined. In all standard pancreatic head resections (e.g., Kausch-Whipple, Longmire-Traverso, Beger), it is possible to fillet open the pancreatic ductal system in its entire course and perform a side-to-side instead of end-to-side pancreaticojejunostomy to drain the ducts completely. An alternative approach combining the classic longitudinal pancreaticojejunostomy with subtotal coring of fibrous pancreatic head tissue was proposed by Frey and Smith in 1987. Because the neck of the pancreas is not transected completely over the superior mesenteric vein, portal hypertension is not a contraindication for this operation as it is for a classic Kausch-Whipple resection.

Technically, the pancreas is exposed in the same manner as in other types of pancreatic surgery (Table 8.3). Briefly, the hepatic flexure of the colon is mobilized, a Kocher maneuver is performed (Fig. 8.1) and the lesser sac is opened by transection of the gastrocolic ligament. In our experience, it seems more advantageous to resect the enlarged pancreatic head subtotally instead of only partially coring it out. For this reason, the gastroduodenal artery is ligated and transected at the superior margins of the pancreas using 4/0 monofilamentous non-resorbable sutures (Prolene®, Ethicon). To prevent damage to the superior mesenteric and portal veins during pancreatic head resection, these vessels must be identified and kept under direct vision. The main pancreatic duct is incised in the body of the organ (Fig. 8.5). This ductal incision is extended as far as possible in both directions to the splenic hilum and the duodenum. All strictures must be incised and all calculi removed carefully to achieve effective drainage of the ductal system. The pancreatic head is resected subtotally using a cautery needle. We preserve about 6–8 mm of pancreatic tissue near the duodenum and about 5 mm of pancreas near the superior mesenteric and portal veins, respectively (Fig. 8.6a). In contrast to other types of anatomic resections of the

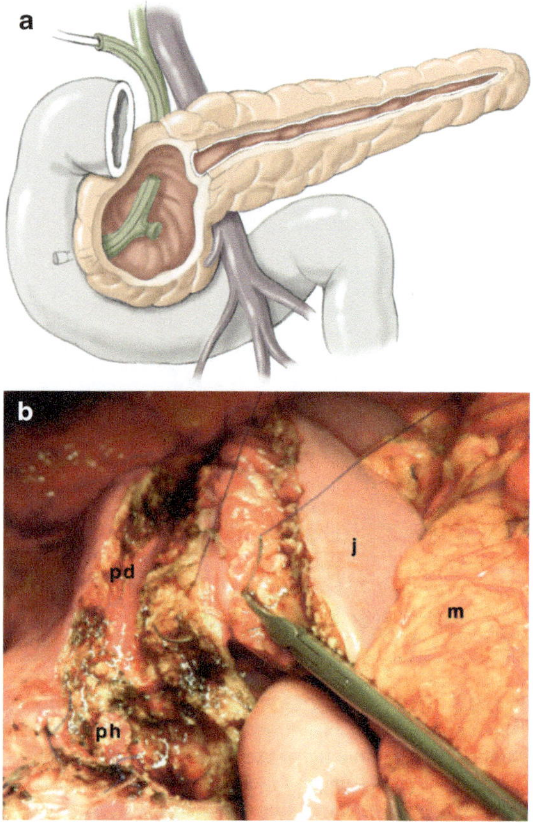

Fig. 8.6 (**a**, **b**) In the Frey procedure, the pancreatic head is resected subtotally so that the bile duct becomes visible at the ground of the resection cavity (**a**). A Teflon or metal probe inserted via the cystic duct may help to identify the course of the bile duct. For reconstruction, side-to-side pancreaticojejunostomy (**b**) using a Y-Roux loop is performed with one layer of running suture of monofilamentous, resorbable material (*ph* resected pancreatic head, *pd* opened pancreatic duct, *j* jejunum, *m* mesocolon transversum)

pancreatic head, the pancreas is not transected completely. Monofilamentous absorbable 4/0 sutures (PDS®, Ethicon) are used for hemostasis when bipolar coagulation is ineffective. As in the Beger and Berne procedures, the bile duct may be incised in its intrapancreatic portion and drained into the resection cavity. A one-layer, longitudinal pancreaticojejunostomy is performed with 50-cm long Roux-en-Y limb using running 4/0 monofilamentous absorbable sutures (PDS®, Ethicon) (Fig. 8.6b). Finally, an end-to-side jejunojejunostomy is performed in two layers (4/0 Vicryl®, Ethicon). One silicone drain (Easy Flow Drainage, P. J. Dahlhausen & Co., GmbH, Cologne, Germany) is placed alongside the pancreaticojejunostomy.

Duodenum-preserving pancreatic head resection (Beger procedure) and the *Berne technique* are described in other chapters as well as the technique of *Left-sided, distal pancreatectomy*.

8.2.2 Drainage Procedures

Surgical drainage procedures have been performed much less frequently in recent years due to excellent endoscopic techniques for drainage. For problematic cases, primary ductal procedures are safe and efficient. The indication for operative care should be discussed with an interdisciplinary approach.

Lateral Pancreaticojejunostomy is performed to drain enterically a dilated pancreatic duct in patients without chronic inflammatory enlargement of the pancreatic head, using the Partington and Rochelle procedure. To expose the entire anterior surface of the pancreas, the gastrocolic ligament is divided, and both colonic flexures are mobilized. Fibrous adhesions between the pancreas and the posterior surface of the stomach are cut. When dilated, the main pancreatic duct can usually be visualized or palpated as a soft fluctuant depression or trough in the body of the gland. If the duct cannot be localized, intraoperative ultrasonography can aid localization of the duct. Once the duct is identified, it is incised longitudinally alongside the needle (which is left in place to aid this ductal incision) using a cautery needle. Once the duct is entered, its precise course is determined using a Teflon probe or an Overholt clamp. To identify all pathologic findings, it is important to unroof the pancreatic duct over its entire length from as close as possible to its entry into the duodenum out to the splenic hilum. Care is taken to avoid injury to the gastroduodenal and pancreatoduodenal arcade. In the head of the pancreas, both the duct of Wirsung and the duct of Santorini are unroofed and drained (Fig. 8.7). Bleeding from the cut edges of the pancreas can

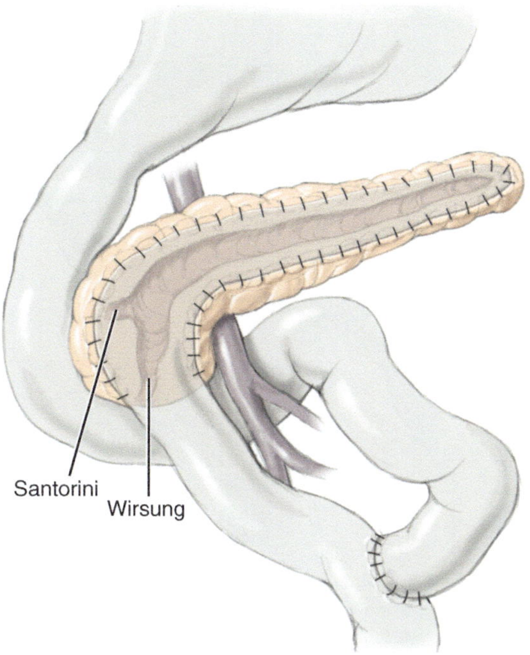

Fig. 8.7 Techniques of pancreatic duct drainage procedure by latero-lateral pancreaticojejunostomy. In the case of a dilated pancreatic duct, both the duct of Wirsung and the duct of Santorini are unroofed and freed from stones and strictures

be controlled by bipolar coagulation. Suture ligatures of 5/0 monofilamentous non-resorbable material (Prolene PDS®, Ethicon) are needed on occasion. Stones are removed meticulously using forceps or an Overholt clamp. In general, we avoid creating a short anastomosis of the pancreatic duct but rather plan on a long pancreaticoenteric anastomosis. For reconstruction, the jejunum is transected approximately 45 cm distal to the ligament of Treitz using a linear cutter (TLC 75 Proximate®, Ethicon). A defect is created in the avascular space of transverse mesocolon to the right of the middle colonic vessels through which the jejunal limb is passed. The stapled end of the distal jejunum is positioned at the splenic hilum and jejunum opened along its anterior mesenteric border. A single layer, side-to-side pancreaticojejunostomy is performed with running sutures of 4/0 monofilamentous resorbable material (PDS®, Ethicon) starting at the splenic flexure. The caudal inferior portion of the anastomosis is performed first (Fig. 8.8) followed by the rostral

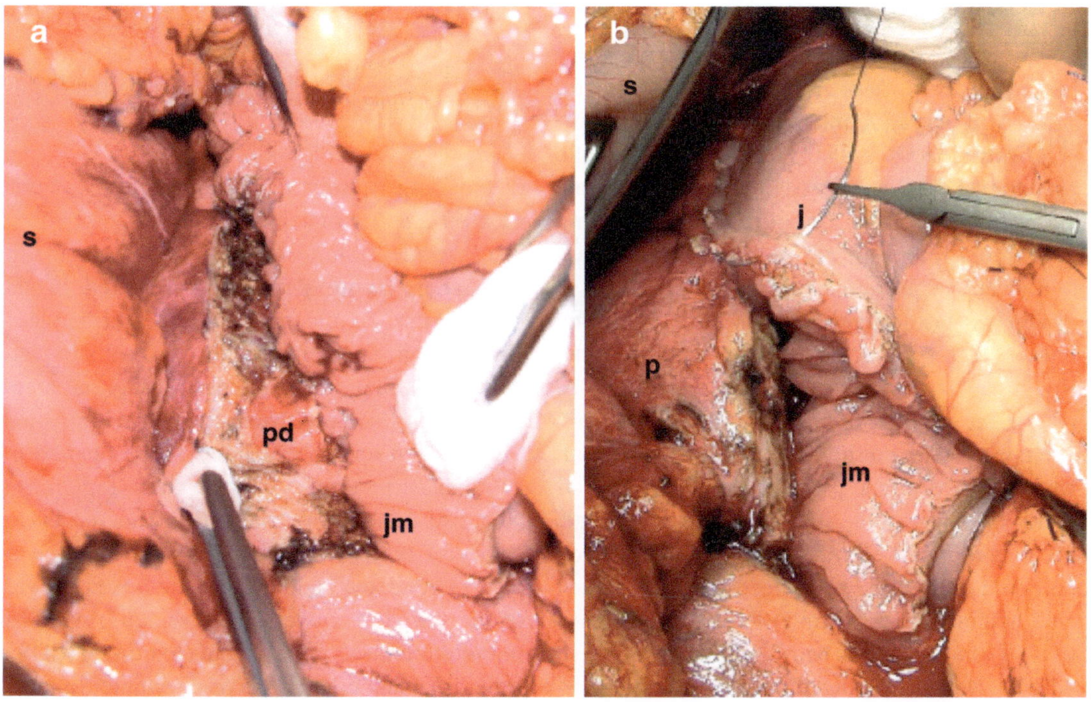

Fig. 8.8 (**a**, **b**) A jejunal Y-Roux limb is used for reconstruction in laterolateral pancreaticojejunostomy. The inferior portion of the anastomosis is performed first (**a**) followed by the superior portion (**b**) (*pd* pancreatic duct, *jm* jejunal mucosa, *s* stomach, *j* jejunum, *p* pancreas)

superior portion. Sutures are passed through the serosa and muscularis of the jejunum (i.e., extramucosally) but through the full thickness of pancreatic parenchyma between fibrous capsule and unroofed duct. We do not attempt necessarily to perform mucosa-to-mucosa apposition. An end-to-side jejunojejunostomy is performed 50 cm distal to the pancreaticojejunostomy to re-establish intestinal continuity (4/0 Vicryl PDS®, Ethicon). One silicone drain (Easy Flow Drainage, P. J. Dahlhausen & Co., GmbH, Cologne, Germany) is placed alongside the length of the pancreaticojejunostomy. In the case of pancreatogenic pain in patients with a non-dilated main pancreatic duct, so-called "small duct disease", longitudinal V-shaped resection of the ventral part of the pancreas may be performed as proposed by Izbicki.

Lateral Pancreaticogastrostomy has only rare indications. This form of enteric drainage may be performed in selected patients of massive adhesions or unsuspected pancreatic necrosis found at operation. Technically, such an operation should follow the same rules as lateral pancreaticojejunostomy.

(Pseudo) cystojejunostomy is performed in similar fashion to a lateral pancreaticojejunostomy (Fig. 8.9). A pre-requisite for safe, successful operative internal drainage of a pancreatic pseudocyst is a mature fibrous wall of the pseudocyst. In general, a wide incision (at least 3 cm) is made in the pseudocyst wall allowing for exploration of the entire cavity and evacuation of any sequestered material (Fig. 8.10). A frozen section to exclude malignancy is done intraoperatively. A one-layer, side-to-side, Roux-en-Y pseudocysto-jejunostomy with 4/0 resorbable monofilamentous sutures (PDS®, Ethicon) is our method of choice. In general, we do not drain a pseudocyst enterically if there is a previous history of hemorrhage, because this will eliminate the self-tamponade potential in the case of rebleeding. Under such circumstances, we prefer resection of the portion of the pancreas bearing the pseudocyst. Alternatively, radiologic embolization or stenting of pseudoaneurysms or operative ligation of bleeding vessels may be appropriate to prevent rebleeding in selected patients.

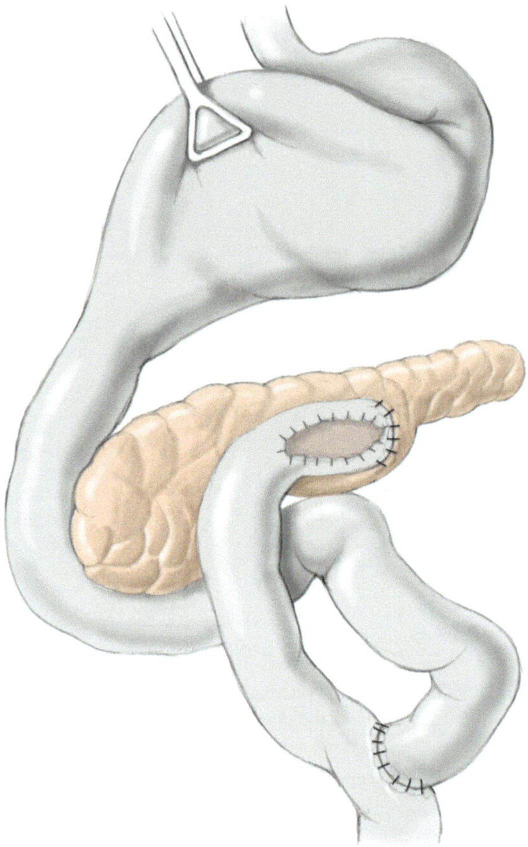

Fig. 8.9 Pseudocystojejunostomy using a one-layer side-to-side Roux-en-Y anastomosis

(Pseudo) cystogastrostomy may be suitable for patients with pseudocysts located in the body or tail of the pancreas with firm adherence to the posterior wall of the stomach. A longitudinal, anterior gastrotomy is made using electrocautery. Next, the posterior wall of the stomach and the pseudocyst are opened by a transgastric transcystic incision (Fig. 8.11). Necrotic material is evacuated, and the entire cavity of the pseudocyst is explored. The wall of the pseudocyst adherent to the posterior wall of the stomach is oversewn ("reefed") with 4/0 monofilamentous resorbable material (PDS®, Ethicon) using continuous or interrupted sutures. Alternatively, an anastomosis may be created

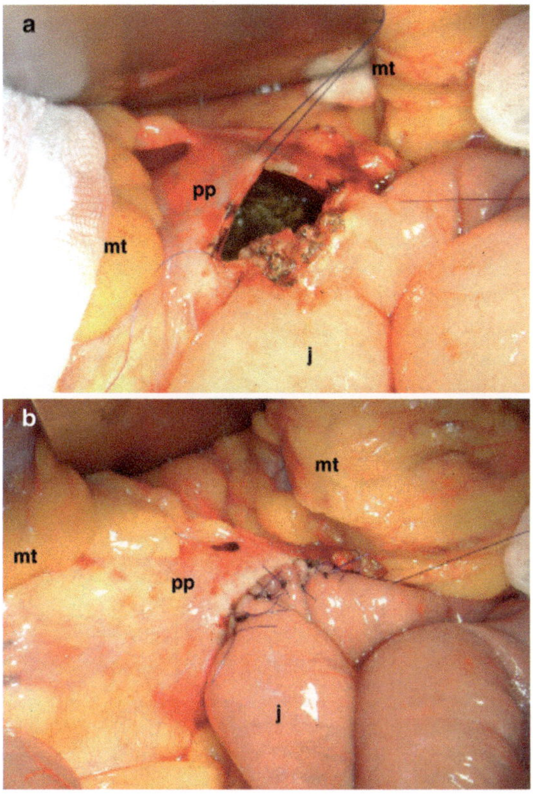

Fig. 8.10 (**a**, **b**) Drainage procedure of a pseudocyst in the pancreas tail (pseudocystojejunostomy) using a jejunal loop and a transmesocolic approach. Single-layer continuous suture (PDS 4/0) at the posterior wall (**a**) and single layer interrupted sutures (PDS 4/0) for the anterior wall (**b**) were used (*pp* pancreatic pseudocyst, *j* jejunum, *mt* mesocolon transversum)

using a circular stapler of 33 mm diameter (ILS-33, Ethicon Endo-Surgery, Norderstedt, Germany). Finally, the incision in the anterior wall of the stomach is closed using 2–3 firings of a linear stapler (TLC 75 Proximate®, Ethicon).

8.3 Additional Medications and Procedures

- Single dose perioperative antibiotic prophylaxis is given intravenously about 30 min prior to skin incision. Because infectious complications after pancreatic surgery originate from bowel flora, the antibiotic chosen must cover the range

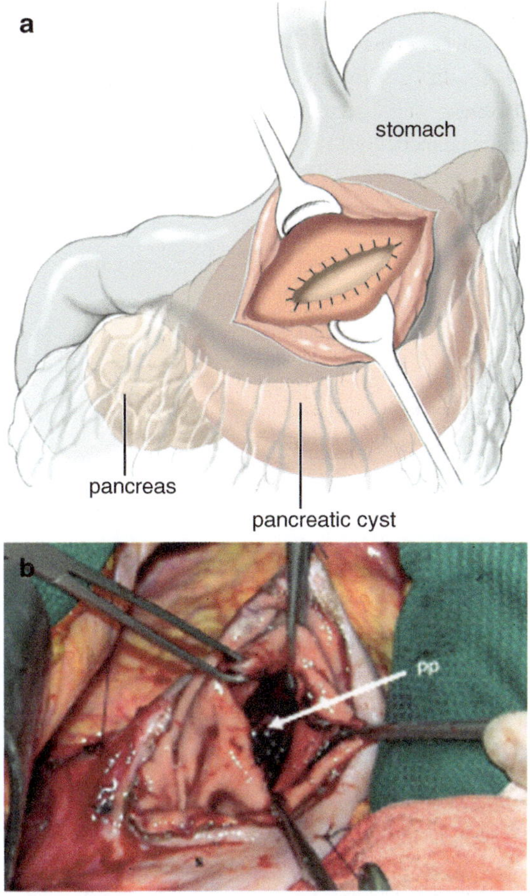

Fig. 8.11 (**a**, **b**) Pseudocystogastrostomy using a longitudinal anterior gastrotomy. The pseudocyst is opened by a transgastric incision. The wall of the pseudocyst is anastomized with the posterior wall of the stomach with 4/0 PDS using interrupted or continuous sutures (*s* anterior gastric wall, *pp* opened pancreatic pseudocyst containing sequestered necrotic material)

of suspected bowel microorganisms. In addition, specific hospital-acquired bacteria and the capacity for pancreatic penetration of the compound should be considered when choosing an antibiotic. In our experience, a combination of 4 g mezlocillin (Baypen®, Bayer, Leverkusen, Germany) and 1 g sulbactam (Combactam®, Pfizer, Karlsruhe, Germany) is effective. In patients with penicillin allergy, we use 1 g imipenem (Zienam®, MSD, Munich, Germany). For lengthy operations, a second antibiotic dose is given 4–5 h after the first application.

Table 8.4 Patients with chronic pancreatitis who underwent pancreatic resection (2006, 2007)

Parameter	Number	%
Patients	42	100
Hospital mortality	3	7.1
Hospital stay (median, days)	17.2 (7–59)	
Relaparotomy	7	16.7
Death without local complications	1	2.4
Kausch-Whipple procedure	4	9.6
Traverso-Longmire procedure	17	40.4
Frey procedure	1	26.2
Beger procedure	2	4.8
Berne procedure	2	4.8
Pancreatic left resection	5	1.8
Total pancreatectomy	1	2.4
Postoperative local morbidity		
Postoperative bleeding[a]	1	2.4
Delayed gastric emptying[b]	7	16.7
Pancreatic fistula[c]	5	11.8
Biliary fistula[d]	2	4.8
Wound infection	5	11.8
Other (i.e. abscess, pleural effusion)	8	19.0
Postoperative systemic morbidity		
Systemic complications[e]	6	14.3

[a]Need for relaparotomy
[b]Nasogastric intubation >10 days, or its reinsertion because of vomiting, or the inability to tolerate a solid diet after the 14th postoperative day. *Other definitions*: No normal oral feeding after 10 postoperative days; intolerance to oral intake and need for nasogastric decompression after the seventh postoperative day
[c]Drain output of any measurable volume of fluid on or after the third postoperative day with an amylase content greater than three times the serum amylase activity. *Other definitions*: Persistent drainage of more than 30 ml amylase-rich fluid (>5,000 units) per day for more than 10 days; drainage of more than 30 ml amylase-rich fluid (at least three times the upper normal limit of serum amylase concentration) per 24 h after the fifth postoperative day
[d]Bilirubin-rich fluid was drained for more than 5 days
[e]Cardiopulmonary, renal, sepsis, neural, other

Table 8.5 Patients with chronic pancreatitis who underwent drainage operation (2006, 2007)

Parameter	Number	%
Patients	10	100
Hospital mortality	0	0
Hospital stay (median, days)	12.4 (9–22)	
Relaparotomy	0	0
Death without local complications	0	0
Pancreaticojejunostomy	1	10
Pancreaticogastrostomy	1	10
Pseudocystojejunostomy	4	40
Pseudocystogastrostomy	4	40
Postoperative local morbidity		
Postoperative bleeding[a]	0	0
Delayed gastric emptying[b]	0	0
Pancreatic fistula[c]	0	0
Biliary fistulad	0	0
Wound infection	1	10
Other (i.e. abscess, pleural effusion)	0	0
Postoperative systemic morbidity		
Systemic complications[e]	0	0

[a]Need for relaparotomy
[b]Nasogastric intubation >10 days, or its reinsertion because of vomiting, or the inability to tolerate a solid diet after the 14th postoperative day. *Other definitions*: No normal oral feeding after 10 postoperative days; intolerance to oral intake and need for nasogastric decompression after the seventh postoperative day
[c]Drain output of any measurable volume of fluid on or after the third postoperative day with an amylase content greater than three times the serum amylase activity. *Other definitions*: Persistent drainage of more than 30 ml amylase-rich fluid (>5,000 units) per day for more than 10 days; drainage of more than 30 ml amylase-rich fluid (at least three times the upper normal limit of serum amylase concentration) per 24 h after the fifth postoperative day
[d]Bilirubin-rich fluid was drained for more than 5 days
[e]Cardiopulmonary, renal, sepsis, neural, other

- In surgery for chronic pancreatitis, inhibitors of pancreatic secretion, such as somatostatin or octreotide, are not given routinely, because the postoperative fistula rate is low due to the hard texture of fibrotic pancreatic parenchyma.
- If possible, patients get an epidural catheter for postoperative pain control.
- During operation, all patients receive a nasogastric tube, which is removed at the completion of anesthesia.
- Enteral nutrition is started on the first postoperative day.
- All patients are given prophylaxis against deep vein thrombosis with a low molecular

weight heparin (enoxaparin, Clexane®, 40 mg, Sanofi-Aventis, Frankfurt, Germany) once daily starting on the evening of the admission day and until discharge.
- Prophylaxis against gastric stress ulcer and anastomotic ulcer is given using 40 mg pantoprazole daily as an intravenous injection (Pantozol®, Nycomed, Constance, Germany).
- Postoperative ICU admission with invasive monitoring is routine.
- The intraoperative drain(s) is removed 48 h postoperatively unless drainage volume is >50 ml/day. Drain output is not measured routinely for amylase activity. Only when the output is high or the color is typical for pancreatic fistula the fluid is checked for amylase activity. In the case of fistula, the drain is maintained in place until the output volume has decreased. In the case of a persistent pancreatic fistula (>3 weeks) without clinically relevant symptoms, the drain is removed incrementally on an every day basis (2–3 cm/day). Usually, the fistula is controlled by a dermal drainage bag and will close by itself over time. In the case of clinical symptoms (e.g., pain, fever, leukocytosis), an abdominal CT should be obtained to exclude gross peripancreatic fluid collection or an abscess, which would require some form of interventional drainage. Reoperation is rarely necessary because of a pancreatic fistula. A biliary fistula requires reoperation if the output is high. Patient discharge with drains in situ is appropriate in patients tolerating enteric or oral nutrition and without signs of organ dysfunction.

8.4 Results

The results of pancreatic surgery in chronic pancreatitis are contained in Tables 8.4 and 8.5.

Commentary

9

David B. Adams and Katherine A. Morgan

9.1 Relevant Basic Information

The indications for surgery in the management of chronic pancreatitis are well formulated: suspicion of cancer, biliary stenosis, duodenal stenosis, arterial erosion, splenic vein occlusion, internal pancreatic fistulae, and pancreatic pseudocyst. There is no doubt, however, that the chief indication for surgical management of chronic pancreatitis in our experience is intractable pain. Patients with chronic pancreatitis and intractable pain are marginalized and stigmatized by health care providers because of the assumption that patients with chronic pancreatitis are responsible for their own pain and suffering due to a character flaw associated with chronic alcoholism and narcotic drug dependence. Mechanisms of pain in chronic pancreatitis remain poorly understood. The ductal hypertension theory of Puestow, the parenchymal hypertension theory of Reber, and the perineural inflammation theory of Bockman and Keith have improved our understanding of pain in chronic pancreatitis but have not elucidated more successful surgical therapies in the management of intractable pain associated with chronic pancreatitis.

The operative complications of bleeding, obstruction, and perforation associated with chronic pancreatitis have anatomic operative solutions in most instances. Remediation of intractable pain due to chronic pancreatitis has been managed less successfully with operations to correct underlying anatomic disorders. Nevertheless, many useful insights into the mechanisms of pancreatic pain have been discovered in the last decade. Pancreatic neurocellular pain pathways operate more like webs than highways, and there are multiple redundancies and alternate routes that bypass operative attempts to inhibit pain pathways. There is evidence that chronic pancreatitis induces changes in pathways of visceral pain with spinothalamic and central re-organization of brain centers that process pain. Central spinal neuropathy, central cerebral neuroplasticity, peripheral extrapancreatic nociception, and pancreatic neuropathy are all part of a synergistic disorder in patients who suffer from intractable, maladaptive pain associated with chronic pancreatitis. Early operative intervention in the management of intractable pain associated with chronic pancreatitis has been suggested as a means to prevent the development of irreversible pain from these visceral and central pain pathways.

Though pancreatic drainage procedures have lesser complication rates than resection procedures, resecting inflamed parenchyma has the potential to achieve better outcomes in pain control. The observation that changes at the cellular level in chronic pancreatitis result in augmentation of synthesis of pancreatic peptides that are known pain transmitters is another argument to

D.B. Adams, M.D. (✉) • K.A. Morgan, M.D.
Department of Surgery,
Medical University of South Carolina,
Charleston, USA
e-mail: adamsdav@musc.edu

R. Mantke et al. (eds.), *International Practices in Pancreatic Surgery*,
DOI 10.1007/978-3-540-74506-8_9,

favor resection over drainage procedures. In our view, total pancreatectomy for chronic pancreatitis has emerged as a selective approach for the early management of chronic pancreatitis without ductal dilation, avoiding the complication of brittle diabetes by combining this procedure with islet auto-transplantation.

9.2 The Puestow Procedure

The principles that Puestow delineated in his 1957 Archives of Surgery report have remained unchanged. The pancreatic ductotomy is carried as far to the right and to the left as possible, and the jejunal limb is passed through the transverse mesocolon to the right of the middle colic vessels. The gastroduodenal artery is divided and ligated at the rostral margin of the neck of the pancreas when necessary. The anastomosis is done in a single layer of interrupted 3-0 silk. The Penrose drain that was utilized by Puestow has been replaced by a single, closed suction drain and a biopsy of the pancreas should be sent for pathologic examination, as Puestow did. If the patient has associated splenic vein occlusion, a splenectomy is performed concomitantly. Terminal biliary stenosis is managed with a choledochoduodenostomy in order to separate the biliary and pancreatic anastomoses and prevent the commingling of pancreatic and biliary secretions if there is an anastomotic leak.

The Puestow procedure can be performed laparoscopically in selected patients. The technique is similar to the open approach, with the exception of the method of anastomosis, which is accomplished more easily with a running technique. In our experience, the laparoscopic Puestow is best applied in patients with a very large pancreatic duct.

In our decades old report of lateral pancreaticojejunostomy (LPJ) for chronic pancreatitis in 85 patients reported from 1977 until 1991, the health of the 62 survivors was good-to-fair in a small majority of the patients (Adams et al. 1994), but 45 % of patients judged their health status to be poor. Notable in this study was that 22 patients were deceased at the time of follow-up, which ranged from 1 to 60 years. Sixty percent of patients required rehospitalizations for medical disorders, usually for management of pain or recurrent pancreatitis. Other disorders that patients developed were drug and alcohol abuse, malnutrition, diabetes, heart disease, esophagitis, gastritis, psychiatric disorders, trauma, pneumonia, and anemia, highlighting the fact that surgery for chronic pancreatitis is palliative surgery.

9.3 The Puestow Procedure in Small Duct Chronic Pancreatitis

Our initial interest in the role of LPJ in patients without dilated pancreatic ducts was tested in the late 1990s when we undertook LPJ in patients with a pancreatic ductal diameter less than 7 mm (Rios et al. 1998). In the follow-up period, which ranged from 3 to 16 months, 59 % of these patients required rehospitalization for pain or pancreatitis, 76 % had emergency room visits and noted that their pain was the same or worse. Sixty-five percent viewed their health status as poor. In those patients who had good outcomes, the pancreatic duct diameter approached 7 mm in diameter and the pancreas was notable for marked fibrosis with pancreatic "encapsulation"; the LPJ was seen to relieve the capsular parenchymal hypertension.

9.4 The Puestow Procedure Combined with Electrohydraulic Lithotripsy of the Ascending Pancreatic Duct

The pathologic key to failure of LPJ is failure to address disease localized to the head of the pancreas. A solution to this shortcoming is combining LPJ with localized head resection as described by Frey. We have avoided head resection and improved the drainage of the head of the pancreas by combining LPJ with electrohydraulic lithotripsy of the ascending pancreatic duct; this technique leads to better eradication of intraductal lithiasis in patients with a heavy stone burden in the ascending pancreatic duct. Using intraoperative

Table 9.1 Outcome in 120 patients with SOD or PD associated with chronic pancreatitis (Morgan et al. 2008)

	SOD	PD	Chronic pancreatitis	Previous gastric surgery	Prior ERCP/ES
Good outcome (%)[a]	66	54	37.5	90	54.3
Multivariate *p* value	NS	NS	0.02	NS	NS

[a]Defined by subject response (pain is somewhat better, much better, or completely gone since surgery) and no further operative therapy performed
NS not statistically significant, *SOD* sphincter of Oddi dysfunction, *PD* pancreas divisum, *ES* endoscopic sphincterotomy

pancreatoscopy with electrohydraulic lithotripsy, the ascending pancreatic duct can be cleared and transampullary access into the duodenum can be obtained with the operating choledochoscope. In our experience in 20 patients with ductal lithiasis and ductal dilation, 90 % of patients achieved good or fair health status with no re-operations for chronic pancreatitis in the follow-up (Rios et al. 2001).

9.5 Major and Minor Duct Sphincteroplasty

Our experience in the management of 68 patients with small duct chronic pancreatitis associated with sphincter of Oddi dysfunction (SOD) or pancreas divisum was reported in 2008 (Morgan et al. 2008). Sixty-eight patients managed from 2001 to 2005 had their outcomes evaluated with the utilization of the SF-36, Version 2, Quality- of- life survey. Good outcome was achieved in 66 % of patients with SOD and 54 % of patient with pancreas divisum. Multivariate analysis showed no significant difference in those who had prior ERCP and endoscopic sphincterotomy, but those who had evidence of chronic pancreatitis on imaging studies fared poorly (Table 9.1). Our clinical impression remains that major and minor duct sphincteroplasty have an important role in patients with chronic pancreatitis associated with pancreas divisum or SOD who have not undergone previous endoscopic sphincterotomy. Operative transduodenal sphincteroplasty and pancreatic septoplasty is warranted in patients with SOD who had initial successful endoscopic treatment with late recurrent ampullary stenosis not associated with radiologic evidence of chronic pancreatitis. Operative sphincteroplasty of the minor papilla has limited long-term success, because the minor sphincter's muscular configuration is minimal. Open operative sphincterotomy rarely extends or improves the effect of a technically satisfactory endoscopic sphincterotomy.

For transduodenal biliary sphincteroplasty with pancreatic ductal septoplasty, a generous Kocher maneuver is employed for optimal anterior mobilization of the duodenum and inspection of the head of the pancreas. An oblique duodenotomy is created overlying the ampulla of Vater. Stay sutures are used at the edges of the duodenal incision for atraumatic exposure. The ampulla is located and the biliary orifice identified and cannulated with a lacrimal duct probe. The duodenal mucosa is not handled with the tips of the forceps and the suction tip is not allowed to make contact with the mucosa to prevent bleeding or hematoma which may obscure visualization. The needle tipped cautery is used to make a generous biliary sphincterotomy, dividing the duodenal mucosa, sphincter muscle, and bile duct over a lacrimal duct probe until there is free flow of bile into the duodenum. The pancreatic duct opening is identified and cannulated. The septum between the biliary and pancreatic ducts is divided with cutting current needle-knife electrocautery. Interrupted 5-0 absorbable monofilament sutures approximating the duodenal mucosa to the bile duct and the pancreatic duct to the bile duct are placed to maintain patency of the sphincteroplasty and septoplasty. A 5-Fr, 2 cm Geenen stent can be left behind selectively in the pancreatic duct to decrease the risk of postprocedural pancreatitis. We then close the duodenum obliquely in a running fashion with 3-0 absorbable monofilament suture.

A number of factors make resection of the head of the pancreas an effective strategy in the surgical management of chronic pancreatitis. The problem is in the head of the pancreas in the majority

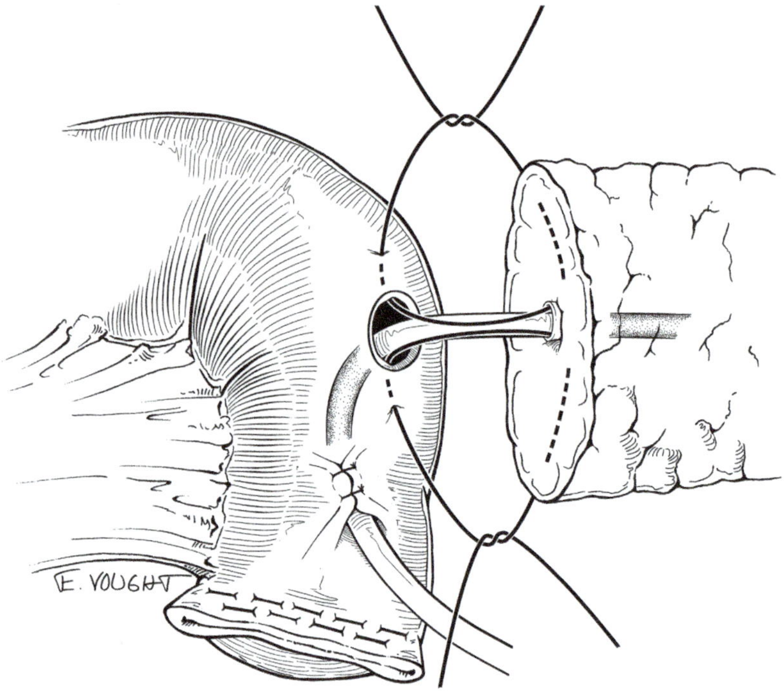

Fig. 9.1 Illustration demonstrating suture placement in back row of interrupted single layer pancreaticojejunal anastomosis over stent

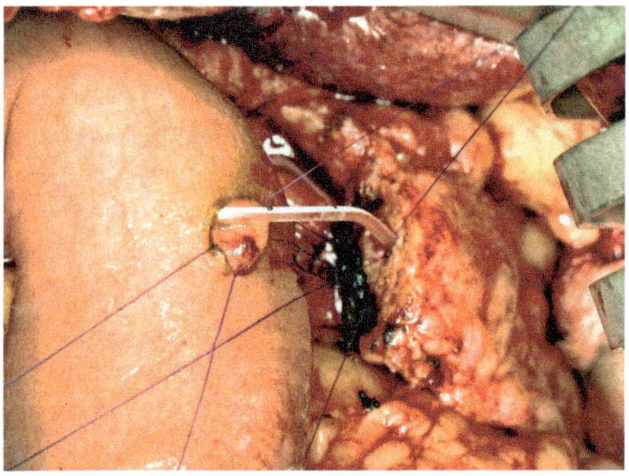

Fig. 9.2 *Posterior row* of pancreaticojejunal anastomosis contructed over >5-Fr silastic stent (Bard pediatric feeding tube) utilizing single layer 5-0 monofilament suture technique. Three posterior interrupted sutures have been placed between full thickness jejunum to full thickness pancreatic duct and capsule

of patients, and parenchymal and neuronal inflammation, the source of the pain, may be eradicated with resection. In addition to relief of pain, obstruction and bleeding complications can be achieved with resection, as well as dealing with the inflammatory mass in the head of the pancreas. Although we have utilized the classic Whipple procedure, the pylorus-preserving Whipple, the duodenal-preserving resection of the head of the pancreas, and the Frey Procedure performed through an upper midline incision, we prefer the classic Whipple procedure for chronic pancreatitis. Also we resect the pylorus routinely because of work demonstrating that pancreatic fibrosis correlates with impaired gastroduodenal motility. When gastric emptying is impaired, resection of the pylorus may improve gastric emptying with limited side effects. We have utilized the Frey procedure in patients with large duct pancreatitis who have widespread calcification within the head of the pancreas encompassing Santorini and Wirsung ducts and the duct to the uncinate process.

There are a variety of methods to construct the pancreatic anastomosis after pancreatic head resection (Adams 2009). The senior author's preferred technique in the at-risk pancreas is a single layer, end-to-side pancreaticojejunostomy with interrupted 5-0 absorbable mono filament suture incorporating full thickness pancreatic duct and capsule to full thickness jejunum (Figs. 9.1 and 9.2). The anastomosis is constructed over an internal-external pancreatic anastomotic Stent (a 5 Fr pediatric feeding tube) which exits the

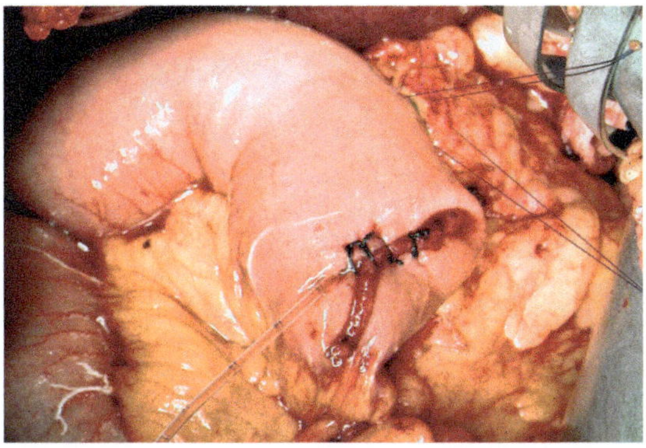

Fig. 9.3 Anterior and posterior interrupted sutures have been placed. >The *posterior row* has been secured and cut and the *anterior row* of >sutures are not tied. The stent exits the end jejunum through a Witzel tunnel

jejunum though a Witzel tunnel (Figs. 9.1–9.3). Closed bulb suction is applied to the Stent.

Our experience with resection of the head of the pancreas in the management of chronic pancreatitis has not necessarily matched the successful outcomes reported from other centers. In pancreatic head resection in patients with small duct chronic pancreatitis, the late complication of pancreaticojejunostomy anastomotic obstruction remains problematic, related probably to the exaggerated fibrosis associated with chronic pancreatitis. Our attempts at revision of stenotic end-to-side pancreaticojejunostomy in chronic pancreatitis are notable for our poor outcomes with recurrent stenosis, pain and pancreatic exocrine (Morgan et al. 2010).

9.6 Distal Pancreatectomy

Although a less common pattern of disease, fibrosis localized to the body and tail of the pancreas may be managed effectively with distal pancreatectomy. Splenic preservation is ideal; however, in many patients with chronic pancreatitis, the plane between the splenic vessels and the pancreas is obliterated by fibrosis, precluding vessel sparing splenic preservation. We have not had success in splenic preservation dependent on the short gastric vessels. In patients with splenic vein thrombosis, splenectomy is carried out routinely. In our patient population, laparoscopic distal pancreatectomy is uncommonly a safe surgical approach in severe chronic pancreatitis because of the anatomic distortion and loss of tissue planes characteristic of fibrosing pancreatitis. When feasible, the laparoscopic approach is challenging but has measurable and gratifying benefits to patients.

9.7 Surgical Outcomes After Operative Drainage and Partial Resection Procedures for Chronic Pancreatitis

Patient selection for operation has never been clear and simple, a recognition that chronic pancreatitis is a protean disease with multiple etiologic factors and variable physiologic and anatomic pathology. Prior to 2009, our algorithm for the management of chronic pancreatitis was the following:

In patients with dilated ducts and no stones, a Puestow-like procedure was undertaken. In patients with ductal lithiasis in the pancreatic head, a lateral pancreaticojejunostomy was undertaken, either with use of the electrohydraulic lithotripsy of the ascending pancreatic duct or a Frey procedure. Patients with a mass in the head of the pancreas underwent a Whipple procedure with lateral pancreaticojejunostomy when a chain-of-lakes ductal configuration was present.

Patients with small duct chronic pancreatitis and a mass in the head underwent the Whipple procedure. Patients with primarily tail disease underwent distal pancreatectomy. Those with pancreas divisum or SOD without evidence of chronic parenchymal and ductal changes underwent an initial attempt at sphincteroplasty. Patients who had sphincteroplasty failure underwent a Whipple procedure.

Our outcome with this strategy (excluding the aforementioned analysis of patients who underwent transduodenal sphincteroplasty) was reported in 2007, identifying 372 patients whose ages range from 14 to 74 years (Schnelldorfer et al. 2007). The most common risk factor for chronic pancreatitis was alcohol abuse with idiopathic pancreatitis, pancreas divisum, gallstones, SOD, and autoimmune disorders identified in the remainder. Preoperative ERCP noted pancreatic ductal strictures in 44 %, pancreatic ductal stones in 27 %, pancreatic pseudocysts in 35 %, and pancreatic ductal fistula in 9 %. Twenty percent of these

Table 9.2 The results of operative therapy in 372 patients with chronic pancreatitis (Schnelldorfer et al. 2007)

	LPJ (n=184) (%)	PD (n=97) (%)	DP (n=91) (%)
Morbidity	*22*	*51*	*29*
Intra-abdominal complications	*13*	*46*	*22*
Intra-abdominal abscess	2	14	16
Delayed gastric emptying	3	14	2
Pancreatic fistula	4	12	5
Others	3	20	3
Extra-abdominal complications	*11*	*11*	*10*
Wound infection	4	6	2
Pneumonia	2	2	2
Respiratory failure	2	1	2
Others	4	4	7
Mortality	*1*	*1*	*2*

Table 9.3 Pain control in 171 survivors available for follow-up (Schnelldorfer et al. 2007)

	LPJ (n=72) (%)	PD (n=42) (%)	DP (n=57)	Combined (n=171) (%)
Pain control in survivors				
Pain-free	20	10	40	24
Good pain control	28	24	21	25
Poor pain control	52	66	39	51

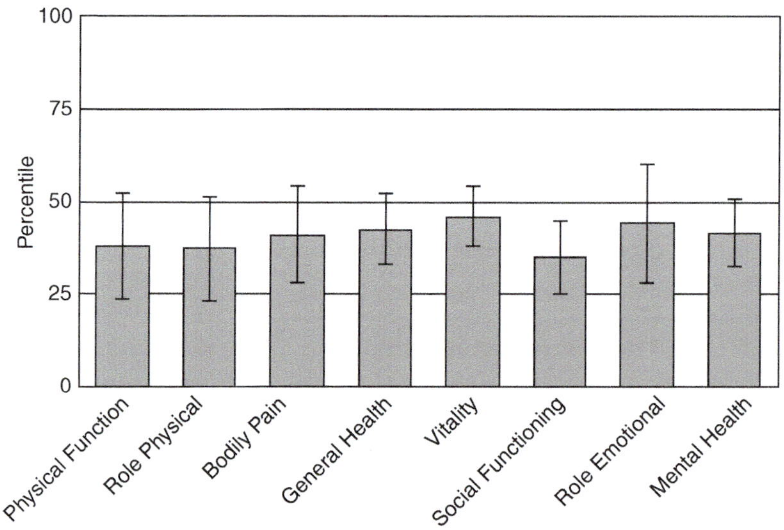

Fig. 9.4 Quality of life SF36,version 2 in survivors (Schnelldorfer et al. 2007)

patients had terminal biliary stenosis, and 8 % had duodenal stenosis. Patients who underwent pancreatoduodenectomy had a 51 % complication rate and those with distal pancreatectomy had a 29 % complication rate compared to LPJ, which had the lowest complication rate of 22 % (Table 9.2). Intraabdominal complications were most prevalent after pancreatoduodenectomy. Outcome as evaluated by pain control was good in only 48 % of those who underwent an LPJ, 34 % of those who underwent a pancreatoduodenectomy, and 61 % of those who underwent a distal pancreatectomy (Table 9.3). Poor pain control was associated with preoperative narcotic dependence and the number of previous abdominal operations. Quality of life assessed by the SF-36 in 171 patients showed that they were below population norms, most notably for social function (Fig. 9.4).

9.8 The Radical Cure of Chronic Pancreatitis

Because of the relatively poor outcome associated with this treatment strategy, we have adopted recently a more radical approach of undertaking a total pancreatectomy with islet auto-transplantation in patients with small duct chronic pancreatitis who have failed endoscopic or operative sphincteroplasty, aborting the previous step of pancreatoduodenectomy. The basic strategy is outlined in Table 9.4. The potential advantages of this approach are elimination of long-term destruction of the pancreas with endocrine and exocrine insufficiency and aborting the development of chronic neuropathic pain syndromes. Avoidance of recurrent emergency room visits and hospitalizations for pain and nausea management are attainable goals that correlate well with outcome metrics of quality of life. Long-term pain relief and excellent islet engraftment in the liver may improve with early radical resection and transplantation.

Table 9.4 The radical cure of chronic pancreatititis

Dilated ducts
No stones – Puestow procedure
Stones – Frey procedure
Head mass – Whipple with lateral pancreaticojejunostomy
Non-dilated ducts
Head mass – Whipple
Body/tail stricture/disruption – distal pancreatectomy/splenectomy
Pancreas divisum with prior endoscopic therapy – total pancreatectomy with islet-auto transplantation
SOD – biliary sphincteroplasty with pancreatic ductal septoplasty if no prior endoscopic therapy and no evidence of chronic pancreatitis on imaging studies. If prior failed endoscopic therapy with evidence of chronic pancreatitis, then total pancreatectomy with islet auto-transplantation

Total pancreatectomy with islet isolation is begun with an upper abdominal midline incision. The lesser sac is entered through the gastrocolic ligament and the gastrocolic, duodenocolic, and splenocolic ligaments are divided. The short gastric vessels are divided as well resulting in wide exposure of the pancreas. A generous Kocher maneuver is performed. The superior mesenteric vein is identified and the plane between this vessel and the neck of the pancreas is dissected from the anterior border of the pancreas. The common bile duct is encircled and divided, followed by division of the proximal duodenum. The distal duodenum is divided at the ligament of Treitz and the mesentery is taken with the harmonic scalpel. The gastroduodenal artery is ligated at its origin from the common hepatic artery and the pancreas is divided at the neck over the portal vein. The head of the pancreas and uncinate pancreas are then mobilized off of the portal vein laterally, dividing tributaries of substance with care. This dissection is carried around the vein circumferentially to the superior mesenteric artery. The harmonic scalpel is then utilized to dissect the pancreas off of the superior mesenteric artery. Metallic clips are utilized for branching arterial hemostasis. The pancreatic head is placed in cold balanced electrolyte solution. Attention is then turned to the body and tail of the pancreas. The inferior and superior borders of the pancreas are defined. During the dissection of the inferior border, the inferior mesenteric vein is sought and divided with care. The splenic artery and vein are then circumferentially dissected and ligated. The spleen is mobilized medially and the pancreas and spleen are taken en bloc to the back table.

On the back table, the organs are placed on slush made from balanced electrolyte solution. The pancreas is perfused with balanced electrolyte solution. The nonpancreatic tissue (duodenum, spleen, and associated fatty material) are separated from the pancreas. The main pancreatic duct is cannulated with a 20-gauge angiocatheter on both head and tail segments and sutured into place. The pancreas is then packaged in sterile, cold solution on ice for transport to the clean cell lab.

After foregut reconstruction and abdominal closure, the patient is transported sedated and intubated to an intensive-care unit room awaiting transportation to the interventional radiology suite when the islet preparation is completed.

In the lab, the prepared pancreas is hand injected with Liberase® enzymes (Roche Applied Science) into the main pancreatic duct and placed into a temperature controlled perfusion circuit to allow optimal enzymatic activity, while being subjected to mechanical agitation. The progress is periodically evaluated with examination of samples from the circuit and when the islets are found to be optimally separated, the circuit is cooled and diluted. The islets, now largely separated from the exocrine and connective tissue, are recovered. They are placed in albumin solution with heparin (70 U per kilogram patient weight) and antibiotic (cefazolin, 1 g). They are then transported again on ice to the interventional radiology suite, where the patient awaits.

Percutaneous transhepatic access to the patient's portal vein is obtained in the interventional radiology suite under fluoroscopic guidance (Fig. 9.5). A Seldinger technique is utilized to place a 5-Fr catheter into the main portal vein distal to its bifurcation. The islets are infused by gravity through the catheter. Portal venous pressures are measured initially, at the midpoint of transplantation, and at the completion of infusion. At the end of the procedure, the intraparenchymal access catheter tract is ablated routinely with hemostatic material.

Routine postoperative care is employed. Specifically, these patients are watched closely for signs of bleeding (due to postoperative heparinization and the possibility of transient portal hypertension), portal vein thrombosis (the islets are thrombogenic and can increase portal venous pressure during infusion), and systemic inflammatory response (tissue thromboplastin and other non-described vasoactive substances are released by the islets).

Outcomes in our early experience with these challenging patients have been promising. Morbidity is acceptable with complications specific to islet transplant including portal vein thrombosis occurring rarely. Transplanted islet function is good and clinically relevant pain relief is obtained in most patients. What we believe will be the measure of success in this approach will be improvement in quality of life, not narcotic analgesia and insulin utilization. We have utilized both the SF 36 and the SF 12 metrics to evaluate patient outcomes. Elevating a patient from below 1.5 standard deviations below the norm to within norms for physical and mental components is considered a clinically relevant, successful result. Patients who were isolated socially from family and friends are able to be restored to physical and emotional function that permits resumption of careers and a family and social life. They are able to avoid the multiple emergency room visits and hospitalizations that characterized their preoperative condition. The rehabilitation involves at least the year-long work of a multi-disciplinary team of behavioral psychologists, nurse practitioners pain specialists, and pancreatic surgeons.

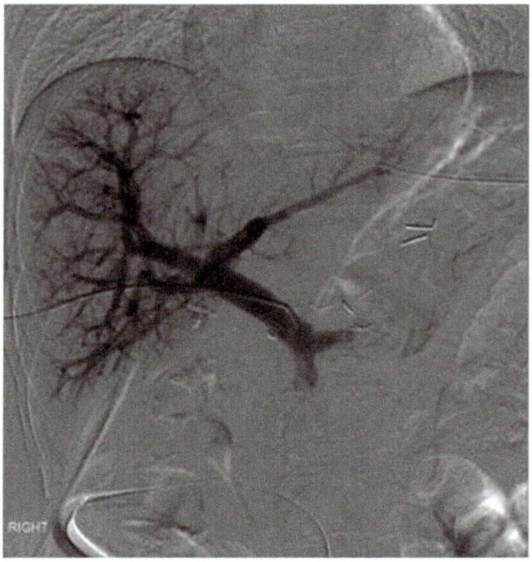

Fig. 9.5 Percutaneous transhepatic access to the patient's portal vein is obtained in the interventional radiology suite under fluoroscopic guidance

Our nascent experience with total pancreatectomy with islet auto-transplantation is promising and suggests that it is an effective means of pain relief in selected patients with debilitating pain secondary to chronic pancreatitis. Ideal patient selection is paramount, because early intervention can prevent the development of central pain processes that are recalcitrant to end organ-directed therapies. Long term follow-up is needed to determine appropriate criteria for patient selection as well as data to provide analysis of cost-effectiveness.

References

Adams DB (2009) The pancreatic anastomosis: the danger of a leak, which anastomotic technique is better? J Gastrointest Surg 13:1182–1183

Adams DB, Ford MC, Anderson MA (1994) Outcome after lateral pancreaticojejunostomy for chronic pancreatitis. Ann Surg 219:481–489

Morgan KA, Romagnuolo J, Adams DB (2008) Transduodenal sphincteroplasty in the management of sphincter of Oddi dysfunction and pancreas divisum in the modern era. J Am Coll Surg 206:908–917

Morgan KA, Fontenot BB, Harvey NR, Adams DB (2010) Revision of anastomotic stenosis after pancreatic head resection for chronic pancreatitis: is it futile? HPB (Oxford) 12(3):211–216

Rios GA, Adams DB (2001) Does intraoperative electrohydraulic lithotripsy improve outcome in the surgical management of chronic pancreatitis? Am Surg 67:533–537

Rios G, Yeoh KG, Tarnasky PR, Cunningham JT, Hawes RH, Cotton PB, Adams DB (1998) Outcome of lateral pancreaticojejunostomy in the management of chronic pancreatitis with non-dilated pancreatic ducts. J Gastrointest Surg 2:223–229

Schnelldorfer T, Adams DB, Lewin DN (2007) Operative management of chronic pancreatitis: long-term results in 372 patients. J Am Coll Surg 5:1039–1047

Commentary 10

P.C. Bornman and J.E.J. Krige

10.1 Selection

While most patients with uncomplicated chronic pancreatitis (CP) can be managed conservatively, operative treatment offers good results in carefully selected patients, especially those who have intractable pain and are at risk for opioid dependency. Operative intervention should only be undertaken when conservative measures including endoscopic interventions have been exhausted. In the alcohol-induced group, patients should be required to undergo a rehabilitation programme before operative intervention is undertaken.

When counselling patients for operation, several factors should be stressed. First, while the reported success rate is 70–80 %, there are substantial risks associated with these operations, and complete or substantial, clinically improve pain relief cannot be guaranteed in the individual patient. Second, pancreatic function, in particular steatorrhoea, occurs frequently even after parenchymal-preserving operations, and the risk of endocrine dysfunction is greatest when a distal pancreatectomy is required. Third, abstinence from alcohol and cessation of smoking are crucial factors that determine the long-term success of operative treatment of chronic pancreatitis.

10.2 Pre-operative Evaluation

Operative procedures for chronic pancreatitis are technically complex and should only be undertaken by surgeons with specialised training in pancreatic surgery working in a multi-disciplinary team. A careful evaluation of the patient's psychologic and social profile, as well as fitness for operative intervention should be undertaken. All patients need assessment of their nutritional status and the degree of pancreatic insufficiency. Some patients will benefit from hospitalisation if they have poorly controlled diabetes, malnutrition, or intractable pain. The response to aggressive supportive therapy may help to select appropriate candidates for operative intervention.

A complete, detailed evaluation of the morphologic status of the pancreas is imperative. Multi-slice CT and in selected cases CT angiography are the most important imaging investigations. MRI/MRCP is often useful to delineate further the changes in the pancreatic and bile ducts. In addition, specific care should be taken to identify associated portal hypertension related to splenic and portal vein occlusion which may have an important bearing on the decision to

P.C. Bornman, FRCS [Ed], FCS [SA], FRCS(Glasg) M.Med Surg (✉)
Surgical Gastroenterology, Department of Surgery, Groote Schuur Hospital, University of Cape Town, Cape Town, South Africa

E23 GIT Clinic, Groote Schuur Hospital, Cape Town, South Africa
e-mail: philippus.bornman@uct.ac.za

J.E.J. Krige, M.Sc., FACS, FRCS [Ed], FCS [SA]
Surgical Gastroenterology, Department of Surgery, Groote Schuur Hospital, University of Cape Town, Cape Town, South Africa

R. Mantke et al. (eds.), *International Practices in Pancreatic Surgery*,
DOI 10.1007/978-3-540-74506-8_10, © Springer-Verlag Berlin Heidelberg 2013

Table 10.1 The most common surgical options for chronic pancreatitis (Bornman et al. 2010)

Procedures	Indications
Resection:	
Pancreatoduodenectomy	Suspicion of malignancy
Distal pancreatectomy	Disease confined to the body and tail of the pancreas
Duodenal preserving resection of the head of the pancreas	Inflammatory mass of the head of the pancreas with or without a dilated pancreatic duct
Pancreatico-jejunostomy	Dilated pancreatic duct without inflammatory mass in the head of the pancreas

operate and the choice of operative procedure. ERCP is now used much less frequently as part of the work-up for operative treatment but may be helpful in combination with EUS and biopsy in patients in whom there is concern about an underlying malignancy. CA 19-9 may help to identify patients with cancers, but false positive values occur frequently, even in the absence of associated obstructive jaundice.

10.3 Surgical Approach

Current operative strategy is based on the principle of maximum preservation of exocrine and endocrine pancreatic function. This strategy involves a paradigm shift away from the standard resection procedures, such as the classic pancreatoduodenal resection, to lesser resections which preserve pancreatic parenchyma and duodenal integrity, such as the Frey operation and its hybrid modifications. Table 10.1 provides a basic outline of the choice of operative procedures based predominantly on the changes in the pancreatic parenchyma and ducts (Bornman et al. 2010). With the exceptions of patients in whom there is concern about a malignancy or when there is predominant disease in the tail of the pancreas, the authors prefer the Frey operation, including those patients with associated complications. The key components of this operation include preservation of the pancreatic neck as well as the capsule of the pancreas of the posterior pancreatic head (Anderson and Frey 2010) which provides the following advantages over the other parenchyma preserving procedures:

1. The operation avoids dissection outside the confines of the pancreas which decreases the risk of both arterial and portal venous injuries.
2. It is the safest operation in the presence of segmental portal hypertension.
3. Compared to the Beger operation, it is technically easier, less hazardous, and achieves the same results in terms of pain relief and parenchymal preservation (Strate et al. 2005).

10.4 Technical Details of the Frey Procedure

A bilateral sub-costal incision is our preferred approach when combined with a fixed mechanical retractor which provides excellent exposure.

10.4.1 Exploration of the Pancreas

Full exposure of the pancreas is obtained utilising the following steps:

(i) Full Kocherisation of the duodenum and pancreatic head is important to ensure an effective and safe coring out of the head of the pancreas.

(ii) An ultrasound dissector is a useful tool for dissection, particularly in the presence of active inflammation.

(iii) The lesser sac is entered by dividing the gastro-colic omentum outside the gastro-epiploic vascular arcade. The opening into the lesser sac should be extended far enough to the left to expose the entire body and tail of the pancreas. To the right, mobilisation of the hepatic flexure of the colon allows optimal exposure of the head of the pancreas.

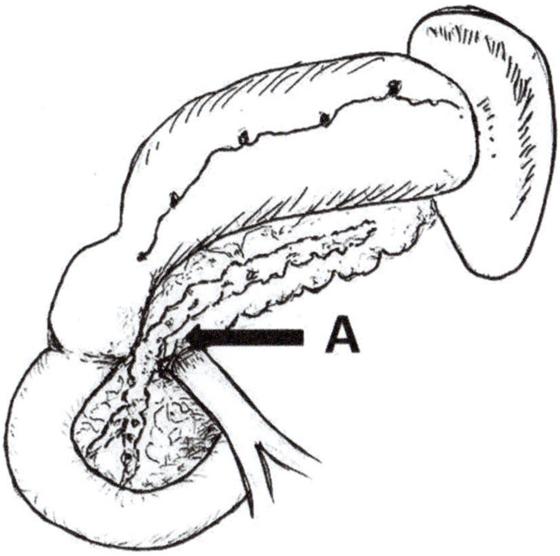

Fig. 10.1 Exposure of the pancreas neck inferior to the duodenum [A]

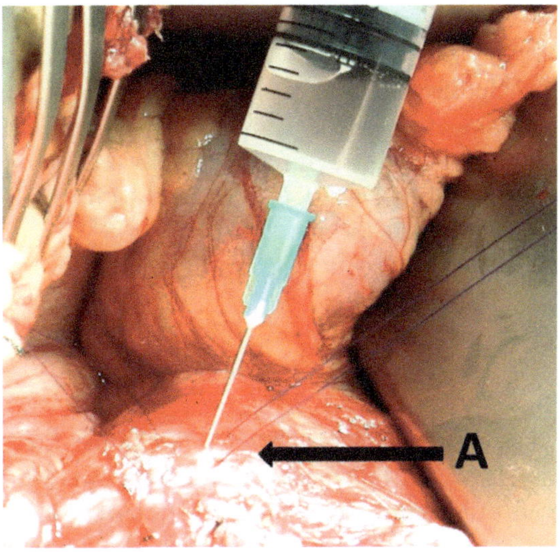

Fig. 10.2 Aspiration of the pancreatic duct between two stay sutures [A]

(iv) Adhesions between the posterior wall of the stomach and the neck, body, and tail of the pancreas should be divided carefully to expose the superior and inferior borders of the pancreas. In addition, it is useful to divide the gastro-hepatic ligament in the region of the antrum and to place a tape around the antrum for rostral traction of the stomach.

(v) Further exposure of the head and in particular the uncinate process is achieved by dissecting in the groove between the right border of the superior mesenteric vein and the uncinate process.

(vi) It is important that both the rostral and caudal neck of the pancreas is exposed adequately to safeguard against vascular injuries, in particular the SMV during incision of the pancreatic duct towards the head (Fig. 10.1). To achieve this, it may be necessary to divide the gastro-epiploic vascular pedicle where it emerges at the inferomedial border of the first part of the duodenum and to expose the SMV caudal to the inferior border of the pancreatic neck. We then ligate the gastro-duodenal artery at this stage with 3/0 monofilament suture where it crosses the anterior surface of the pancreas.

10.4.2 Identifying the Pancreatic Duct

Identification of the pancreatic duct is best done in the neck of the pancreas. The following techniques facilitate identification of the duct.

(i) Palpation and ballottement with the right index finger while gently squeezing the neck of the pancreas between the index finger and thumb of the left hand may locate the dilated duct. Often, a trough-like depression is evident.

(ii) While performing the above manoeuvre, a 17 gauge needle and syringe are used to confirm the lumen of the main pancreatic duct (Fig. 10.2). When this is achieved, it is important not to aspirate too much fluid, because this may decompress the duct and hamper the ability to fillet open the duct.

(iii) With the needle still in the duct localising the position of the duct, two 3/0 monofilament stay sutures are placed above and below the puncture site which will facilitate exploration of the pancreatic duct.

(iv) While pulling up on the two stay sutures, a diathermy needle is use to cut down alongside the needle until the duct is entered.

(v) Even with the needle in the duct, the pancreatic duct can be missed; cutting too deeply may result in bleeding from the underlying splenic vessels. This disaster can be avoided by gently probing with a curved dissector to locate the duct which usually lies more superficial in the pancreas than anticipated.

(vi) Intra-operative ultrasonography can be a useful tool when it is difficult to indentify the pancreatic duct.

10.4.3 Exploration of the Pancreatic Duct

The pancreatic duct is explored first in the direction of the tail. Filleting of the duct distally is done with a diathermy blade, cutting between the blades of a curved dissector positioned inside the duct. The ductotomy is accomplished in short increments, and placement of haemostatic and stay sutures assists with further exposure of the pancreatic duct. The surgeon should make all attempts to remove as many pancreatic duct calculi as possible (Fig. 10.3a,b). Calculi in side ducts may be particularly difficult to extract and often need to be crushed before removal. It may be difficult to explore and open the entire duct due to strictures, stones, and narrowing of the duct toward the tail of the pancreas. Detailed pre-operative imaging of the pancreatic duct will guide the surgeon during this stage of the operation. Intra-operative ultrasonography may be useful to indentify the pancreatic duct pathology. In some instances, a cut down into the parenchyma will help to get across a stricture into the distal duct. Although the general recommendation is to explore and incise the entire duct to the tail, this manoeuvre may not be feasible and may be potentially dangerous in some cases. If there are no strictures or stones in the tail, it may not be necessary to extend the exploration to the very end of the pancreatic tail.

10.4.4 Coring Out of the Head

This part of the operation is often the most difficult. Mature judgement and experience are necessary to achieve the objectives of the operation while minimising the risks of bleeding and injury to surrounding structures. The placement of sutures at the

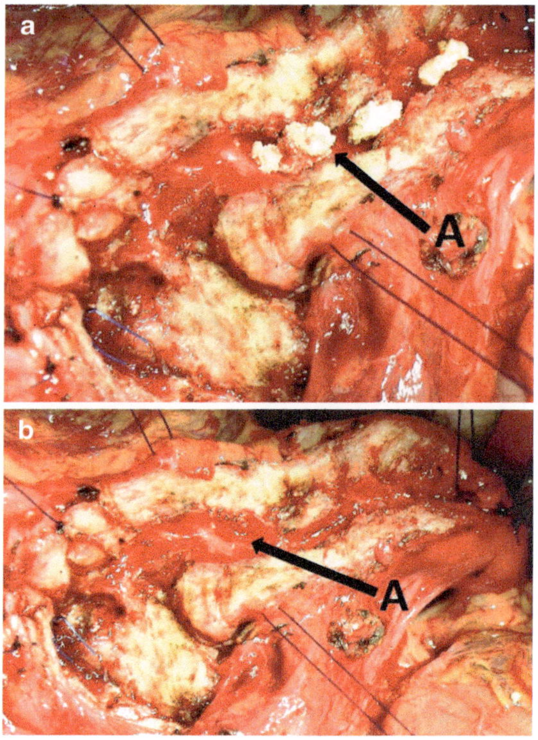

Fig. 10.3 (**a**) Multiple calculi in main duct and (**b**) as many as possible of the calculi are removed from the main and side ducts [A]

planned margin of the resection in the head and uncinate process is useful to avoid injury to the duodenum and to achieve haemostasis (Fig. 10.4). Holding the head of the pancreas in the surgeon's hand during this stage of the operation is of great assistance in guiding the dissection. The safest method of opening the proximal aspect of the pancreatic duct in the head of the gland and performing the coring out procedure is with the guidance of a curved dissector positioned in the main pancreatic duct (Fig. 10.5). As in the dissection in the body of the pancreas, the dissection in the neck and head of the pancreas proceeds incrementally with the placement of haemostatic sutures as the duct is gradually opened and the forceps is advanced.

The coring out procedure is done in a piecemeal fashion using a diathermy blade with a blend setting (Fig. 10.6). The objective is to open and decompress all the side ducts with removal of any stones present (Figs. 10.6 and 10.7). The extent of the resection will vary, but as little pancreatic

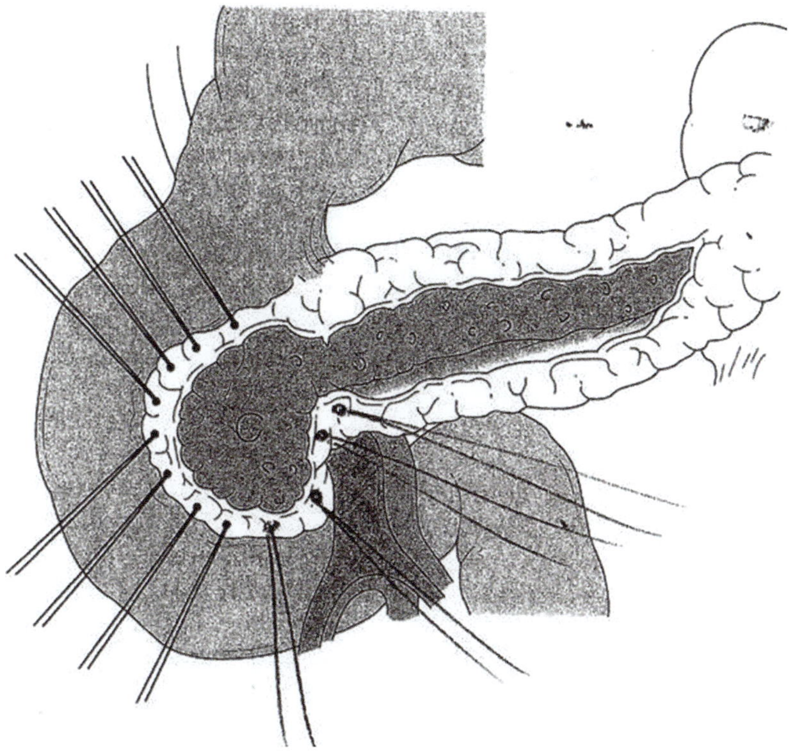

Fig. 10.4 Placement of haemostatic sutures at the envisaged resection margins in the head to avoid injury to the duodenum and surrounding vascular structures

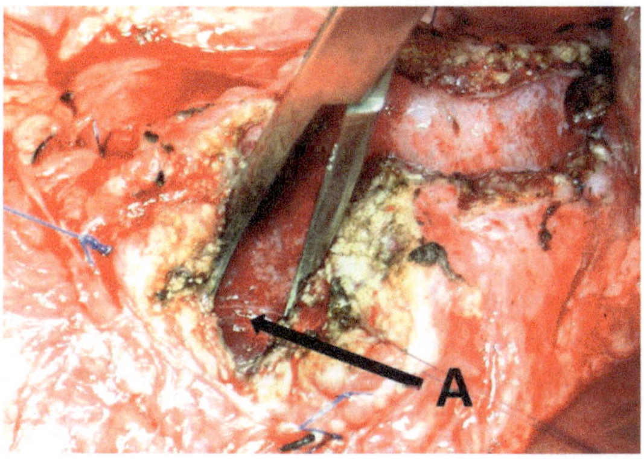

Fig. 10.5 Exploring the pancreatic duct towards the head by cutting down with diathermy between the blades of a curved forceps [A]

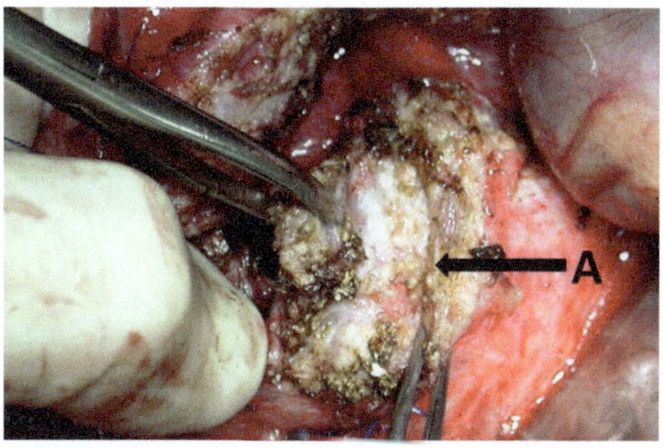

Fig. 10.6 Coring out of the head and uncinate process with diathermy blade [A] while holding the pancreatic head in the surgeon's hand

tissue as possible should be left behind, being careful not to break through the capsule posteriorly or to injure the bile duct (Fig. 10.8). It is not so much the amount of pancreatic tissue that is removed but the remnant that is left behind that matters. Palpation with the fingers behind and the thumb in front of the head of the pancreas provides the best way of judging the safety, adequacy, and depth of the resection. Meticulous haemostasis must be achieved at this stage of the operation using diathermy and suture ligation.

10.4.5 Pancreatico-Jejunostomy

A Roux-en Y limb is fashioned from the proximal jejunum about 20 cm distal to the duodeno-jejunal

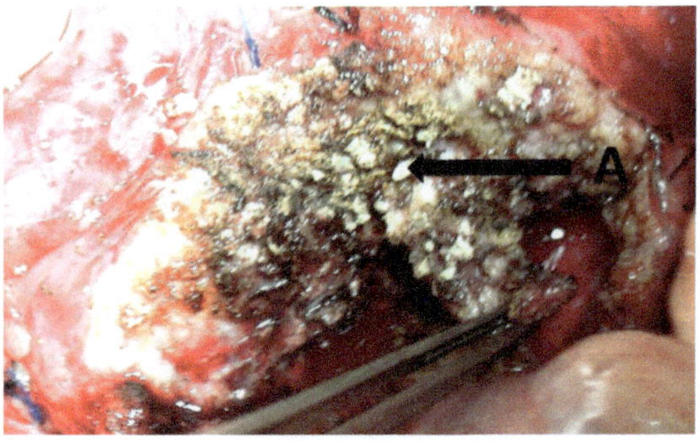

Fig. 10.7 Studded side-duct calculi in the head and uncinate process of the pancreas [A]

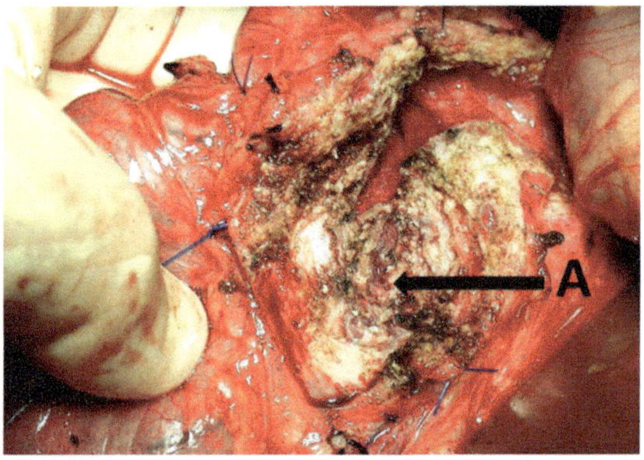

Fig. 10.8 Coring out of the head of the pancreas leaving as little as possible of the diseased pancreas [A]

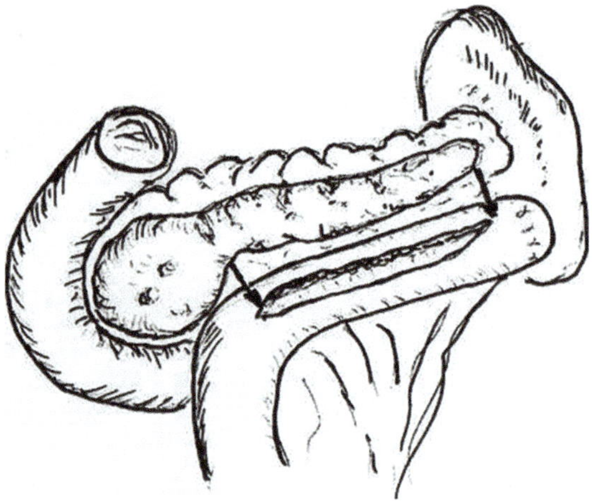

Fig. 10.9 The length of the incision into the jejunal limb is measured from the neck to the tail of the pancreas

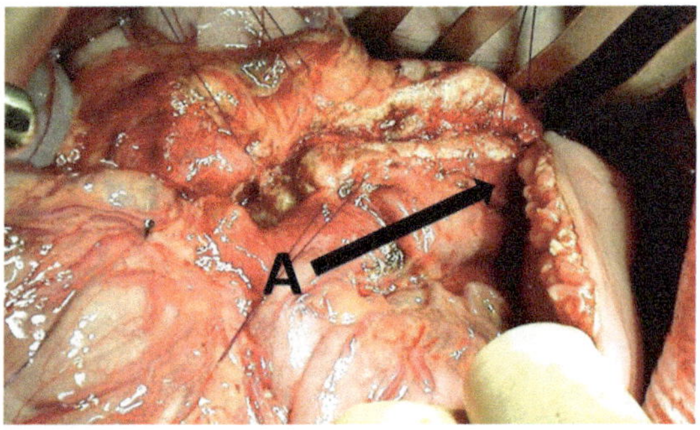

Fig. 10.10 The pancreatico-jejunostomy is carried out with a continuous monofilament 3/0 suture starting at the apex of the incision into the tail of the pancreas [A]

junction using a staple device. The Roux limb is brought retrocolically through the right transverse mesocolon near the hepatic flexure. This approach provides the best site for the position of the jejunal limb for the pancreatic anastomosis and when bile duct drainage is also necessary.

Judging the length of the jejunal incision for the pancreatic anastomosis is important. There is a tendency to make the incision in the jejunum too long, in which case technical difficulties may occur with the pancreatic anastomosis. As a rule of thumb, the initial enterotomy in the jejunum should be slightly less than and not exceed the length of the opened pancreatic duct as measured from the neck to the tail (Fig. 10.9). In most instances, this initial length should be adequate to complete the pancreatico-jejunostomy.

The anastomosis is performed with a single, continuous, 3/0 monofilament suture starting at the apex of the incision into the pancreatic duct in the tail (Fig. 10.10). The first suture for the inferior part of the anastomosis is placed from inside-out through the jejunum and outside-in through the pancreas. For the anterior layer, the suture is placed outside-in through the pancreas and inside-out through the jejunum. The two short ends are then tied together. The inferior anastomosis is first completed with careful placement of the sutures while the jejunal loop is gently pulled inferiorly and laterally to provide maximum exposure. When possible, the anastomosis can be done to the edge of the pancreatic duct, but this is not essential or advisable if the pancreatic duct is situated deeply in the pancreatic parenchyma and when the gland parenchyma is hard. The anterior anastomosis is completed in a similar fashion. Interrupted buttressing sutures may be required to ensure a water tight anastomosis.

We then place a suction drainage system in the lesser sac near the anastomosis.

10.4.6 Frey Procedure in Patients with Associated Complications

(i) *Intra pancreatic pseudocyst*: The Frey procedure is also suitable for patients in whom there is an associated intra-pancreatic pseudocyst in conjunction with a dilated pancreatic duct. In such cases, the procedure may be started in the head especially when the pancreatic duct is not grossly dilated. The coring out procedure is easier in the presence of a cyst; if biliary obstruction is present, the coring out process will usually be sufficient to decompress the biliary obstruction, thereby obviating the need for a formal biliary bypass.

(ii) Associated bile duct obstruction: Bile duct obstruction in chronic pancreatitis is often low grade and has a benign natural history. In such patients, no additional biliary drainage procedure is usually required when a Frey procedure is performed for pain. A biliary bypass is only indicated when there is a high grade stricture as evidenced by persistent obstructive jaundice with or without cholangitis or in the absence of jaundice, when there is a grossly dilated bile duct with markedly increased Alkaline Phosphatase and Gamma Glutamyl Transferase activities. The best operative procedure to decompress the bile duct obstruction is by a hepatico-jejunostomy using the same Roux limb as used for the pancreatico-jejunostomy; the biliary anastomosis should be distal to the pancreatic anastomosis. We remove the gallbladder during this operation to avoid later complications related to gallbladder stasis. In some cases, the bile duct may be entered during the coring out procedure in which case, the edges of the open bile duct can be marsupialised to the surrounding pancreatic tissue and drained enterically via the pancreatico jejunostomy.

There is a subgroup of patients with minimal pain in whom jaundice is the predominant reason for operative intervention. The decision to perform a Frey procedure in addition to the biliary bypass remains controversial. Those in favour argue that a substantial number of these patients will develop severe pain and that the addition of the Frey procedure does not add much to the risks of the operation; however, there should be a low threshold not to proceed with a Frey procedure if there are adverse factors such as a small pancreatic duct, the presence of an active inflammatory process, or associated segmental portal hypertension.

References

Anderson DK, Frey CF (2010) The evolution of the surgical treatment of chronic pancreatitis. Ann Surg 251:18–32

Bornman PC, Botha JF, Ramos JM, Smith MD et al (2010) Guidelines for the diagnosis and treatment of chronic pancreatitis. S Afr Med J 100(12):847–859

Strate T, Taherpour Z, Bloechle C, Mann O et al (2005) Long term follow up of a randomized trial comparing the Beger and Frey procedures for patients suffering from chronic pancreatitis. Ann Surg 241:591–598

Commentary

11

Thilo Hackert and Markus W. Büchler

11.1 Relevant Basic Information, Indication, and Contraindication

From the pathophysiologic point of view, operative therapy of chronic pancreatitis (CP) includes primarily drainage procedures and resection of chronically-inflamed tissue which must be considered in the context of two aspects. First, ductal or pseudocyst drainage without resection is the maximal, parenchyma-sparing approach which offers – at least theoretically – preservation of all residual endocrine and exocrine function. Second, the remaining fibrotic tissue may be responsible for ongoing symptoms, especially pain. Besides, drainage alone offers only limited functional benefit if the tissue preserved has been subjected to long-lasting inflammation and maintains an ongoing, increased risk of malignant transformation. The generation of pain as the leading symptom in CP is highly complex and not fully understood. It is generally accepted that pancreatic ductal and possibly parenchymal hypertension and perineural inflammation are the two main mechanisms of pain generation in CP. From the clinical course, pain is an early symptom in patients with CP who manifest an increasing tendency toward ongoing and escalating pain in the long term, despite any new obvious parenchymal changes or new stimuli (e.g. pseudocysts, enlargement, etc.) (Vardanyan and Rilo 2010). Thus, pain management should be started as early as possible to avoid the end stage of chronic and irreversible pain.

One of the most important pathophysiologic concepts of CP is the concept of neuroimmunologic inflammation (Friess et al. 1999). This concept implies the interaction of immunologic changes and resultant neural modulation that lead to reactive changes in nerve diameter, density, and function leading to a growing pain intensity in the long term in one subset of patients with CP. In a recent study, tissue samples of 141 patients who underwent resections for CP were investigated with regard to these neuroimmunologic interactions (Ceyhan et al. 2009). Clinical pain severity correlated with both the inflammatory changes associated with tissue fibrosis but also with the increase in nerve diameter and density in the resected tissue. A highly significant correlation between these parameters and the clinical pain score was found, suggesting that the long-lasting inflammatory changes exert a neuromodulatory role in the generation of pancreatic pain. This intense pain character is understood not only as a result of morphologic changes, but also as a progressive course of stimulus-independent pain with characteristics of an autonomous pain syndrome due to a neural plasticity and memory function of the peripheral and

T. Hackert
Department of Surgery, University of Heidelberg, Im Neuenheimer Feld 110, 69120 Heidelberg, Germany

M.W. Büchler, M.D. (✉)
Professor of Surgery, Chair, Department of Surgery, University of Heidelberg, 69120 Heidelberg, Germany
e-mail: markus_buechler@med.uni-heidelberg.de

R. Mantke et al. (eds.), *International Practices in Pancreatic Surgery*,
DOI 10.1007/978-3-540-74506-8_11, © Springer-Verlag Berlin Heidelberg 2013

central nervous system that develops over time (Drewes et al. 2008; Sakorafas et al. 2007). This neural dysregulation may be related to hyperexcitability of dorsal root neurons combined with a decreased descending inhibition; these chronic changes in neural function can lead to changes in gut "sensitivity" and "viscerotomes" as the corresponding projection areas represented in the CNS, leading to a chronic pain syndrome. The long-term effect is explained by irreversible changes in the brain with cortical reorganization that results in the clinical observation of the severe, unrelenting stimulus-independent, neuropathic pain of CP (Drewes et al. 2008).

Because these changes often become evident early during CP, it is of utmost importance to "break" this cycle of pain generation and chronification as early as possible (Strobel et al. 2009). Therefore, definitive operative therapy through resection of this altered tissue is the most effective treatment and should be considered before end-stage refractory pain has developed (Strobel et al. 2009). Indeed, we maintain that operative intervention should be undertaken in selected patients early after failure of conservative treatment and should be considered in many patients at the same time as endoscopic therapies are discussed.

From a technical point of view, pancreatic resection for CP can be complicated by mechanical compression of the portal vein or occlusion with subsequent extrahepatic portal, mesenteric, or splenic venous hypertension with extensive development of venous collaterals. In this situation, dissection of the portal vein and subsequent pancreatic resective procedures may be difficult. Drainage operations that achieve the goal of pancreatic duct decompression can be helpful to cope with these difficulties and can be combined with a hepaticojejunostomy to resolve concomitant extrahepatic biliary obstruction if necessary. Furthermore, limited and parenchyma-sparing operations, such as the Bern modification of the duodenum-preserving pancreatic head resection that is described below, offer a suitable approach to CP without addressing the portal vein pathology directly. Indeed, the approach we describe may itself "decompress" the obstructed retropancreatic portomesenteric system and reverse the portal hypertension.

11.2 Operative Technique

In most patients with CP, the major pathologic changes are focused on the head of the pancreas with an inflammatory mass and/or calcifications; these changes lead to subsequent stenosis of the pancreatic and/or bile duct (Keck and Marjanovic 2009) (Fig. 11.1). The operative goal in the majority of patients with CP is, therefore, some form of pancreatic head resection.

The best technique for the operative treatment of pancreatic head lesions in CP is still under debate. Partial pancreatoduodenectomy with or without preservation of the pylorus has served as the primary, resectional procedure for many years. These resections, however, are less satisfactory in terms of late morbidity, with an incidence of diabetes mellitus of up to 48 % postoperatively (Sakorafas et al. 2000). The original, duodenum-preserving pancreatic head resection (DPPHR) introduced by Beger in 1972 (Beger et al. 1989) has undergone several modifications and, in many institutions, is considered the standard procedure for non-malignant head lesions in CP (Diener et al. 2008). Whenever possible and depending on the extent of the calcified and fibrotic lesions, we prefer the "Berne modification" as the best, tissue-sparing approach (Fig. 11.2). The procedure starts with an extensive Kocher maneuver of the pancreatic head to permit full palpation of the head of the pancreas during the resection but also to allow control of any bleeding by compression during the resection phase. The anterior aspect of the pancreatic head should be exposed after dissection of the right gastroepiploic vessels and ligation of the gastroduodenal artery – if possible – to minimize blood loss during excision of the head. In those patients with severe peripancreatic inflammation, it may be necessary to ligate the gastroduodenal and/or pancreatoduodenal artery during excision of the pancreatic head. With this operation, it is not necessary to tunnel under the neck of the pancreas but above the mesenteric vein (as with the Beger procedure), because this is often difficult and potentially dangerous due to the chronic inflammatory adherence of the parenchyma to the portomesenteric venous confluence. The resection margin should be

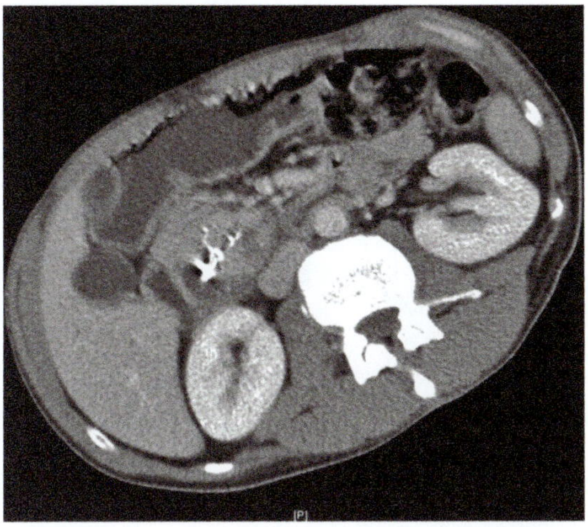

Fig. 11.1 High-resolution CT scan, hydro technique with 30° right-sided position of the patient showing an inflammatory head mass with calcifications as a typical finding in CP patients

defined by circular stay sutures (e.g. 4-0 polypropylene) around the altered tissue area, which also decreases bleeding during excision of the pancreatic head. The head region is excised sharply by scalpel. To minimize bleeding and avoid perforation of the posterior parenchyma layer, all thee steps are controlled by the left hand positioned behind the pancreatic head. As much fibrotic and calcified tissue as possible should be removed; in addition, the pancreatic duct must be opened and inspected to extract stones and ensure free drainage from the left side of the gland into the resection cavity.

Special attention has to be paid to the bile duct. In patients with preoperative biliary obstruction and/or endoluminal biliary stents, the bile duct needs to be opened widely, and the orifice should be sutured open into the resection cavity to avoid postoperative recurrence of bile duct stenosis (Gloor et al. 2001). Hemostasis in the resection cavity is achieved by selective suture ligation with nonabsorbable, monofilament sutures (e.g. 5-0 polypropylene). The operation is completed by a retrocolic, side-to-side pancreatojejunostomy to a Roux-en-Y jejunal limb constructed approximately 40 cm distal to the ligament of Treitz and passed through the right mesocolon. The pancreatojejunostomy is constructed by a two-layer, running suture using 4-0 PDS and incorporating the duodenal wall in the outer anterior seromuscular layer if necessary. An end-to-side jejunojejunostomy with a

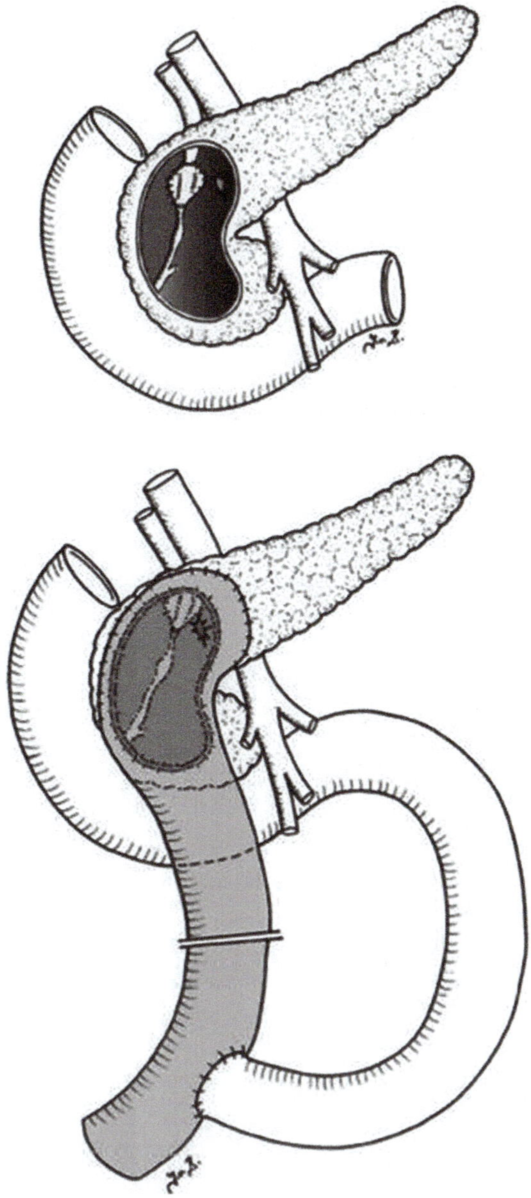

Fig. 11.2 Duodenum-preserving pancreatic head resection, Berne modification. Excavation of the pancreatic head without preparation of the portal vein. The bile duct is incised and reinserted in patients with cholestasis (*above*). Reconstruction by side-to-side pancreatic-jejunostomy (*below*)

two-layer, running PDS 5-0 suture completes the operation.

As in all our pancreatic resections, we place drains at the site of the pancreatic anastomosis to recognize and manage the development of an anastomotic leak. The DPPHR procedure is widely accepted nowadays and has been shown to be equally effective as the classic pancreatoduodenectomy in terms of long-term pain relief, morbidity, and mortality, but has less intraoperative blood loss, a shorter hospital stay, more postoperative weight gain, less exocrine insufficiency, better occupational rehabilitation, and a similar quality of life (Beger et al. 1989; Diener et al. 2008; Gloor et al. 2001; Büchler et al. 1995; Farkas et al. 2006; Klempa et al. 1995; Izbicki et al. 1995). The methodologic quality of these studies, however, especially with regard to long-term outcomes, is not sufficient to define the best type of pancreatic head resection in CP based on level I evidence. For this reason, the CHROPAC trial was initiated in 2009 (Diener et al. 2010). In this study, partial duodenopancreatectomy is compared to DPPHR in patients with CP in a randomized, double-blind, multicenter approach. The primary outcome parameter will be evaluation of quality of life in the long-term follow-up. Data on this study are expected in 2013.

Rarely, symptoms arise from CP limited to the pancreatic body and tail of the pancreas. In these cases, fibrosis, calcification, and pseudocysts are the most important findings, while small duct disease limited to this region is rather rare. For these patients, distal pancreatectomy as described elsewhere can be performed. For patients with disease limited to the neck or proximal body of the gland, a middle or central pancreatectomy can be used as a parenchyma-sparing procedure (Müller et al. 2006); however, this procedure is extremely rare in patients with CP (Fig. 11.3).

In this procedure midline or transverse laparotomy is followed by opening of the lesser sac by division of the gastrocolic ligament under preservation of the gastroepiploic vessels. The anterior aspect of the pancreas is exposed by dividing the adhesions between the posterior surface of the stomach and the pancreas. After a Kocher maneuver, the superior mesenteric, portal, and splenic veins are dissected free from the posterior aspect of the pancreas. All small side branches to the pancreas are divided by clips or bipolar coagulation. The segment of altered tissue can afterwards be resected. Pancreatic transection can either be carried out proximally with a stapler or by scalpel and by scalpel towards the distal margin. Bleeding vessels on either margin are ligated by 5-0 monofilament sutures. The sharply cut margin towards the head is afterwards primarily closed similar to the procedure during distal pancreatectomy (Fig. 11.4). Subsequently, the distal stump of the pancreas is further mobilized from the splenic vein and artery, with ligation of small tributaries, over 2 cm lateral to the cut end. Reconstruction is accomplished with a 50- to 60-cm retrocolic Roux-en-Y loop of the jejunum. An end-to-side

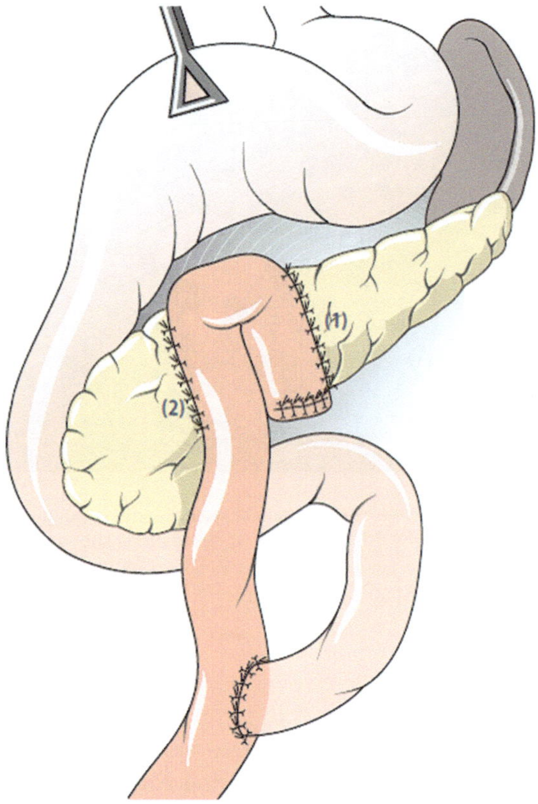

Fig. 11.3 Middle pancreatectomy. Segmental tissue resection and reconstruction by pancreatico-jejunostomy towards the pancreatic tail (*1*) and covering of the cut surface towards the head after closure with a seromuscular jejunum patch (*2*)

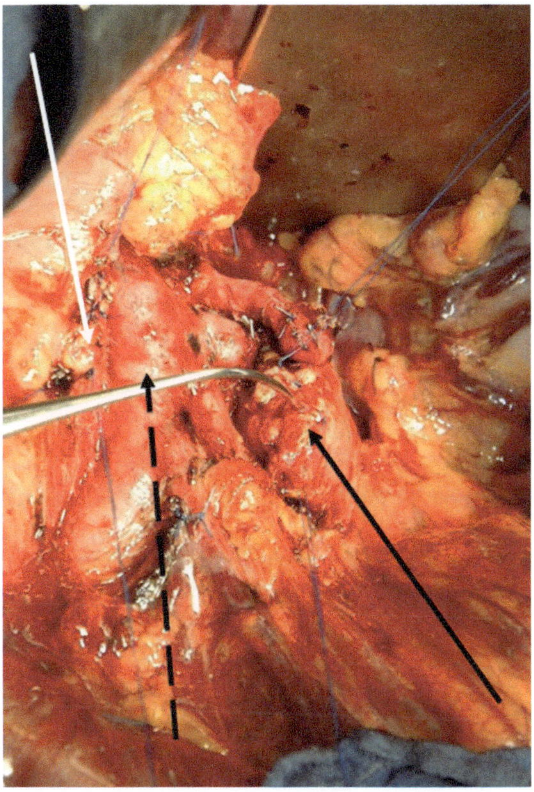

Fig. 11.4 Intraoperative situs during middle pancreatectomy. Cut margin of the pancreatic head (*white arrow*) and the pancreatic tail with probe inserted into the pancreatic duct (*black arrow*). Transection above the portal vein (*broke black arrow*)

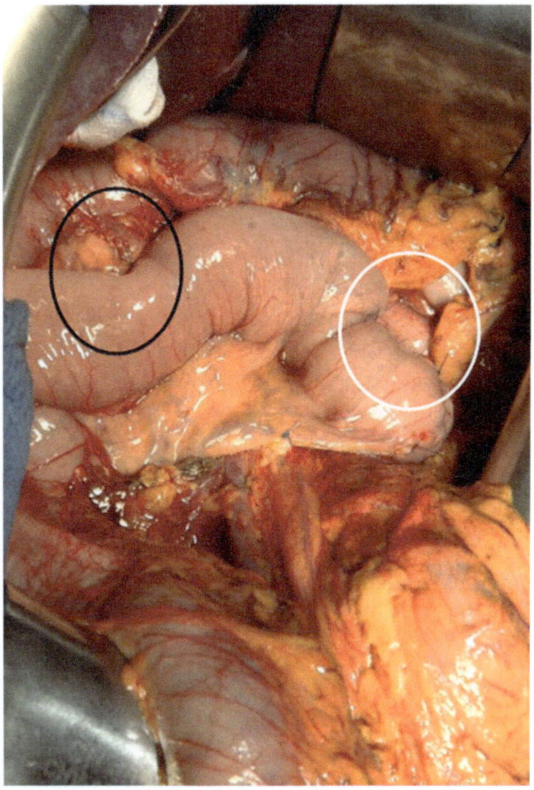

Fig. 11.5 Final intraoperative situs during middle pancreatectomy. Pancreatico-jejunostomy towards the pancreatic tail (*white circle*) and closed cut surface towards the head (*black circle*)

pancreaticojejunostomy is performed using a double layer of interrupted monofilament absorbable sutures (PDS 5-0). The technique used in our institution is identical to that used in the Whipple procedure. The inner layer of this anastomosis includes three ventral and three dorsal pancreatic duct to mucosa stitches as described in the chapter of partial duodeno-pancreatectomy. The already closed pancreatic head remnant is finally covered with the same jejunal loop using interrupted absorbable monofilament sutures (PDS 5-0) between the seromuscular layer of the jejunum and the capsule of the pancreas (Fig. 11.5). No fibrin glue or other sealants are required. Reconstruction is completed by an end-to-side Roux-Y enteroenterostomy 20–25 cm distal to the ligament of Treitz (Müller et al. 2006). At present, fistula rates between 8 and 63 % are reported for middle pancreatic resection, which is explained by the different underlying pathologies with lowest rates achieved in CP patients (Müller et al. 2006; Bassi 2007; Adham et al. 2008; Christein et al. 2006).

Operative enteric drainage of a pseudocyst is a procedure performed less frequently in patients with CP than other operative measures. We suggest operative drainage in patients with symptomatic pseudocysts (most frequently pain and gastrointestinal discomfort caused by compression of the stomach, duodenum, or the proximal small bowel) as well as for pseudocysts complicated by rupture or bleeding, which usually correlates with the size of the pseudocyst. Pseudocysts with a diameter less than 5 cm rarely cause symptoms or complications. Although most pseudocysts can be managed successfully by endoscopic therapy, those pseudocysts with bleeding or hematoma need to be approached operatively. Furthermore, patients with unsuccessful prior endoscopic or interventional therapy should undergo operative management. We prefer to use a cystojejunostomy to create the draining site at the most caudal point of the cyst, which is more difficult with a cystogastrostomy. For cystojejunostomy, the lesser sac is opened, and the anterior aspect of the pseudocyst is exposed after lysis of the inflammatory adhesions to the posterior wall of the stomach. In other patients, the pseudocyst extends to and through the transverse mesocolon, thereby allowing a transmesocolic approach. To ensure pseudocyst localization, needle puncture of the pseudocyst can localize the most caudal point of the pseudocyst. With operative enteric drainage, the cystic wall is incised by electrocautery, fluid and solid material evacuated, and cystotomy is extended as wide as possible. A frozen section of the wall of the pseudocyst is required to exclude the unexpected malignancy. Then the edges of the cystotomy can be "reefed" to control bleeding by oversewing the edges with a non-resorbable, monofilament suture (e.g. Prolene 4-0). A side-to-side transmesocolic, "retrocolic" cystojejunostomy to a Roux limb is performed using a double layer of running monofilamentabsorbable4-0PDS.Reconstruction is completed by an end-to-side jejunojejunostomy, 20–25 cm distal to the pancreatic anastomosis.

When patients with CP are operated on with the procedures as described above, it has to be underlined that if there is any suspicion of malignancy, the planned operative procedures need to be identical to those for pancreatic cancer.

The perioperative management in patients with CP is similar to that in patients who undergo pancreatic resection for other indications with regard to prophylactic antibiotics (mezlocillin or ciprofloxacin in case of penicillin allergy and metronidazole) as a single dose before the start of the operation. We do not use prophylactic, perioperative octreotide routinely in patients with CP. Usually, pancreatic anastomoses in these patients are uncomplicated due to the fibrotic tissue with very low rates of pancreatic fistulas.

Results from Heidelberg 01/2006-12/2008

Parameter	Number	%
Patients	233	100
DPPHR	74	31.7
Pylorus-preserving Whipple	97	41.6
Classical pancreatoduodenectomy	13	5.6
Total pancreatectomy	10	4.3
Distal pancreatectomy	27	11.6
Others	12	5.2
30-day mortality	2	0.9
Hospital stay (median, IQR)	9 (5–11)	
Morbidity		
Postoperative bleeding	9	3.9
Pancreatic fistula (grade B + C)	10	4.3
DGE	30	13.1
Wound infection	11	4.7

References

Adham M, Giunippero A, Hervieu V, Courbière M, Partensky C (2008) Central pancreatectomy: single-center experience of 50 cases. Arch Surg 143:175–180, discussion 180–181

Bassi C (2007) Middle segment pancreatectomy: a useful tool in the management of pancreatic neoplasms. J Gastrointest Surg 11:726–729

Beger HG, Buchler M, Bittner RR et al (1989) Duodenum-preserving resection of the head of the pancreas in severe chronic pancreatitis. Early and late results. Ann Surg 209:273–278

Büchler MW, Friess H, Muller MW et al (1995) Randomized trial of duodenumpreserving pancreatic head resection versus pylorus-preserving Whipple in chronic pancreatitis. Am J Surg 169:65–69

Ceyhan GO, Bergmann F, Kadihasanoglu M, Altintas B, Demir IE, Hinz U, Müller MW, Giese T, Büchler MW, Giese NA, Friess H (2009) Pancreatic neuropathy and neuropathic pain – a comprehensive pathomorphological study of 546 cases. Gastroenterology 136(1):177–186

Christein JD, Smoot RL, Farnell MB (2006) Central pancreatectomy: a technique for the resection of pancreatic neck lesions. Arch Surg 141:293–299

Diener MK, Rahbari NN, Fischer L et al (2008) Duodenum-preserving pancreatic head resection versus pancreatoduodenectomy for surgical treatment of chronic pancreatitis: a systematic review and meta-analysis. Ann Surg 247(6):950–961

Diener MK, Bruckner T, Contin P, Halloran C, Glanemann M, Schlitt HJ, Mössner J, Kieser M, Werner J, Büchler MW, Seiler CM (2010) ChroPac-trial: duodenum-preserving pancreatic head resection versus pancreatoduodenectomy for chronic pancreatitis. Trial protocol of a randomised controlled multicentre trial. Trials 11:47

Drewes AM, Krarup AL, Detlefsen S, Malmstrøm ML, Dimcevski G, Funch-Jensen P (2008) Pain in chronic pancreatitis: the role of neuropathic pain mechanisms. Gut 57(11):1616–1627. Epub 2008 Jun 19. Review

Farkas G, Leindler L, Daroczi M et al (2006) Prospective randomised comparison of organ-preserving pancreatic head resection with pylorus-preserving pancreaticoduodenectomy. Langenbecks Arch Surg 391:338–342

Friess H, Zhu ZW, di Mola FF, Kulli C, Graber HU, Andren-Sandberg A, Zimmermann A, Korc M, Reinshagen M, Büchler MW (1999) Nerve growth factor and its high-affinity receptor in chronic pancreatitis. Ann Surg 230(5):615–624

Gloor B, Friess H, Uhl W, Büchler MW (2001) A modified technique of the Beger and Frey procedure in patients with chronic pancreatitis. Dig Surg 18(1):21–25

Izbicki JR, Bloechle C, Knoefel WT et al (1995) Duodenum-preserving resection of the head of the pancreas in chronic pancreatitis. A prospective, randomized trial. Ann Surg 221:350–358

Keck T, Marjanovic G, Fernandez-del Castillo C, Makowiec F, Schäfer AO, Rodriguez JR, Razo O, Hopt UT, Warshaw AL (2009) The inflammatory pancreatic head mass: significant differences in the anatomic pathology of German and American patients with chronic pancreatitis determine very different surgical strategies. Ann Surg 249(1):105–110

Klempa I, Spatny M, Menzel J et al (1995) Pancreatic function and quality of life after resection of the head of the pancreas in chronic pancreatitis. A prospective, randomized comparative study after duodenum preserving resection of the head of the pancreas versus Whipple's operation. Chirurg 66:350–359

Müller MW, Friess H, Kleeff J et al (2006) Middle segmental pancreatic resection: an option to treat benign pancreatic body lesions. Ann Surg 244:909–918, discussion 918–920

Sakorafas GH, Farnell MB, Nagorney DM et al (2000) Pancreatoduodenectomy for chronic pancreatitis: long-term results in 105 patients. Arch Surg 135:517–523

Sakorafas GH, Tsiotou AG, Peros G (2007) Mechanisms and natural history of pain in chronic pancreatitis: a surgical perspective. J Clin Gastroenterol 41(7):689–699. Review

Strobel O, Büchler MW, Werner J (2009) Surgical therapy of chronic pancreatitis: indications, techniques and results. Int J Surg 7(4):305–312. Epub 2009 Jun 6

Vardanyan M, Rilo HL (2010) Pathogenesis of chronic pancreatitis-induced pain. Discov Med 9(47):304–310

12 Commentary

Michael B. Farnell and Ashleigh L. Levendale

12.1 Relevant Basic Information, Indications, and Contraindications

The approach to the surgical management for patients with chronic pancreatitis at Mayo Clinic is very similar to that outlined by the Magdeburg group. The majority of patients operated for chronic pancreatitis have undergone a formal anatomic resection. I agree that surgery for patients with chronic pancreatitis should be reserved for those patients with intractable pain, local complications, or when there is suspicion of malignancy. About 60 % of patients in the last 2 years have undergone resection and about 40 % either drainage alone or a combination of drainage and coring out of the head of the pancreas (Frey operation).

My approach to patients with chronic pancreatitis is very straightforward. When there is an inflammatory mass in the head of the pancreas associated with biliary or duodenal stenosis, intractable pain, and/or suspicion of malignancy, my preference is pancreatic head resection. For those less common patients with large duct disease and no inflammatory mass, my preference is to perform a drainage procedure. In the past, my approach was the lateral pancreaticojejunostomy after the Partington-Rochelle technique. In the last few years I have been employing the Frey operation for those patients with large duct disease (≥7 mm in diameter). I consider the Frey operation as an extended drainage procedure rather than a resection. While I agree that distal pancreatectomy has a limited role in patients who have chronic pancreatitis involving the entire gland, there is a subset of patients with focal chronic pancreatitis who are managed best with distal pancreatectomy. This subset has a history of acute pancreatitis who go on to develop strictures or complete occlusion of the pancreatic duct, resulting in focal obstructive pancreatitis of the left pancreas or a "disconnected duct syndrome". These patients typically present with intractable pain, a disconnected segment of pancreas, or with a focal stenosis of the pancreatic duct. It is worth noting that the number of patients who undergo surgery for chronic pancreatitis over the last few years has decreased because of the myriad of endoscopic therapies now available.

The development of portal hypertension as a result of the inflammatory mass in the head of the pancreas is a contraindication to resection in my hands. I have no substantive experience with performing pancreatic head resection in an effort to relieve portal hypertension as has been described by some groups. In contrast, patients with a disconnected duct syndrome who have splenic vein thrombosis, sinistral hypertension, and bleeding gastric varices may be managed by distal pancreatectomy/splenectomy which both relieves the

M.B. Farnell, M.D. (✉) • A.L. Levendale
Division of Gastroenterologic and General Surgery, Department of Surgery,
Mayo Clinic, College of Medicine,
200 First Street SW, Rochester, MN 55905, USA
e-mail: farnell.michael@mayo.edu

R. Mantke et al. (eds.), *International Practices in Pancreatic Surgery*,
DOI 10.1007/978-3-540-74506-8_12,

pain associated with the disconnected portion of pancreas as well as prevents future episodes of gastric hemorrhage.

Celiac artery stenosis either due to atherosclerotic disease at its origin or secondary to median arcuate ligament syndrome should be sought in every patient being considered for pancreatic head resection. While stenosis can be identified in the sagittal views of the superior mesenteric artery, suspicion of celiac artery stenosis should be raised by seeing a plethora of collateral arteries coursing through the head of the pancreas on the arterial phase of the abdominal CT on the axial and coronal images. In such patients, if resection is to be undertaken, a plan for dealing with the celiac artery stenosis should be developed prior to operation; options include either preoperative catheter-based angioplasty, intraoperative median arcuate ligament release, celiac artery angioplasty, or bypass.

In addition to chronic alcohol abuse, most of the patients who I see with chronic pancreatitis and intractable pain also have long-standing narcotic usage and most have chemical dependency. Accordingly, management of pain in the perioperative period is a substantial challenge, and we engage a dedicated, pain management service to help not only with postoperative pain control but also with a postoperative program for controlled substance withdrawal to address long-term the narcotic dependence.

With regard to preoperative investigations, my preference is to utilize a pancreas protocol CT to assess both the morphology of the pancreas as well as the surrounding vasculature. I prefer endoscopic retrograde cholangiopancreatography to determine the anatomy of the bile duct and pancreatic duct. In those cases where the papilla cannot be cannulated successfully or if obstruction in the pancreatic head precludes opacification of the pancreatic duct in the neck, body, and tail, we have found magnetic resonance cholangiopancreatography (MRCP) to be very helpful. Endoscopic ultrasonography (EUS) is used selectively. While the EUS allows for fine needle aspirate or if possible a core biopsy of the pancreas, if there is suspicion of malignancy, a negative biopsy does not exclude the presence of cancer, and, therefore, resection may be indicated.

While I agree with the Magdeburg group that prophylactic pancreatic resections in patients with hereditary pancreatitis are not appropriate, I do tend to offer total pancreatectomy and islet autotransplantation for those patients with hereditary pancreatitis and intractable pain earlier in the course of their disease than I did in the past. Previously I would perform targeted resection or drainage in those patients; however, with the current possibility of islet autotransplantation, I have utilized total pancreatectomy in such patients as primary therapy in selected circumstances. Early in our experience at Mayo Clinic, the harvested islets were injected into the portal system using a percutaneous, transhepatic route in interventional radiology postoperatively. More recently, we place a catheter via the recanalized umbilical vein for infusion into the portal circulation in the postoperative period in the intensive care setting. The catheter is removed 48–72 h postoperatively. The postoperative infusion of islets has negated the necessity of leaving the patient's abdomen open on the operating table for the approximate 4-h period required to prepare the islets for infusion.

12.2 Major Operative Technique

12.2.1 Incision and Exposure

Many patients with chronic pancreatitis are quite thin and in such patients with a high costal arch, I approach the pancreas via a midline incision, while those who have a broad costal arch are approached with a bilateral subcostal incision. I use a fixed, self-retaining upper abdominal retractor to facilitate exposure.

12.2.2 Pancreatic Resection Procedures: Technique

Over the past 2 years, the majority of pancreatic head resections were of the pylorus-preserving type. Only one patient underwent a classic Kausch-Whipple procedure. As noted in the introduction to this commentary, I have included distal pancreatectomy for disconnected duct syndrome.

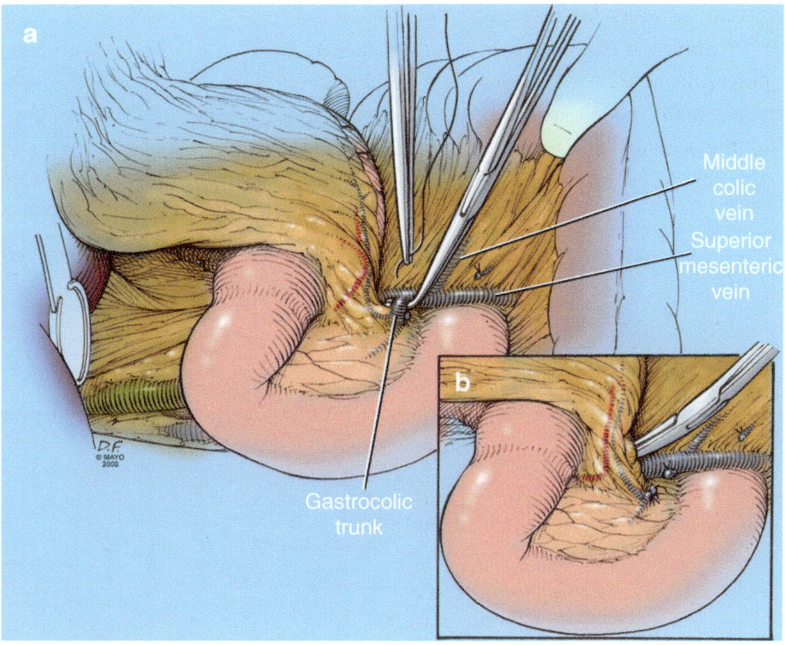

Fig. 12.1 (**a**) The superior mesenteric vein is identified beneath the neck of the pancreas. The gastrocolic venous trunk is ligated in continuity with 3-0 silk and divided. (**b**) A plane is developed between the neck of the pancreas anteriorly and the superior mesenteric vein/portal vein confluens posteriorly. A Shallcross right angle is used to develop gently this plane. Care is taken to perform this in a very delicate manner lest there be injury to the venous system and resultant severe hemorrhage (Reproduced with Permission of Mayo Foundation for Medical Education and Research. All Rights Reserved)

Typically, a splenectomy is performed with the procedure because of the intense inflammatory reaction surrounding the spleen and tail of the pancreas. Splenic preservation in this setting may be difficult to impossible. Moreover, performing splenectomy in the setting of sinistral hypertension will help to prevent or ameliorate bleeding from gastric varices. Total pancreatectomy is being performed more frequently and earlier in patients with idiopathic or hereditary pancreatitis and intractable pain because of the addition of islet autotransplantation.

12.2.2.1 Pylorus-Preserving Pancreatoduodenectomy

The pylorus-preserving pancreatoduodenectomy begins with a Kocher maneuver and mobilization of the hepatic flexure of the colon inferiorly to open up the right upper quadrant and enhance access to the pancreas. Rather than dividing the greater omentum, my preference is to free the omentum from the transverse colon in an avascular plane and allow the omentum to remain attached to the stomach. Adhesions between the pancreas and the back wall of the stomach are lysed to expose the anterior surface of the pancreas. This opens the lesser sac completely and provides access to the entire pancreas for both inspection and palpation. Next, the superior mesenteric vein (SMV) is identified by locating the cleft between the uncinate process of the pancreas posteriorly and the transverse mesocolon anteriorly at the level of the transverse duodenum. By identifying this cleft and further developing it, the SMV is identified. The SMV is followed cephalad to the gastrocolic venous trunk which is now ligated in continuity and divided (Fig. 12.1a). Next, a plane is developed between the neck of the pancreas anteriorly and the superior mesenteric vein/portal vein (SMV/PV) posteriorly (Fig. 12.1b). In some patients with chronic pancreatitis, this maneuver may be difficult and, if so, it is better not to persist in these efforts lest troublesome or even very severe bleeding from the portal vein posterior to the neck of the pancreas ensues. I agree with the Magdeburg group that it is not particularly helpful to try and gain proximal and distal control of the SMV below and the portal vein above the neck of the pancreas at this stage in the procedure; any bleeding that occurs is still being supplied by the splenic vein, the inferior mesenteric vein, and the first jejunal branch, as well as other small tributaries, and proximal and distal control will simply not stop

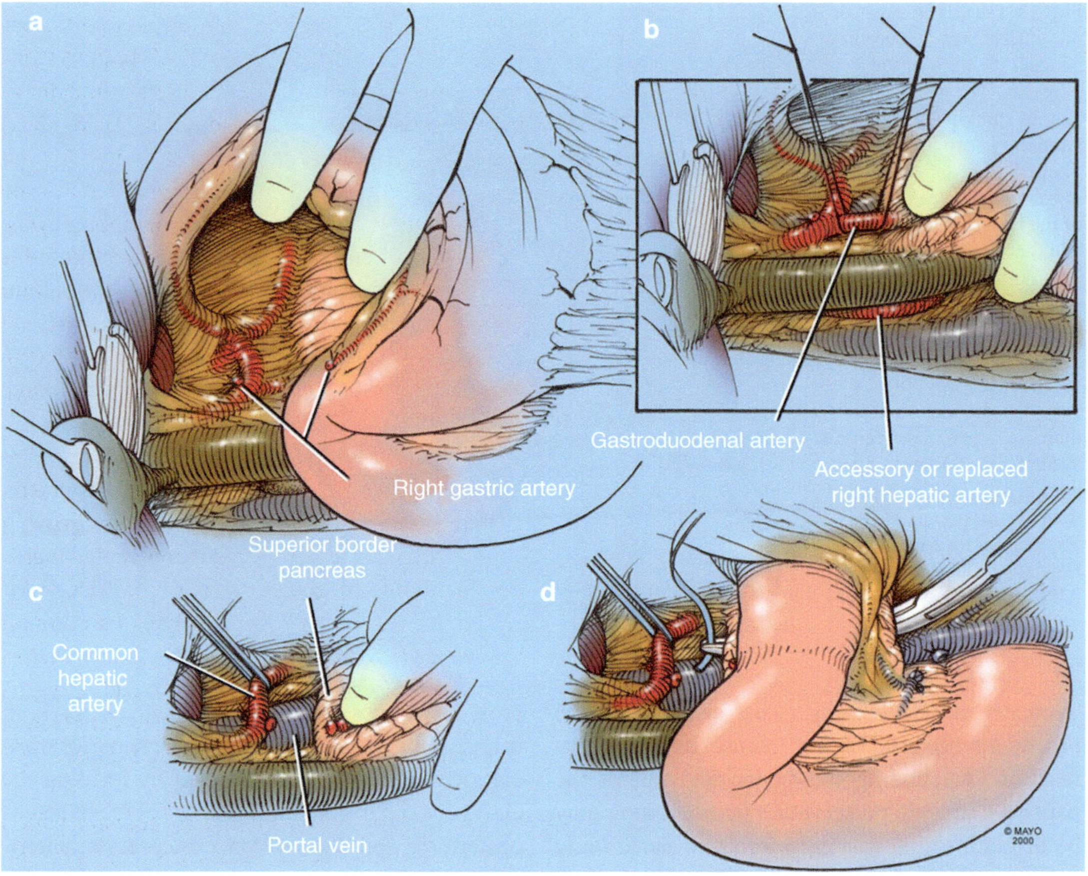

Fig. 12.2 (**a**) The right gastric artery is clamped, divided and ligated with 3-0 silk. (**b**) The common hepatic artery is identified; after skeletonizing the gastroduodenal artery, it is ligated in continuity with 2-0 silk supplemented with a transfixing suture of 3-0 silk and divided. Arterial pulsation posterior to the bile duct is a tip-off to a replaced right hepatic artery. (**c**) The portal vein is identified rostral to the rostral border of the pancreas and the tunnel completed beneath the neck of the pancreas. (**d**) An umbilical tape is placed around the neck of the pancreas (Reproduced with Permission of Mayo Foundation for Medical Education and Research. All Rights Reserved)

the bleeding. Packing of the space posterior to the neck of the pancreas with gauze or compressing the head of the pancreas and SMV/PV with the surgeon's left hand, with the thumb anteriorly and the fingers posteriorly, will help to tamponade any bleeding so that additional maneuvers can be performed to deal with the hemorrhage. At times it may be difficult or virtually impossible (and dangerous) to identify the proper plane between the pancreas and the portal vein; if an improper plane is chosen, the portal vein may be delaminated resulting in a very thin-walled portal vein that is at risk for tearing during the later phases of the operation. It is better to abandon attempts at getting under the neck of the pancreas if the plane is not friendly enough.

Next, attention is directed rostral to the neck of the pancreas. The right gastric artery is clamped, divided, and ligated with 3-0 silk (Fig. 12.2a). Typically the hepatic artery lymph node is identified rostral to the neck of the pancreas. This area is mobilized and the common hepatic artery identified beneath. The investing tissue around the common hepatic artery is incised and the gastroduodenal artery identified. At this juncture, it is appropriate to palpate the space posterior to the bile duct. A replaced right hepatic artery arising from the superior mesenteric artery courses posterior to the bile duct and the arterial pulsation will be palpable in this region. It is important to recognize this variant before encircling and dividing the common hepatic duct. The gastroduodenal artery is ligated

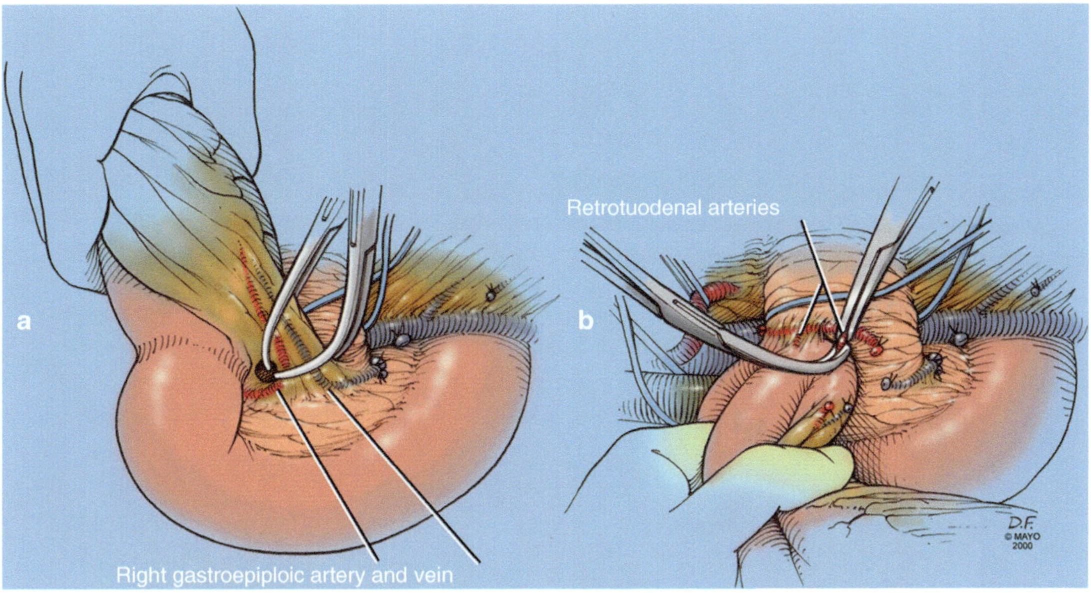

Fig. 12.3 (**a**) The right gastroepiploic artery and vein are clamped, divided, and ligated with 2-0 silk. (**b**) Any retroduodenal arteries are clamped, divided and ligated with 3-0 silk mobilizing approximately 3 cm of duodenum beyond the pylorus (Reproduced with Permission of Mayo Foundation for Medical Education and Research. All Rights Reserved)

in continuity with 2-0 silk supplemented with a suture ligature of 3-0 silk and divided (Fig. 12.2b, c). An umbilical tape is then placed posterior to the neck of the pancreas if the space was developed successfully (Fig. 12.2d). Next, the gallbladder is removed from its fossa from above downward. I then mobilize the cystic duct as far distally as possible. The common hepatic duct is then mobilized above the entrance of the cystic duct, care being taken to avoid injury to the portal vein and also to protect a replaced right hepatic artery if present. Likewise, an umbilical tape is passed around the common hepatic duct. The gallbladder is allowed to remain attached to the common duct. Next, the right gastroepiploic artery and vein are clamped, divided, and ligated with 2-0 silk (Fig. 12.3a). The retroduodenal arteries are clamped, divided, and ligated with 3-0 silk, skeletonizing the duodenum for approximately 3–4 cm beyond the pylorus (Fig. 12.3b). Next, attention is directed below the mesocolon to the infracolic compartment. The ligament of Treitz is taken down. The jejunal mesentery is transilluminated and an appropriate arcade chosen approximately 20 cm distal to the ligament of Treitz. This distance is chosen in order to provide adequate length on the mesentery of the jejunal biliopancreatic limb such that it can be brought through the mesocolon to the right of the middle colic vessels. The mesentery of the jejunum is clamped, divided, and ligated with 3-0 silk. More recently I have used a LigaSure® device (Covidien Inc, Mansfield, Massachusetts, USA) to divide the small vessels in the jejunal mesentery. Dissection of these small vessels is carried proximally until the uncinate process of the pancreas becomes visible. The uncinate process indicates the proximal extent of the dissection of the duodenojejunal mesentery (Fig. 12.4a–d). The jejunum is then divided with a linear stapling device. The jejunum is passed posterior to the superior mesenteric artery into the right supracolic compartment. The stapled end of the jejunum to be retained for reconstruction is imbricated with interrupted 3-0 silk. The defect at the ligament of Treitz is closed with running 3-0 absorbable polyglactin suture. The duodenum is transected and stapled with a linear stapler approximately 3 cm distal to the pylorus.

Next, a bulldog clamp is placed on the proximal common hepatic duct and the common hepatic duct transected. I typically harvest the margin from the common hepatic duct for frozen section. Next, a Satinsky clamp is placed posterior to the

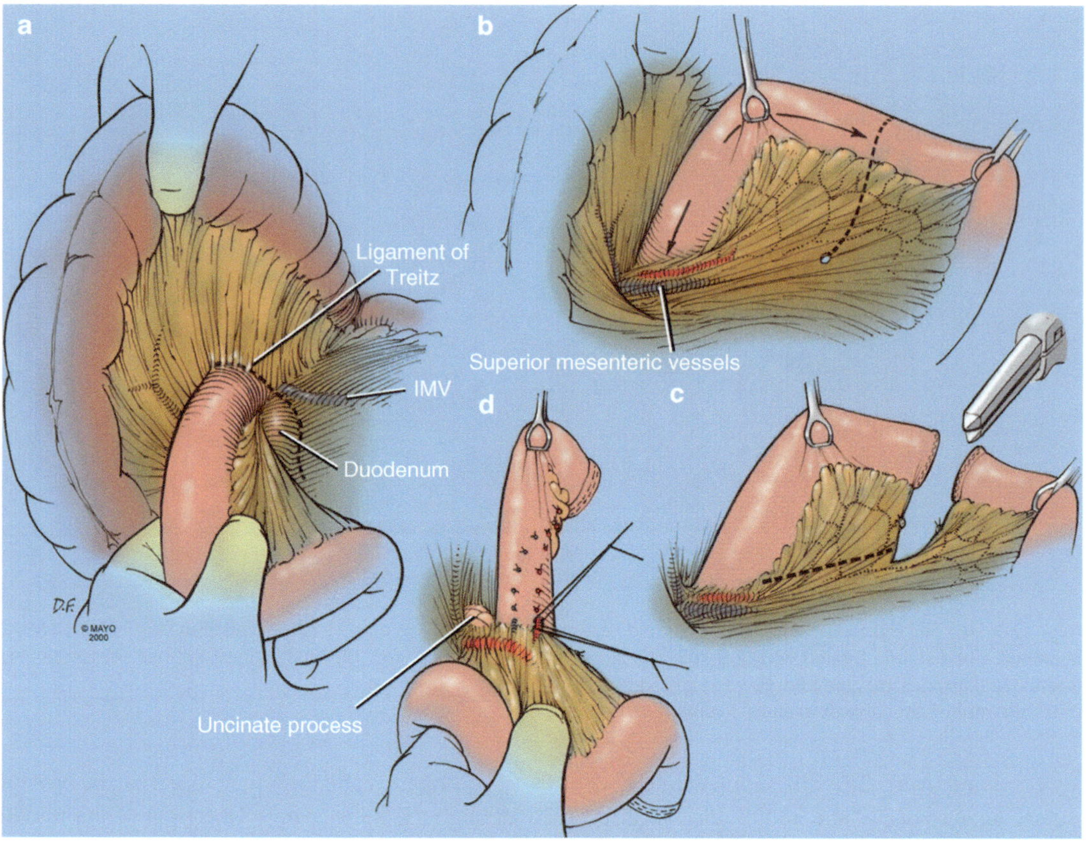

Fig. 12.4 (**a**) Attention is directed to the infracolic compartment. The ligament of Treitz is taken down being careful to protect the inferior mesenteric vein. (**b**) After the jejunum is transilluminated, an appropriate arcade chosen for dividing the mesentery of the jejunum approximately 20 cm beyond the ligament of Treitz. The jejunal mesentery is clamped, divided and ligated with 3-0 silk. (**c**) The bowel is transected with a GIA stapler. The jejunal/duodenal vessels are ligated in continuity with 3-0 silk and divided. Alternatively, a LigaSure® device may be used for this step. (**d**) Dissection is carried proximal until the uncinate process is visible (Reproduced with Permission of Mayo Foundation for Medical Education and Research. All Rights Reserved)

neck of the pancreas. I divide the pancreas not to the right of the SMV but either over the mid portion or slightly to the left (Fig. 12.5a). This is an important step, because the pancreatic duct courses quite posteriorly in the pancreas as it approaches the right side of the SMV/PV confluens. In order to have the pancreatic duct centered in the pancreatic remnant, it is my preference to divide it slightly further to the left than described by the Magdeburg group. After harvesting the margin from the neck of the pancreas for frozen section analysis, the SMV/PV is teased from the portal vein groove of the pancreatic head. Venous tributaries are ligated in continuity with 3-0 silk and divided (Fig. 12.5b). The first jejunal branch is often quite large and is very short. If this branch courses to the right of the superior mesenteric artery, it will need to be divided and ligated to facilitate a periadvential dissection of the superior mesenteric artery. Accordingly, this vessel is mobilized carefully and ligated in continuity with 2-0 silk supplemented on the superior mesenteric vein side with a suture ligature of 4-0 polypropylene and then divided (Fig. 12.5c). Next, a periadventitial dissection of the superior mesenteric artery is undertaken. I currently use the LigaSure® device for this dissection, except for the inferior pancreaticoduodenal artery, which I identify and ligate in continuity with 3-0 silk supplemented with a 4-0 suture of polypropylene (Fig. 12.5d).

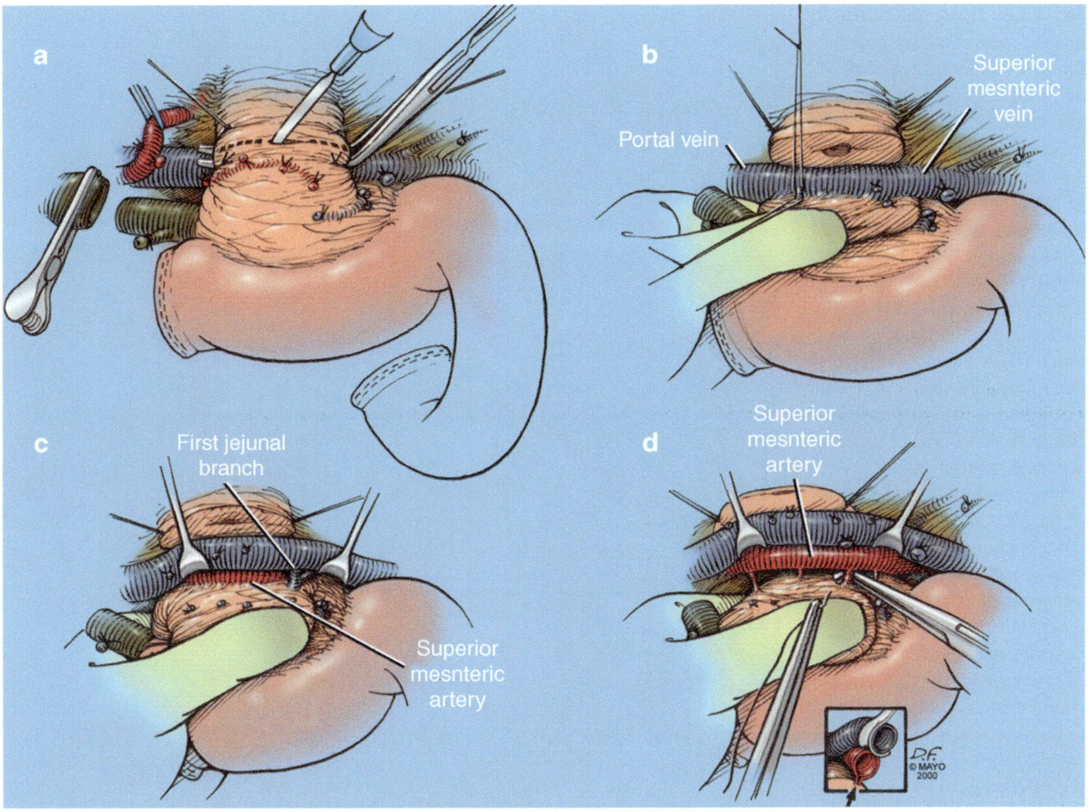

Fig. 12.5 (**a**) A bulldog clamp is applied to the common hepatic duct and the common hepatic duct transected sharply. The neck of the pancreas is divided with cautery. (**b**) Venous tributaries of the portal vein are ligated in continuity with 3-0 silk and divided freeing the portal vein from the portal vein groove. (**c**) The first jejunal venous branch is ligated in continuity with 2-0 silk supplemented with a suture ligature of 4-0 polypropylene and divided. (**d**) A periadventitial dissection of the SMA is undertaken using a LigaSure® device, however, the inferior pancreatoduodenal artery is ligated individually in continuity with 3-0 silk and divided (Reproduced with Permission of Mayo Foundation for Medical Education and Research. All Rights Reserved)

After the specimen is removed, the bed of resection is checked for hemostasis. Areas of problematic hemostasis include the jejunal mesentery as well as the area of the periadventitial dissection of the superior mesenteric artery. Hemostasis in these sites should be ensured carefully.

To initiate reconstruction, an opening is made in the mesocolon to the right of the middle colic vessels through which the jejunum is brought. Using optical magnification (2.5×), an end-to-side pancreaticojejunostomy is fashioned splinted temporarily with an 8 French Silastic® catheter. This catheter is used temporarily to ensure that the sutures placed in the small opening in the jejunum do not obliterate the anastomosis. After placement of the anterior row of 6-0 polyglactin in the mucosa-to-mucosa anastomosis, a nerve hook is used to remove the Silastic catheter and the 6-0 sutures are tied. Next, the anterior row of interrupted 4-0 silk suture from the capsule and parenchyma of the pancreas to the seromuscular layer of the jejunum are placed and tied (Fig. 12.6a–c). About 3–4 in. downstream, an end-to-side hepaticojejunostomy is fashioned with continuous 5-0 polyglactin (Fig. 12.6d). Two sutures are used, one each anteriorly and posteriorly, in order to prevent purse-stringing of the anastomosis. Those patients who have a small bile duct, particularly if it is thin-walled, are best managed with an interrupted anastomosis using interrupted 6-0 polydioxanone. The traversing jejunal limb is secured to the mesocolon with interrupted

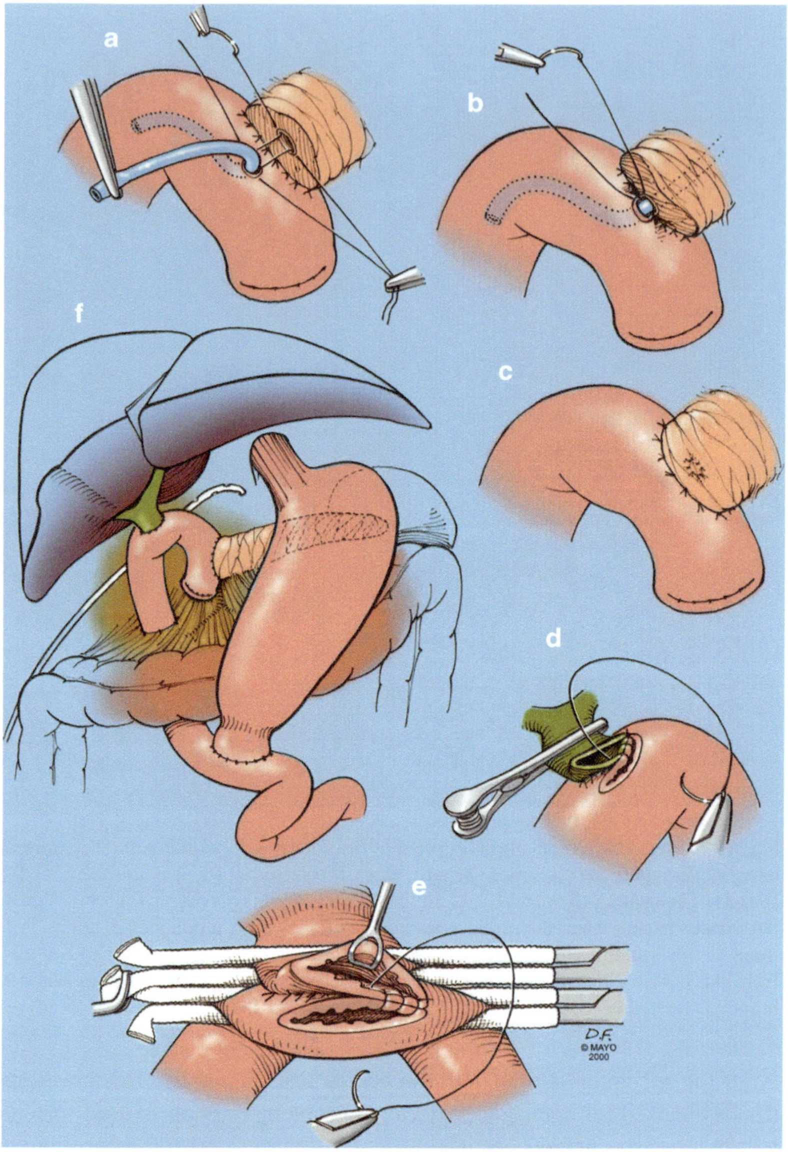

Fig. 12.6 (**a**) A mucosa-to-mucosa pancreaticojejunostomy is fashioned with an outer layer of interrupted 4-0 silk and an inner layer of inner layer of interrupted 6-0 polyglactin. (**b**) An 8 French Silastic® catheter is used as a temporary stent but removed prior to tying the anterior row of 6-0 polyglactin. (**c**) Completed mucosa-to-mucosa pancreaticojejunostomy. (**d**) An end-to-side hepaticojejunostomy is fashioned with two sutures of continuous 5-0 vicryl using a separate suture for the anterior and posterior portion of the anastomosis to prevent purse-stringing. (**e**) Lastly, an end-to-side duodenojejunostomy is fashioned with an inner layer of running 3-0 polyglactin and an outer layer of interrupted 3-0 silk. (**f**) A single drain is placed adjacent to the pancreatic and biliary anastomoses (Reproduced with Permission of Mayo Foundation for Medical Education and Research. All Rights Reserved)

3-0 silk, and 20–30 cm distally, an antecolic, end-to-side duodenojejunostomy is fashioned with an inner layer of running 3-0 polyglactin and an outer layer of interrupted 3-0 silk (Fig. 12.6e). If the blood supply to the duodenal cuff is suboptimal, I respect additional duodenum until the mucosa appears pink and viable. I have no problem with performing a pylorojejunostomy if necessary in order to ensure adequate blood supply at the anastomosis. A single drain is my current preference. It is placed in Morison's pouch with the drain posterior to the pancreaticojejunostomy (Fig. 12.6f).

12.2.2.2 Left-Sided Distal Pancreatectomy

Distal pancreatectomy/splenectomy is one of the more common operations in my practice for patients who have chronic obstructive pancreatitis. I agree with the Magdeburg group that for patients with true chronic pancreatitis involving the entire gland, a left-sided resection is rarely indicated. In those patients who have prior attacks of necrotizing pancreatitis with critical stenoses or complete obliteration of the pancreatic duct, a "disconnected duct syndrome" may ensue, and resection of the remnant pancreas may be indicated. I have not found it to be a durable solution to anastomose a Roux-en-Y limb to these disconnected segments, because the anastomosis tends to stenose in these patients with development of intractable pain. Accordingly, I usually recommend resection in such cases; however, one has to recognize that this procedure is technically difficult due to the surrounding inflammation and fibrosis around the remnant pancreas. Collateral damage to surrounding organs is a possibility, and care must be taken relative to the posterior wall of the stomach, the transverse colon, the fourth portion of the duodenum, the left kidney, and the adrenal gland. I approach the distal pancreatectomy by freeing the omentum from the splenic flexure of the left transverse colon and entering the lesser sac, hemisecting the omentum, and then serially clamping, dividing, and ligating the short gastric vessels all the way up to the gastroesophageal junction; this initial maneuver frees the stomach from the disconnected pancreatic segment. The splenocolic and splenorenal ligaments are incised and a plane developed between the spleen and tail of the pancreas anteriorly and the left kidney and adrenal gland posteriorly. Dissection is then carried medially where the splenic artery and vein sought, each ligated in continuity with 2-0 silk supplemented with a transfixing suture of 3-0 silk, and divided, allowing the specimen to be removed. Typically, when there is a complete disconnection, there is no need to oversew the stump of the remaining proximal pancreas.

12.2.2.3 Total Pancreatectomy

At Mayo we have performed five total pancreatectomies as primary surgical therapy for chronic pancreatitis in the last 2 years. As noted in the introduction to this commentary, we have been employing total pancreatectomy and islet autotransplantation in selected patients with intractable pain due to hereditary or idiopathic pancreatitis. The operative exposure for total pancreatectomy is very similar to that for a pylorus-preserving pancreatoduodenectomy; however, the omentum is freed completely from the transverse colon, releasing both the hepatic and splenic flexures inferiorly to expose the pancreas all the way from the head to the tail. I have performed spleen-sparing total pancreatectomy in some patients but often due to the surrounding fibrosis, it is not possible to preserve the spleen. I will not describe the total pancreatectomy step by step but will make a few technical points worth noting.

First, in patients with heredity pancreatitis and intractable pain selected earlier in the course of their disease for pancreatectomy due to the availability of islet autotransplantation, the peripancreatic inflammatory reaction is typically less than seen in patients with more long-standing disease and dissection around the SMV/PV confluens and superior mesenteric artery is more straightforward.

Second, it is important to preserve the blood supply to the pancreas to the very terminal stages of the procedure to minimize the warm ischemia time. I do this by preserving both the splenic artery and splenic vein until the last step in the operation. This maneuver is accomplished by mobilizing the head, neck, and body of the pancreas sufficiently such that the venous tributaries of the SMV/PV confluens can be ligated in continuity and divided freeing the portal vein from the portal vein groove and the superior mesenteric artery from the uncinate process of the pancreas. The splenic artery and vein are only then ligated in continuity doubly with 2-0 silk with a transfixing suture of 3-0 silk and divided, minimizing the warm ischemia time. An example of a total pancreatectomy with preservation of the splenic artery and vein to the terminal step is shown in Fig. 12.7.

One of the potential problems with the pylorus-preserving total pancreatoduodenectomy and splenectomy is adequate venous drainage of the stomach. If the spleen is taken with the total pancreatoduodenectomy, the only venous drainage of the stomach will be via the coronary vein. It is important to preserve the coronary vein during the dissection. Another trick is to take the short gastric vessels as close to the splenic hilum as possible to preserve as much venous capacitance within the stomach and greater omentum as possible. In my experience, this approach results in less venous congestion of the stomach. If the stomach develops

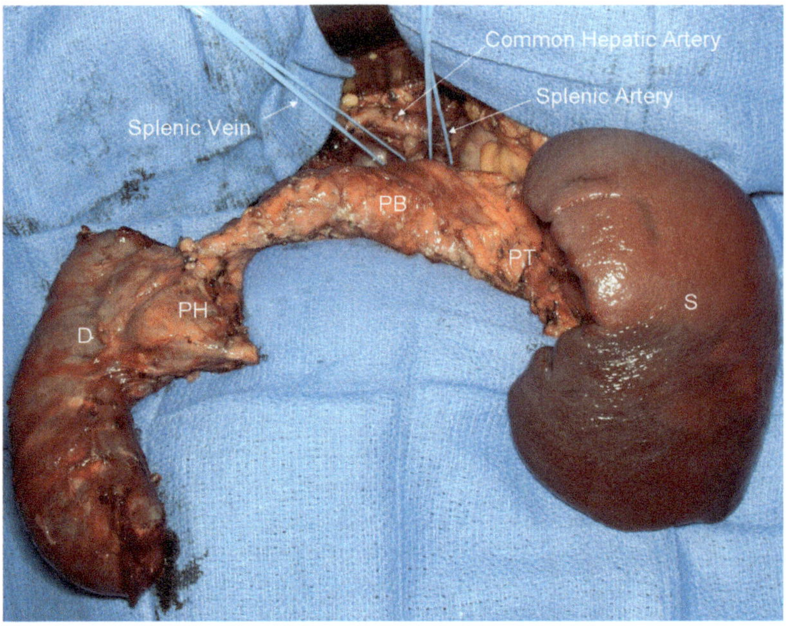

Fig. 12.7 Pylorus-preserving total pancreatoduodenectomy and splenectomy with preservation of the blood supply to the pancreatic remnant via the splenic artery and splenic vein. The blue vessel loops encircle the splenic artery and the splenic vein. Ligation of the splenic artery and the splenic vein is preserved at the very final step in the procedure. Note that other than the lower pole of the spleen, the specimen is well perfused. The warm ischemia time in this case was 2 min 8 s (*D* duodenum, *PH* pancreatic head, *PB* pancreatic body, *S* spleen, *PT* pancreatic tail)

marked venous congestion after an attempt at a total pancreatoduodenectomy/splenectomy, distal gastrectomy may be necessary.

12.2.3 Drainage Procedures: Technical Notes

12.2.3.1 Frey Procedure

The Frey procedure is being employed increasingly when the patient has large duct disease and pancreatic drainage is entertained. My approach to the procedure is very similar to that described by the Magdeburg group. I find it advantageous to remove the gallbladder when present and place a biliary Fogarty catheter through the cystic duct, into the bile duct and ultimately into the duodenum to allow precise identification of the bile duct during the non-anatomic part of the resection of the tissue in the head of the pancreas. I prefer not to expose the bile duct during the course of the subtotal resection of the pancreatic head. I agree that it is important to extend the filleting of the pancreatic duct as far as possible both proximally and distally in the pancreas. I find bleeding from the subtotal resection of the pancreatic head to be troublesome when performing this operation. I use cautery but also use suture ligatures of 4-0 and 5-0 polypropylene for hemostasis liberally. Hemostasis needs to be done carefully, because bleeding from the pancreatic head into the jejunal limb can be problematic in the postoperative period. I bring the limb through the mesocolon to the right of the middle colic vessels with the toe of the limb oriented toward the hilum of the spleen and the heel in the head of the pancreas. My preference is to perform the anastomosis with a single layer of interrupted 3-0 silk. The sutures are placed full thickness on the bowel and into the leathery parenchyma of the pancreas. While a mucosa-to-mucosa anastomosis is ideal, it is not possible in every patient. I leave a closed suction drain adjacent to the pancreatic anastomosis.

12.2.3.2 Lateral Pancreaticojejunostomy

Lateral pancreaticojejunostomy is utilized in those patients who have large duct chronic pancreatitis without either an inflammatory mass in the head of the pancreas or multiple calculi in the side branches of the head and uncinate process of the gland. My technique is almost exactly like that described by the authors in the chapter. I have not found it necessary to use ultrasonography to identify the pancreatic duct. Needle aspiration or ballottement of the enlarged, tense pancreatic duct allows identification of the

Table 12.1 Patients with chronic pancreatitis who underwent drainage procedures at Mayo Clinic, Rochester, MN, USA (2009, 2010)

Drainage/other		
Parameter	Number	%
Patients	*13*	
Hospital mortality	0	0
Hospital stay (median, days)	9 (2–33)	
Frey procedure	5	39
Lateral pancreaticojejunostomy	3	23
Biliary/duodenal bypass	2	15
Biliary bypass, gastrojejunostomy, cyst jejunostomy	1 each	
Postoperative local morbidity		
Relaparotomy	1	0
Wound infection	2	15
Delayed gastric emptying	2	15
Postoperative bleeding, pancreatic fistula, biliary fistula	0	0
Postoperative systemic morbidity		
Systemic complications	0	0

Table 12.2 Patients with chronic pancreatitis who underwent resection at Mayo Clinic, Rochester, MN, USA (2009, 2010)

Resection		
Parameter	Number	%
Patients	*36*	
Hospital mortality	0	0
Hospital stay (median, days)	17 (5–65)	
Distal pancreatectomy with splenectomy	14	40
Pylorus-preserving pancreatoduodenectomy	13	36
Total pancreatectomy	5	14
Kausch-Whipple procedure	1	
Beger procedure	1	
Distal pancreatectomy	1	
Central pancreatectomy	1	
Postoperative local morbidity		
Relaparotomy	4	11
Delayed gastric emptying	12	33
Pancreatic fistula	6	17
Biliary fistula	4	11
Wound infection	6	17
Postoperative bleeding	1	
Other (i.e. abscess, pleural effusion)	3	8
Postoperative systemic morbidity		
Systemic complications	9	25

pancreatic duct. I use cautery and fillet the pancreatic duct in a longitudinal manner. It is critical to extend the filleting all the way from the splenic hilum to the medial wall of the duodenum and unroof both Santorini's and Wirsung's ducts.

12.3 Results

The results of pancreatic surgery for chronic pancreatitis at the Mayo Clinic for 2009 and 2010 are included in Tables 12.1 and 12.2.

Commentary

13

A. Fingerhut, S.V. Shrikhande, and P.J. Shukla

13.1 Relevant Basic Information

Chronic pancreatitis (CP) is predominantly a chronic inflammatory disease that is being detected with increasing frequency. While chronic alcohol intake is associated with the development of CP, gene mutations have also been linked to both hereditary and possibly tropical forms of the disease. Independent of the etiology, CP is usually discovered at a stage when the morphologic and inflammatory changes are similar in all variants (Shrikhande et al. 2003). Recurrent, often severe, pain is the dominant and classic symptom of CP that necessitates treatment and is the single most important reason for patients to consult the clinician and ultimately the surgeon (Shrikhande et al. 2002).

Routine blood tests do not help in establishing the diagnosis of CP – the diagnosis is more clinical and based on patient symptoms. Upper abdominal pain usually radiating to the back with a previous history of similar such episodes, some requiring hospitalization, and relief of pain with analgesics are clues to a definitive diagnosis. Some patients also have a history of previous attacks of acute pancreatitis. While alcohol is responsible for alcoholic CP in the western world, there are hereditary, tropical, and other variants seen in the east, particularly in India. Patients with tropical CP are usually young and present early with florid clinical symptoms and radiologic findings of the disease. A number of patients suffer from diabetes mellitus and also report steatorrhoea.

CP is confirmed primarily by a combination of careful patient history and radiologic imaging – i.e. contrast enhanced computed tomography (CT) and magnetic resonance imaging/magnetic resonance cholangio-pancreatography (MRI/MRCP). These imaging modalities help both in disease documentation and localization, as well as for treatment planning.

13.2 Indications for Surgery

The primary indication for operative intervention is longstanding, intractable pain (Shrikhande et al. 2000) which becomes progressively uncontrollable by analgesics that have been used in a stepwise pattern. Apart from uncontrolled pain, the other indications for operative intervention are for complications associated with CP, such as:

1. Pancreatic pseudocysts
2. Common bile duct obstruction
3. Duodenal obstruction
4. Suspected pancreatic cancer
5. Dilated main pancreatic duct without pain in young uncontrolled diabetics

A. Fingerhut (✉) • P.J. Shukla
Department of Digestive Surgery,
Centre Hospitalier Intercommunal,
Poissy, France
e-mail: abefingerhut@aol.com

S.V. Shrikhande
Department of Surgical Oncology, Gastrointestinal and
HPB Surgical Unit, Tata Memorial Hospital,
Mumbai, India

R. Mantke et al. (eds.), *International Practices in Pancreatic Surgery*,
DOI 10.1007/978-3-540-74506-8_13, © Springer-Verlag Berlin Heidelberg 2013

13.3 Contraindications

Absolute
1. Cirrhosis of liver
2. Severe medical conditions

Relative
1. Portal hypertension due to portal venous obstruction

13.4 Operative Technique

13.4.1 Drainage Procedures

13.4.1.1 Lateral Pancreaticojejunostomy

- Wide Kocher maneuver (Valley Lab Cautery, USA)
- Division of gastrocolic omentum (Harmonic Scalpel, Ultracision, Ethicon, USA)
- Exposure of the entire length of pancreas
- Ligation of the gastroduodenal artery (4-0 polypropylene)
- Identification of the dilated main pancreatic duct (by palpation/directed needle puncture)
- Opening the entire length of duct with cautery (>8 cm)
- Extraction of pancreatic calculi
- Side- to-side, duct- to- mucosa pancreaticojejunostomy* (Shrikhande et al. 2004) (3-0 polypropylene/3-0 polydioxanone)
- End to side jejunojejunostomy (4-0 polyglactin or polydioxanone)
- *We believe it is important to perform a duct to mucosa anastomosis. The extensive and progressive fibrosis of CP can obliterate an anastomosis even after years (Shrikhande et al. 2004).

13.4.1.2 Overall Experience with Lateral Pancreaticojejunostomy

- Excellent long term pain control (85–95 %); those who do not get pain relief have causes of pain not correctable by operative intervention (Shrikhande et al. 2001)
- Low morbidity (<5 %)/mortality (<1 %)
- Better/easier control of diabetes (Nealon and Thompson 1993; Evans et al. 1997)
- Perhaps delays ultimate "burnout" of pancreas (Nealon and Thompson 1993)
- Organ-preserving procedure

13.4.1.3 Cystogastrostomy

Retrogastric pseudocysts are often treated best by cystogastrostomy. The edge of the cystogastrostomy can bleed briskly on occasion; moreover, when the cyst wall is immature, anastomosis between stomach and cyst wall can be hazardous. In these situations, we prefer to take a few interrupted sutures of 2-0 polyglactin very early in the course of the procedure i.e. soon after the posterior wall of the stomach is incised and an entry is made into the cyst cavity to oversew the cystogastrostomy.

13.4.2 Resection Procedures

Resectional procedures are tailored according to the location and extent of the disease process. Development of pancreatic cancer in the setting of pre-existing CP is common, especially in the tropical form of CP (Augustine and Ramesh 1992; Chari et al. 1994).

13.4.2.1 CP with Head-Dominant Mass

Pancreatoduodenectomy (PD) has been the standard operative procedure for pain and pancreatic head-related complications of CP. PD is a relatively safe procedure in high-volume centers, where mortality rates are less than 5 %. PD not only achieves excellent pain relief and treats other complications associated with a pancreatic head mass, but PD also eliminates the possibility of cancer in this mass. We rarely perform the duodenum-preserving pancreatic head resection (DPPHR) we use DPPHR only if inflammation around the superior mesenteric vein (SMV) and portal vein (PV) is not severe. In cases where the diagnosis of chronic pancreatitis is unequivocal with severe inflammation around the SMV – PV, we prefer the head coring procedure (Frey procedure). Usually the head coring is combined with a drainage procedure. Most of the initial steps are similar to lateral pancreaticojejunostomy. The head coring is best performed by placing a few 2-0/3-0 polypropylene sutures into the pancreatic parenchyma along the "C" aspect of the duodenum, a few millimeters away from the duodenal wall. With a wide Kocher maneuver already performed, it is easy to control the head mass in the left hand of the operating surgeon while using electrocautery to excise the head mass. We prefer to control bleeding with polypropylene sutures, which tend to hold well in a firm to hard pancreas. The medial extent of the head mass needs special attention where it is crucial to define the SMV along the inferior margin of the pancreas. We also prefer to ligate the gastroduodenal artery prior to beginning the head coring procedure.

Occasionally when the head mass is not very large, we core a small part of the head and later follow the main pancreatic duct from the body/neck region toward the head region with the help of a fine Mixter or Llhey clamp. All the tissue over the clamp is divided with electrocautery – this maneuver lays open the posteriorly dipping ducts in the head region. A meticulous (and often time consuming) dissection to remove all calculi from both the main ducts and also from the side branches is crucial to ensure an optimal drainage and resection procedure.

The Basic Chapter of "Chronic Pancreatitis Surgery" by Hans-Ulrich Schulz, Rene Mantke, and Hans Lippert is illuminating in many respects. The more complex an operation, the more steps that can be modified or altered according to the need for improvement, but also because of personal feelings, beliefs, or experience-based foundations. Rarely has any one operation or the basic principles concerning the resection of the head of the pancreas been modified as much as pancreatoduodenectomy, and rarely has one operation been given a name that does not correspond to the original surgeon who performed or described it. It has been written that Alessandro Codivilla (1861–1912) performed the first pancreatic head resection prior to 1890 and that Walther Kausch (1867–1928) reported the first successful excision of the duodenum and a portion of the pancreas in two stages for ampullary cancer in 1912 (Schnelldorfer et al. 2008).

While the restricted indications for the Kausch-Whipple procedure herein – "typically used in patients with chronic pancreatitis who have had a prior gastric resection for ulcer, in rare situations of extensive adhesions between the pancreatic head and the pyloric region, and if the duodenum stump becomes ischemic during an attempted pylorus preservation" might well explain why the authors performed the Whipple procedure in less than 10 % of the patients undergoing resection in their series, it is of note that many pancreatic surgery specialist do not consider pancreatoduodenectomy for chronic pancreatitis, except when there is an undetermined focal mass in the head and/or the ductal system is not dilated. In contrast, it is difficult to understand why 17 of 42 patients undergoing resection had the Traverso-Longmire procedure if the indication for pylorus-preserving pancreatoduodenectomy was patients who present with "suspicion of cancer or those with combined stenoses of the intra-pancreatic bile duct, pancreatic duct, and duodenum due to inflammatory pancreatic head enlargement." This obviously attests to a particular pattern of recruitment.

Moreover, the use of a loop anastomosis (Braun anastomosis), rather than a Roux-en-Y set-up, as they do in the other resection techniques, as well as the use of two layers for this anastomosis, which they do not do in any other of the enteroenterostomies described in this chapter, are different than our approach. Our attitude is to avoid construction of omega loops with use of an enteroenterostomy and to perform single-layered enteric anastomosis.

Among the different operations proposed and performed in this series (Whipple, Traverso-Longmire, Beger, and Frey), 40 % of the operations were Traverso-Longmire (pylorus-preserving) pancreatoduodenectomies, while less than 10 % were the duodenum-preserving operations (Beger or Frey operations). Clear advantages in terms of quality of life of the duodenum-preserving operations over the Whipple and pylorus-preserving operations have been shown in prospective randomized studies (Diener et al. 2008). Conversely, the 11.8 % fistula rate, greater than the fistula rate usually reported in chronic pancreatitis, might point to the adjunctive albeit controversial role of somatostatin, which has been shown in some studies in Europe to be effective even in the setting of chronic pancreatitis (Friess et al. 1995).

13.5 Summary

Management of CP should be tailored according to the individual patient's symptoms as assessed by objective tests and by modern radiologic imaging which documents the dominant focus of the disease and extent of disease. Mass-forming and small duct CP warrants an approach of resection, while dilated duct disease and pancreatic pseudocysts need drainage procedures. Radical pancreatic resection – PD – provides good results as far as pain management in CP is concerned. These procedures are especially useful when a malignant neoplasm cannot be excluded in small-duct CP with a head-dominant mass. Before undertaking resection for what is largely a benign disease, each surgeon must assess his/her own abilities and experience, because safe pancreatic resections are a prerequisite, and referral to experienced, high-volume centers is recommended generally.

Major resections are associated with the development of brittle diabetes that can be difficult to control and manage. Furthermore, with over 90 % long-term pain relief and results of randomized, controlled trials favoring organ-preserving procedures, every attempt is made to consider a non-anatomic, head coring procedure (DPPHR or Frey procedure) over a head resection in those patients with head-dominant disease. In our practice, we encounter situations commonly where there is a dilated main pancreatic duct without head-dominant disease; here drainage procedures have not only proved to be safe procedures with low morbidity and almost no mortality but have also given excellent long term pain relief. In recent years, the parenchymal-preserving procedures that have combined the advantages of resection with those of drainage procedures have proven advantageous, especially for management of pain in small-duct CP. We do not have much experience with drainage procedures for small duct disease.

References

Augustine P, Ramesh H (1992) Is tropical pancreatitis premalignant? Am J Gastroenterol 87:1005–1008

Chari ST, Mohan V, Pitchumoni CS, Viswanathan M, Madanagopalan N, Lowenfels AB (1994) Risk of pancreatic carcinoma in tropical calcifying pancreatitis: an epidemiologic study. Pancreas 9:62–66

Diener MK, Rahbari NN, Fischer L, Antes G, Buchler MW, Seiler CM (2008) Duodenum-preserving pancreatic head resection versus pancreatoduodenectomy for surgical treatment of chronic pancreatitis: a systematic review and meta-analysis. Ann Surg 247:950–961

Evans JD, Wilson PG, Carver C, Bramhall SR, Buckels JA, Mayer AD, McMaster P, Neoptolemos JP (1997) Outcome of surgery for chronic pancreatitis. Br J Surg 84:624–629

Friess H, Beger HG, Sulkowki U, Beckers H, Hofbauer B, Dennlerp HJ, Buchler MW (1995) Randomized controlled multicenter study of the prevention of complications by octreodie in patients undergoing surgery for chronic pancreatitis. Br J Surg 82:1270–1273

Nealon WH, Thompson JC (1993) Progressive loss of pancreatic function in chronic pancreatitis is delayed by main pancreatic duct decompression. A longitudinal prospective analysis of the modified puestow procedure. Ann Surg 217:458–468

Schnelldorfer T, Adams DB, Warshaw AL, Lillemoe KD, Sarr MG (2008) Forgotten pioneers of pancreatic surgery: beyond the favorite few. Ann Surg 247:191–202

Shrikhande SV, Friess H, Buechler MW (2000) Pathogenesis of pain in chronic pancreatitis. In: Wig JD (ed) The pancreas. Azad Publishers, Chandigarh

Shrikhande SV, Friess H, diMola F, Tempia A, Conejo Garcia J, Zimmermann A, Buechler MW (2001) NK-1 receptor gene expression is related to pain in chronic pancreatitis. Pain 91:209–217

Shrikhande SV, Friess H, Zimmermann A, Ramesh H, Buechler MW (2002) Comparison of alcoholic, idiopathic and tropical chronic pancreatitis on a molecular basis. In: Buechler MW, Helmut F, Waldemar U, Peter M (eds) Chronic pancreatitis: novel concepts in biology and therapy. Blackwell Publishing, Berlin, pp 66–72

Shrikhande SV, Martignoni ME, Shrikhande M, Friess H, Ramesh H, Buechler MW (2003) Inflammatory cell changes in alcoholic, idiopathic and tropical chronic pancreatitis. Br J Surg 90:1565–1572

Shrikhande SV, Friess H, Nande AG, Adyanthaya K, Shrikhande VN, Buechler MW (2004) Novel technique of pancreatojejunal reconstruction following spontaneous closure of previous lateral pancreatojejunostomy. Int Surg 89:46–50

Commentary

14

Michael G.T. Raraty and John P. Neoptolemos

We would agree with the authors that there are two options in terms of surgery for chronic pancreatitis – *vis.* Resection or drainage procedures, however, most of our patients presenting with symptomatic chronic pancreatitis and requiring operative therapy do so with parenchymal disease rather than predominantly main duct obstruction, and, therefore, resection is the mainstay of our practice in the operative management of chronic pancreatitis. Drainage procedures are confined largely to drainage of pancreatic pseudocysts with a Roux-en-Y pseudocyst-jejunostomy. We prefer this option to pseudocyst-gastrostomy in order to minimise the influx of gastric content into the pseudocyst cavity. In many cases, patients present with enlargement of the pancreatic head simulating neoplasia and, therefore, are treated as we would for any suspicious pancreatic head mass and undergo a pancreatoduodenectomy. As many as 20 % of patients undergoing pancreatoduodenectomy for a pancreatic head mass prove subsequently to have chronic pancreatitis or intraductal papillary mucinous neoplasms on histologic examination of the specimen.

M.G.T. Raraty • J.P. Neoptolemos (✉)
Division of Surgery and Oncology,
University of Liverpool,
Liverpool, UK
e-mail: j.p.neoptolemos@liverpool.ac.uk

14.1 Preoperative Assessment

Patients with established chronic pancreatitis may be considered for operative treatment because of intractable pain or complications associated with the disease. These complications include extrinsic compression of the bile duct, duodenum, or portal/superior mesenteric vein. We prefer to operate before the patient is opiate-dependent, although even patients on high doses of morphine may be weaned off opiates after resection. We require patients with alcohol-related chronic pancreatitis to demonstrate that they have stopped drinking before any operative therapy.

All patients are assessed using a high-quality, multi-phase contrast-enhanced CT as the principal modality of imaging. CT is particularly helpful in assessing involvement of the superior mesenteric, portal, and splenic veins and the development of varices. Cavernous transformation of the portal vein with extensive varices around the head of the pancreas is a relative contra-indication to resection of the pancreatic head. The presence of clinically relevant liver disease/cirrhosis is also a relative contra-indication to operative intervention because these patients have a very poor outcome after major surgery.

R. Mantke et al. (eds.), *International Practices in Pancreatic Surgery*,
DOI 10.1007/978-3-540-74506-8_14, © Springer-Verlag Berlin Heidelberg 2013

14.2 Duodenum-Preserving Pancreatic Head Resection

As long as there is no suspicion of cancer, our preferred operative approach is the duodenum-preserving pancreatic head resection, with or without transection of the pancreatic neck (Beger or Frey procedures). The principal aim of this procedure is to remove any inflammatory mass within the pancreatic head and decompress the bile duct, duodenum, and portal vein, whilst retaining normal enteric and biliary anatomy and preserving as much functioning pancreatic tissue as possible. Initial exposure proceeds as for a standard pancreatoduodenectomy with a Kocher maneuver of the duodenum and separation of the greater omentum from the transverse colon. The lesser sac is thus exposed, although in patients with chronic pancreatitis, this space may be largely obliterated by inflammatory adhesions between the anterior surface of the pancreas and the posterior surface of the stomach and transverse mesocolon. The superior mesenteric vein is identified and the inferior border of the pancreas defined, allowing initial assessment of the degree of involvement of the superior mesenteric vein. The gastro-hepatic omentum is then opened to expose the superior border of the pancreas and the portal vein above the pancreatic neck. The stomach and proximal duodenum are lifted away from the neck of the pancreas in order to allow full access to the pancreatic neck from the inferior compartment. We prefer not to ligate the main trunk of the gastroduodenal artery in order to preserve the blood supply to the superior pancreatoduodenal arterial arcades, although some of its lesser branches will be ligated at a later stage in the procedure. The key decision is to determine whether it is possible to safely divide the neck of the pancreas along the line of the SMV/portal vein and perform a classic Beger-type resection. If the neck cannot be separated from the vein, then we would proceed with the Berne modification of the Frey procedure; *i.e.* non-anatomic resection of the pancreatic head alone without formal division of the neck of the pancreas. If the neck can be separated from the portal vein, then it is divided between stays using diathermy in the same way as for a pancreatoduodenectomy. We do not send samples routinely for frozen section analysis; however, if the surgeon is suspicious of the presence of tumour tissue, then core biopsies from the pancreatic head may be sent for frozen section analysis and a formal pancreatoduodenectomy considered.

After transection of the pancreatic neck, the head and uncinate process of the pancreas are outlined with a series of stay sutures running along the edge of the superior mesenteric/portal vein, around the tip of the uncinate process, along the groove between the pancreatic head and duodenum, and across the superior border of the pancreatic head adjacent to the gastroduodenal artery. These stays are placed using 3-0 PDS and abut each other in a contiguous row around the tissue to be resected. They act both for haemostasis and as an aid in reconstruction; where the residual pancreatic tissue is quite soft, these sutures supply added reinforcement for the later anastomosis. Using the left hand placed behind the head of the pancreas, the pancreatic head tissue is cored out using diathermy to cut just inside the row of stay sutures and extending as far as the posterior margin of the pancreatic head – the aim being to remove the full depth of pancreatic tissue whilst retaining a layer of connective tissue posteriorly and to leave only a thin rim of pancreatic tissue around the edges of the cavity. As much diseased tissue as possible is removed. Haemostasis of small vessels is performed with 4-0 sutures as the dissection continues. During dissection of this cavity, the main bile duct is often exposed posteriorly; this intrapancreatic portion of the bile duct is not opened deliberately into the cavity, but if it is or if there is ongoing obstruction, the edges are marsupialised with 4-0 PDS sutures.

For reconstruction, a Roux-en-Y loop of jejunum is fashioned and passed posterior to the colon. The end of this loop is anastomosed to the previously divided pancreatic neck. This pancreatic anastomosis is performed using either the Cattell-Warren technique, or the Blumgart technique, using four 3-0 PDS mattress sutures through the pancreatic body approximately 1 cm away from the cut margin, and taking the jejunum both anteriorly and posteriorly to buttress the sutures. The pancreatic duct is treated in the same way as for the Cattell-Warren technique, using 4-0 PDS. In both techniques, we utilise a fine-bore paediatric feeding tube as a pancreatic duct stent. This stent is cut to a length of approximately 10 cm and placed across the pancreatic anastomosis to discourage stricture formation.

The jejunal loop is then opened longitudinally along the anti-mesenteric border approximately 3 cm away from the pancreatico-jejunostomy. A hole is made sufficiently large to cover the open cavity where the head of the pancreas has been removed and the jejunum sutured around the edges of this cavity, taking sutures through the residual rim of pancreatic tissue. We have found that a continuous suture technique using a double-ended suture of 3-0 PDS or monocryl is the most convenient way of doing this.

Finally, the gallbladder is removed as a prophylactic measure.

We place two simple, corrugated, "passive" drains adjacent to the anastomosis. We prefer not to use suction drains in proximity to bowel due to the risk of injury to the bowel wall.

14.3 Additional Medication and Procedures

All patients receive antibiotic prophylaxis with cefuroxime and metronidazole and octreotide, 100 µg subcutaneously, 3 times a day for 7 days, commencing on the evening before operation.

All patients are admitted routinely to a postoperative critical care unit for the first night postoperatively, but transferred to the Pancreatic Enhanced Recovery Unit the following day, where they remain until fit for discharge on day 7-10.

A nasogastric tube is left routinely in situ postoperatively but is not used routinely for supplemental feeding, instead we encourage early introduction of fluids – sips of water may be taken as soon as the patient has recovered sufficiently from the anaesthetic – and oral intake is gradually increased over the next few days until the patient is taking solids by day 4. Early mobilization is encouraged.

The drains are gradually shortened, commencing on day 3 as long as the output is not excessive and there is no clinical suspicion of an anastomotic leak.

During 2007–2008, we performed 25 duodenum-preserving pancreatic head resections, but also a further 39 pancreatoduodenectomies for suspicious mass lesions within the head of pancreas which on subsequent histology proved to be due to chronic pancreatitis rather than malignancy (compared with 151 for cancer – thus, 20 % of pancreatic resections were for presumed cancer).

14.4 Chronic Pancreatitis Affecting the Body/Tail of Pancreas

14.4.1 Operative Technique

Our operative approach to the pancreatic body/tail is very similar to that described for resection of pancreatic tumours in this area, although in most cases of chronic pancreatitis, we would aim to preserve the spleen.

Initial exposure of the pancreas proceeds as for a pancreatoduodenectomy with separation of the greater omentum from the transverse colon, although for a left-sided resection, this separation is continued across to the splenic flexure.

The duodenum is Kocherized in the same way as we would for a pancreatic head resection in order to allow control of the superior mesenteric and portal veins if necessary. This manoeuvre is particularly important if the pancreas is to be transected formally across the neck. For more distal lesions, it is sometimes possible to transect the pancreas further to the left, however, adequate access for control of the veins is still essential before dissection of the pancreas commences.

After mobilisation of the pancreatic neck in a manner similar to that employed for a pancreatic head resection (although preserving the gastroduodenal artery and right gastro-epiploic vessels), the splenic artery is ligated and divided and the pancreatic neck divided. This may be performed using a stapling device, or using diathermy as described for the pancreatic head resection. In the latter case, the stump is oversewn with 4-0 PDS, taking care to identify and ligate the pancreatic duct separately. The splenic vein is then ligated and divided behind the body of the pancreas, and the pancreatic body mobilised, continuing the dissection up to the splenic hilum, but preserving the short gastric vessels. The splenic hilum is then transected using a vascular stapling device (ATS-45, Ethicon) and the specimen removed.

Postoperative care is similar to that for pancreatic head resection, although often only a single corrugated drain is required.

During 2007–2008, we performed 14 left-sided pancreatic resections for chronic pancreatitis.

14.5 Drainage Procedures

We favour a Roux-en-Y cyst-jejunostomy rather than a cyst-gastrostomy for drainage of pancreatic pseudocysts, and the technique used is as described. Drainage procedures for the pancreatic duct are employed rarely in our practice, because we rarely see patients with isolated duct dilatation in whom such procedures would be appropriate. In most cases, a dilated duct is due to a stricture within the duct in the pancreatic head or disease within the pancreatic head, and therefore, we favour resection of the strictured/diseased portion of the duct in the head rather than drainage of the duct in the tail. If the duct is dilated with no apparent stricture then other pathologies, such as a main-duct IPMN should be considered, and a formal resection is undertaken because of the malignant potential of such lesions.

Part III

Cystic Neoplasms of the Pancreas: SCN, MCN, IPMN

Basic Chapter

15

Thilo Hackert, Stefan Fritz, and Markus W. Büchler

15.1 Relevant Basic Information, Indications and Contraindications

Cystic lesions of the pancreas are frequent findings with an age-dependent incidence of up to 25 % in elderly people as estimated from autopsy findings and from current techniques of imaging (Kimura et al. 1995; Jani et al. 2011). This spectrum of both benign, neoplastic and malignant or potentially malignant lesions must be differentiated from pancreatic pseudocysts as a residual finding after acute or recurrent chronic pancreatitis. Three important cystic neoplasms have to be recognized and differentiated from one another – serous cystic neoplasms (SCN), mucinous cystic neoplasms (MCN), and intraductal papillary mucinous neoplasms (IPMN). The relevant clinical importance of these cystic lesions of the pancreas is the malignant potential arising from MCN and IPMN, and thus, the need to recognize, differentiate, and manage these neoplasms correctly.

SCN, which represent about 15 % of all cystic lesions, are neoplastic cystic lesions found predominantly in women (80–90 %) 60 years of age and older (Matsumoto et al. 2005). Importantly, however, SCN have no relevant malignant potential, and therefore if asymptomatic, most do not require resection.

In contrast, *MCN* represent a potential precursor of pancreatic cancer and show a malignant transformation via an adenoma-carcinoma sequence in up to 30–50 % of all cases (Reddy et al. 2004; Zamboni et al. 1999; Tanaka et al. 2006). Because they are associated with an as yet not well understood hormonal stimulation (Izumo et al. 2003; Thompson et al. 1999), they are observed nearly exclusively in 50–70 year-old women (99 %). Although not impossible to be found in a male, it would be distinctly unusual, and the diagnosis should be questioned; in the past literature, many "MCN" were misdiagnosed and were really IPMN.

IPMN are probably the most important of the cystic pancreas lesions. Originally described as a pathomorphologic finding in 1936 as "villous tumors of the Wirsung duct" (Haban 1936; Hivet et al. 1975) and in later year as "papillary epithelial hyperplasia" (Klöppel et al. 1980), the terminology of IPMN was introduced in the 1990s (Kloppel 1998). More recently, the differentiation between "side-branch" and "main-duct" IPMN has added further knowledge to the pathopysiologic aspects and the potential of malignancy of IPMN with a definite and important impact on the clinical management. To understand the morphology of IPMN as seen on the various forms of imaging, it needs to be emphasized that the visible changes with cystic

T. Hackert • S. Fritz
Department of Surgery, University of Heidelberg, Heidelberg, Germany

M.W. Büchler, M.D. (✉)
Professor of Surgery, Chair, Department of Surgery, University of Heidelberg, 69120 Heidelberg, Germany
e-mail: markus_buechler@med.uni-heidelberg.de

R. Mantke et al. (eds.), *International Practices in Pancreatic Surgery*,
DOI 10.1007/978-3-540-74506-8_15, © Springer-Verlag Berlin Heidelberg 2013

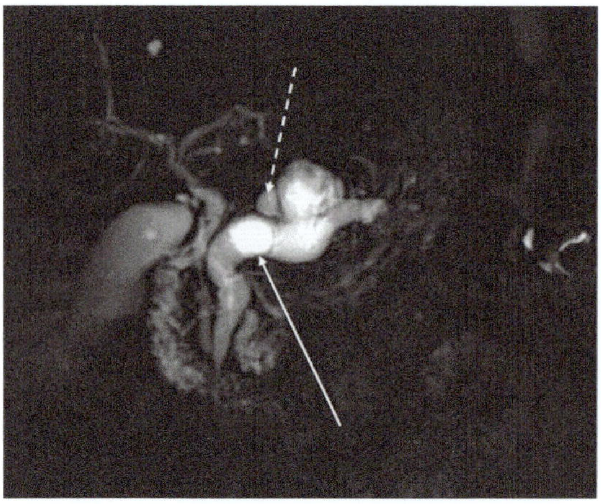

Fig. 15.1 MRCP showing a mixed-type IPMN. Main-duct component (*white arrow*) and branch-duct component (*broken white arrow*)

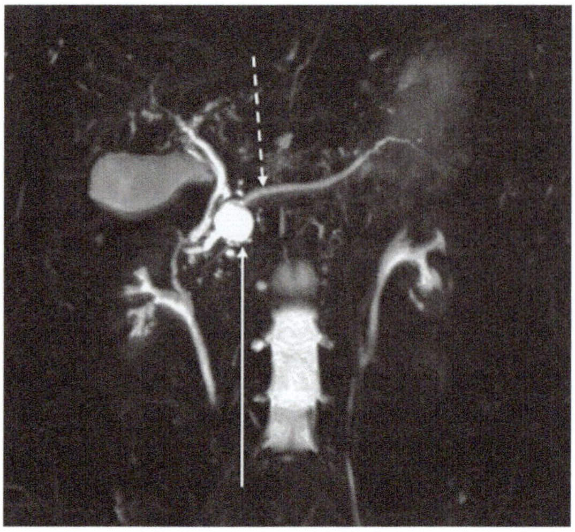

Fig. 15.2 MRCP showing a branch-duct IPMN (*white arrow*), main duct not dilated (*broken white arrow*)

lesions or dilation of the main pancreatic duct are only indirect signs of the epithelial pathology. In IPMN, the abnormal cells produce a very mucinous secretion which is not drained efficiently via the normal pathways due to its high viscosity. Consequently, obstruction of the corresponding ducts leads to a passive dilation, which causes the typical endosonographic or radiologic findings that lead to the diagnosis of IPMN. Malignant transformation of IPMN implies genetic mutations quite common to other pancreatic carcinomas, such as k-ras, p53, p16, and Smad4 (Z'graggen et al. 1997; Iacobuzio-Donahue et al. 2000; Biankin et al. 2004; House et al. 2003; Fritz et al. 2009) and involves an adenoma-borderline-carcinoma sequence. IPMN represent 36 % of all cystic lesions of the pancreas with an increasing frequency of recognition due to improved diagnostics and increased awareness of this disease. About 65 % of all IPMN are located in the pancreatic head and uncinate process, 24 % in the body, and 11 % in the tail of the gland (D'Angelica et al. 2004; Belyaev et al. 2008; Sohn et al. 2004). Main-duct IPMN, characterized by dilation of the pancreatic duct of more than 10 mm (Fig. 15.1), harbors a risk of malignant transformation of about 70 %, which suggests that the diagnosis of main-duct IPMN can be regarded as a general indication for resection (Tanaka et al. 2006). In contrast, branch-duct IPMN (Fig. 15.2) has an overall risk of malignant transformation of about 25 % (Tanaka et al. 2006). There is ongoing discussion about this risk with regard to size, rate of growth, and radiologic features to better discriminate high-risk patients with branch-duct IPMN. Detailed guidelines and recommendations on this topic are given in the "management" section below. In patients with both main-duct and branch-duct IPMN (Fig. 15.1), so called mixed type IPMN, management is identical to the main-duct component as the leading determinant of malignant transformation.

Diagnosis and surveillance of cystic pancreatic lesions is usually made by either endoscopic ultrasonography (EUS), contrast-enhanced computed tomography (CT) or magnetic resonance imaging (MRI). Because EUS requires experience and is highly investigator-dependent, this technique cannot be performed everywhere with reproducible quality (Cone et al. 2011). EUS does, however, offer the opportunity to acquire cyst fluid, cytology, and even biopsies to help to determine the type of cystic lesion when there is any question of the type of cystic lesion. In experienced hands, EUS, although a rather invasive examination for the patient, offers the advantage of a detailed local imaging without any radiation exposure.

Thin slice, contrast-enhanced CT is a suitable imaging modality with the advantage of high-resolution cross sectional imaging, which is especially helpful in evaluating local resectability in cysts suspicious for malignancy (Grenacher 2009). Furthermore, CT is quick, easily read, and is available as a diagnostic tool nearly everywhere. To achieve the best quality and resolution, a pancreas-adapted CT protocol should include the so-called "hydro-technique" with oral water intake (1 l or more) and i.v. infusion of buscopan (10 mg) prior to the examination to achieve a maximum distension of the stomach and duodenum and a negative contrast inside the lumen. The examination is performed in an oblique, 30°, right-sided position (Grenacher 2009).

MRI is a very helpful and accurate diagnostic tool for cystic lesions. MRI has the advantage of imaging not just the cystic changes themselves but equally important, the characteristics of the cyst wall morphology (such as mural nodules and septae within the cyst) and the pancreatic duct, which can be recognized if a synchronous magnetic resonance cholangio-pancreatography (MRCP) is performed as a "non-invasive ductal examination". Moreover, MRI involves no radiation as does CT and is less "invasive" than EUS. Because of the important advantages and lack of radiation, we advocate MRI as the imaging method of choice and should be used especially for younger patients in whom a long-time program of surveillance is planned in the non-operative (or postoperative) management of IPMN (Fatima et al. 2011; Yoon et al. 2009).

In addition to all imaging modalities, the tumor markers CEA and CA 19-9 can be helpful in the clinical evaluation of IPMN. An increased serum CA 19-9 level shows a reasonably good correlation with in situ and invasive IPMN carcinomas (Fritz et al. 2011b).

In addition to the management of the IPMN itself, extrapancreatic neoplasms must be considered and sought in patients with IPMN. According to recent studies, patients with IPMN not only can develop synchronous pancreatic adenocarcinomas (~10 % of all patients) but also extrapancreatic malignancies, such as breast, gastric, colorectal, lung, and prostate cancer, at a greater rate (up to 30 %) than in the general population (Yoon et al. 2008; Reid-Lombardo et al. 2010). These organs-at-risk should be evaluated in the overall surveillance of patients with IPMN. Although evidence-based guidelines are not available currently, several groups recommend colonoscopy, chest X-ray, and careful gynecologic and urologic evaluations during the initial workup of the patient with IPMN and also on a regular basis during future surveillance.

15.2 Operative Management of Cystic Pancreatic Neoplasms

Operative techniques for cystic neoplasms are different for neoplasms with low- and high-risk potential of malignancy. While the latter require formal oncologic resections, including lymphadenectomy, less extensive, local approaches are suitable for selected benign cystic lesions.

15.2.1 SCN

SCN are generally not associated with any significant risk of malignancy; although malignant variants of serous cystic neoplasms have been reported, they are extremely rate. Therefore, most patients with SCN do not require resection unless the SCN causes mechanical complications due to size (usually >4 cm) or shows a growth tendency of more than 2–10 mm/year (Bassi et al. 2003; Tseng et al. 2005). Thus, most of the patients require only surveillance imaging, often at 2–3 year intervals.

15.2.2 MCN

According to the 2006 international consensus guidelines (Tanaka et al. 2006), most MCN should be managed by resection as a potentially malignant neoplasm. This approach implies an oncologic resection, including partial pancreatoduodenectomy or distal pancreatectomy and lymphadenectomy as described in the chapter above for pancreatic cancer. A more recent study

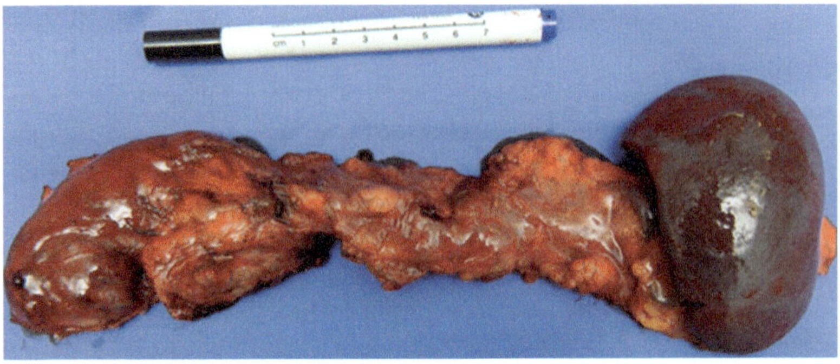

Fig. 15.3 Resection specimen after total pancreatectomy with splenectomy in an extended main-duct IPMN. Final histopathology revealed two synchronous carcinomas (head and tail, T1 and Tis)

published in 2008 (Crippa et al. 2008), however, has re-defined this recommendation, and although resection is still recommended, this report suggested that local approaches (e.g. enucleation, central pancreatectomy, or spleen-preserving distal pancreatectomy) might be appropriate in a small MCN without suspicion of malignancy.

15.2.3 IPMN

Main-duct IPMNs are often extensive lesions that may involve not only just the head, body, or tail of the pancreas, but on occasion (in 15–20 %) may involve much of the entire gland. After the diagnosis is made, operative resection should be entertained in most all patients (Tanaka et al. 2006; Schmitz-Winnenthal et al. 2003). In well-localized main-duct IPMN, an oncologic, partial pancreatoduodenectomy or a formal distal pancreatectomy are suitable procedures; for distal pancreatectomy, a splenectomy is performed as well to ensure adequate clearance of the peripancreatic nodal basin. In all situations, an intraoperative, frozen section should be routine to confirm clear resection margins. It is essential to include the edge of the main pancreatic duct in this examination to achieve an appropriate pathologic evaluation. When IPMN is present at the cut margin, the resection should be extended whenever possible until clear margins are achieved. For extensive main-duct IPMN, a total pancreatectomy (Fig. 15.3) may be necessary (Schmitz-Winnenthal et al. 2003; Müller et al. 2007). This operation can be performed as an en-bloc resection starting with the pancreatic head, similar to partial pancreatoduodenectomy and proceeding to the left without transection of the gland anterior to the portal vein. Obviously, a total pancreatectomy obligates exocrine and endocrine replacement and the not insignificant morbidity of the apancreatic state, and thus not all patients are candidates for this operation because of inability to understand the problem or follow the requisite treatment required.

Management of *branch-duct IPMN* is the subject of ongoing international controversy with regard to the correct timing and extent of operative interventions. Based on the 2006 consensus guidelines (Tanaka et al. 2006), the so-called “Sendai criteria” have been established with the recommendation to resect branch-duct IPMN when they are >3 cm in diameter. IPMN < 3 cm should only be resected when “high-risk” stigmata are present, including mural nodules, positive cytology, symptoms, or a synchronously dilated main duct (>6–8 cm) suggesting the concomitant presence of main duct IPMN, i.e. mixed duct IPMN. Growing evidence, however, suggests that these guidelines are not always sufficient to identify all pre-malignant lesions. In larger series, the incidence of malignant branch-duct IPMN (including both in situ and invasive carcinoma) was approximately 25 % among all IPMN < 3 cm, and there was no reliable cutoff in diameter to differentiate benign from malignant epithelial changes (Jang et al. 2008; Schmidt et al. 2007). The existence of mural nodules as a predictor of malignancy did not always correlate with malignancy (Jang et al. 2008), neither did the existence of clinical symptoms (Lee et al. 2008). Therefore, management of small (<3 cm) and "Sendai-negative" branch-duct IPMN remains a clinical challenge.

From 2004 to 2010, at the University of Heidelberg, a total of 287 patients underwent operative resection for the diagnosis of IPMN (Fritz et al. 2012). Among these, there were 123 branch-duct IPMNs, 91 of which were <3 cm; 69 were "Sendai-negative" IPMNs with a mean diameter of 1.7 cm but a malignant transformation (in situ and invasive carcinoma) was present in 25 %. These findings underline the concept that size alone, as well as currently established image-based markers of potential malignancy (mural nodules, main duct dilation), are not reliable predictors, and even small, branch-duct IPMN (<3 cm) have a relatively high risk of malignant transformation of the lining epithelium. With these considerations in mind, the decision for resection should include all the morphologic and clinical factors (imaging, tumor markers, symptoms, age, progression, and prior patient history), but the decision for each patient is best individualized to offer the best approach at the moment.

15.3 Operative Technique

Our standard operative approach for all suspected, malignant, branch-duct IPMNs is a formal oncologic resection with lymphadenectomy – comparable to other malignant pancreatic neoplasms. Depending on the location of the lesion, either partial pancreatoduodenectomy or distal pancreatectomy (Fig. 15.4) is our accepted procedure. Our approaches are described in detail in the Chap. 1 .

Pancreatic parenchymal-sparing enucleation of a small, branch-duct IPMN offers a limited type of resection with the chance to preserve all normal pancreatic tissue. Enucleations can be performed safely and with oncologically acceptable techniques if the excised lesion is confirmed by intraoperative frozen section to be benign. In case of unexpected malignancy, a more extended resection should be undertaken. One of the most important considerations during enucleation is an accurate localization of the neoplasm or cystic

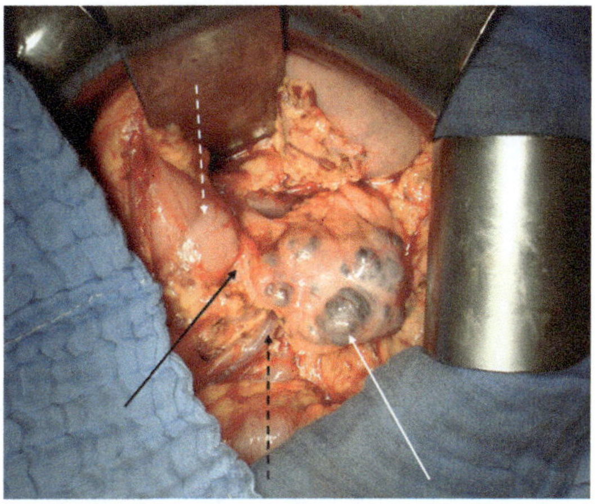

Fig. 15.4 Intraoperative finding of a large SCN in the pancreatic body (*white arrow*). Pancreatic neck (*black arrow*), superior mesenteric vein (*broken black arrow*), stomach with pylorus (*broken white arrow*) before distal pancreatectomy. Indication for resection was epigastric symptoms and growth under surveillance

lesion. Aside from the preoperative imaging, one of the most important aspects of tumor location is the experience of the surgeon performing the exploration (Crippa et al. 2007; Hackert et al. 2011). Mobilization of the pancreas is essential for careful and accurate digital examination of the suspected lesion. Palpation should be supplemented by intraoperative ultrasonography to exclude multifocal lesions. In addition, the relationship to the pancreatic duct can only be clarified intraoperatively by ultrasonography (Lee et al. 2008). We consider a branch duct IPMN of 3 cm as the limit for a safely performed enucleation. In contrast, branch duct IPMNs measuring >3 cm in size have malignant histologic changes significantly more frequently, and thus a local approach is not appropriate; in addition, tissue trauma and the resultant wound surface area after an enucleation of lesions >3 cm reach a critical size that predisposes to development of fistulas or other complications, including bleeding or postoperative pancreatitis (Lee et al. 2008). Enucleation is performed by careful dissection outside the tumor margins using clip ligation or selective suture ligation of vessels supplying the lesion using a thin, atraumatic needle with non-resorbable suture material (e.g. 5-0 polypropylene). Special attention needs to be directed at the connection to the pancreatic duct, because all branch duct IPMNs are in direct communication with the pancreatic ductal system. This communication should be sought specifically and obliterated by clip or suture ligation to avoid development of postoperative fistula. There is no evidence that use of sealants or glue application decreases complications after enucleation. Drain placement remains essential, because currently, fistula rates of 20 % are reported, most of which, however, clinically uncomplicated (Hackert et al. 2011).

Another type of pancreas-sparing local resection for benign IPMN in the body/neck of the pancreas is a segmental or "central" pancreatectomy. The technical aspects of this approach are described in detail in the "chronic pancreatitis" chapter.

15.4 Prognosis

The prognosis of a resected benign IPMN is excellent with 10-year survival rates of >95 % for both main duct and branch duct IPMN (Fernandez-del Castillo and Adsay 2010; Crippa et al. 2010). When IPMN recurs in the pancreatic remnant (about 2–8 %), resection should be entertained as well in appropriately selected patients. The prognosis of resected IPMN-associated carcinomas is generally more favourable than the prognosis of typical ductal pancreatic adenocarcinoma (PDAC). In a study by Wasif et al. (2010), 729 patients with IPMN-carcinomas were compared to 8,082 patients with pancreatic ductal cancer. Overall survival was 34 vs. 18 months, respectively. The most important factor influencing survival was early resection. In tumor stages Tis and T1 of IPMN carcinomas, 5- and 10-year survival rates were 70 and 60 %. Another study including 132 patients with IPMN-carcinoma vs. 1,128 patients with ductal cancer demonstrated that this survival benefit decreased dramatically when the tumor stage exceeded T1 or if lymph node metastases were present, resulting in survival data as poor as for typical ductal cancer (Poultsides et al. 2010). In this situation, even adjuvant therapy failed to improve survival (Turrini et al. 2010), underlining the importance of early resection of IPMN before progression to advanced tumor stages.

IPMN: results from University of Heidelberg, 01/2004-07/2010 (Fritz et al. 2012)

Parameter	Number	%
Patients	287	
Main-duct IPMN	47	16
Mixed-type IPMN	137	48
Branch-duct IPMN	103	36
Partial pancreato-duodenectomy	172	60
Total pancreatectomy	47	16
Distal pancreatectomy	57	20
Enucleation	8	3
Segmental resection	3	1
30-day mortality	3	1
Median hospital stay (IQR)	9 (7–14)	
Morbidity		
Postoperative bleeding	6	2
Pancreatic fistula	11	4
Delayed gastric emptying	37	13
Wound infection	11	4

References

Bassi C, Salvia R, Molinari E, Biasutti C, Falconi M, Pederzoli P (2003) Management of 100 consecutive cases of pancreatic serous cystadenoma: wait for symptoms and see at imaging or vice versa? World J Surg 27(3):319–323. Epub 2003 Feb 27

Belyaev O, Seelig MH, Muller CA, Tannapfel A, Schmidt WE, Uhl W (2008) Intraductal papillary mucinous neoplasms of the pancreas. J Clin Gastroenterol 42(3):284–294. Review

Biankin AV, Kench JG, Biankin SA, Lee CS, Morey AL, Dijkman FP, Coleman MJ, Sutherland RL, Henshall SM (2004) Pancreatic intraepithelial neoplasia in association with intraductal papillary mucinous neoplasms of the pancreas: implications for disease progression and recurrence. Am J Surg Pathol 28(9):1184–1192

Cone MM, Rea JD, Diggs BS, Billingsley KG, Sheppard BC (2011) Endoscopic ultrasound may be unnecessary in the preoperative evaluation of intraductal papillary mucinous neoplasm. HPB (Oxford) 13(2):112–116. doi:10.1111/j.1477-2574.2010.00254.x. Epub 2010 Dec 22

Crippa S, Bassi C, Salvia R et al (2007) Enucleation of pancreatic neoplasms. Br J Surg 94:1254–1259

Crippa S, Salvia R, Warshaw AL, Domínguez I, Bassi C, Falconi M, Thayer SP, Zamboni G, Lauwers GY, Mino-Kenudson M, Capelli P, Pederzoli P, Castillo CF (2008) Mucinous cystic neoplasm of the pancreas is not an aggressive entity: lessons from 163 resected patients. Ann Surg 247(4):571–579

Crippa S, Fernandez-Del Castillo C, Salvia R, Finkelstein D, Bassi C, Dominguez I, Muzikansky A, Thayer SP,

Falconi M, Mino-Kenudson M, Capelli P, Lauwers GY, Partelli S, Pederzoli P, Warshaw AL (2010) Mucin-producing neoplasms of the pancreas: an analysis of distinguishing clinical and epidemiologic characteristics. Clin Gastroenterol Hepatol 8:213–219

D'Angelica M, Brennan MF, Suriawinata AA, Klimstra D, Conlon KC (2004) Intraductal papillary mucinous neoplasms of the pancreas: an analysis of clinicopathologic features and outcome. Ann Surg 239(3):400–408

Fatima Z, Ichikawa T, Motosugi U, Muhi A, Sano K, Sou H, Haradome H, Kiryu S, Araki T (2011) Magnetic resonance diffusion-weighted imaging in the characterization of pancreatic mucinous cystic lesions. Clin Radiol 66(2):108–111. Epub 2010 Nov 18

Fernandez-del Castillo C, Adsay NV (2010) Intraductal papillary mucinous neoplasms of the pancreas. Gastroenterology 139:708–713, 713 e701–702

Fritz S, Fernandez-del Castillo C, Mino-Kenudson M, Crippa S, Deshpande V, Lauwers GY, Warshaw AL, Thayer SP, Iafrate AJ (2009) Global genomic analysis of intraductal papillary mucinous neoplasms of the pancreas reveals significant molecular differences compared to ductal adenocarcinoma. Ann Surg 249(3):440–447

Fritz S, Hackert T, Hinz U, Hartwig W, Büchler MW, Werner J (2011) Role of serum carbohydrate antigen 19–9 and carcinoembryonic antigen in distinguishing between benign and invasive intraductal papillary mucinous neoplasm of the pancreas. Br J Surg 98(1):104–110. doi:10.1002/bjs.7280. Epub 2010 Oct 14

Fritz S, Klauss M, Bergmann F, Hackert T, Hartwig W, Strobel O, Bundi B, Büchler MW, Werner J (2012) Small (Sendai negative) branch-duct IPMNs – not harmless. Ann Surg 256:313–320

Grenacher L, Klauss M (2009) Computed tomography of pancreatic tumors. Radiologe 49(2):107–123. Review

Haban G (1936) Papillomatosis and carcinoma of the ductal system of the pancreas. Virchows Arch A Pathol Anat 297:207–220

Hackert T, Hinz U, Fritz S, Strobel O, Schneider L, Hartwig W, Büchler MW, Werner J (2011) Enucleation in pancreatic surgery: indications, technique, and outcome compared to standard pancreatic resections. Langenbecks Arch Surg 396(8):1197–1203

Hivet M, Maisel A, Horiot A, Conte J (1975) Diffuse villous carcinoma of wirsung's duct. Total pancreatectomy. Med Chir Dig 4:159–623

House MG, Guo M, Iacobuzio-Donahue C, Herman JG (2003) Molecular progression of promoter methylation in intraductal papillary mucinous neoplasms (IPMN) of the pancreas. Carcinogenesis 24(2):193–198

Iacobuzio-Donahue CA, Wilentz RE, Argani P, Yeo CJ, Cameron JL, Kern SE, Hruban RH (2000) Dpc4 protein in mucinous cystic neoplasms of the pancreas: frequent loss of expression in invasive carcinomas suggests a role in genetic progression. Am J Surg Pathol 24(11):1544–1548

Izumo A, Yamaguchi K, Eguchi T, Nishiyama K, Yamamoto H, Yonemasu H, Yao T, Tanaka M, Tsuneyoshi M (2003) Mucinous cystic tumor of the pancreas: immunohistochemical assessment of "ovarian-type stroma". Oncol Rep 10(3):515–525

Jang JY, Kim SW, Lee SE, Yang SH, Lee KU, Lee YJ, Kim SC, Han DJ, Choi DW, Choi SH, Heo JS, Cho BH, Yu HC, Yoon DS, Lee WJ, Lee HE, Kang GH, Lee JM (2008) Treatment guidelines for branch duct type intraductal papillary mucinous neoplasms of the pancreas: when can we operate or observe? Ann Surg Oncol 15(1):199–205. Epub 2007 Oct 2

Jani N, Bani Hani M, Schulick RD, Hruban RH, Cunningham SC (2011) Diagnosis and management of cystic lesions of the pancreas. Diagn Ther Endosc 2011:478913. Epub 2011 Aug 22

Kimura W, Nagai H, Kuroda A, Muto T, Esaki Y (1995) Analysis of small cystic lesions of the pancreas. Int J Pancreatol 18(3):197–206

Kloppel G (1998) Clinicopathologic view of intraductal papillary-mucinous tumor of the pancreas. Hepatogastroenterology 45:1981–1985

Klöppel G, Bommer G, Rückert K, Seifert G (1980) Intraductal proliferation in the pancreas and its relationship to human and experimental carcinogenesis. Virchows Arch A Pathol Anat Histol 387(2):221–233

Lee CJ, Scheiman J, Anderson MA, Lee CJ, Scheiman J, Anderson MA et al (2008) Risk of malignancy in resected cystic tumors of the pancreas <or =3 cm in size: Is it safe to observe asymptomatic patients? A multi-institutional report. J Gastrointest Surg 12:234–242

Matsumoto T, Hirano S, Yada K, Shibata K, Sasaki A, Kamimura T, Ohta M, Kitano S, Kashima K (2005) Malignant serous cystic neoplasm of the pancreas: report of a case and review of the literature. J Clin Gastroenterol 39(3):253–256. Review

Müller MW, Friess H, Kleeff J, Dahmen R, Wagner M, Hinz U, Breisch-Girbig D, Ceyhan GO, Büchler MW (2007) Is there still a role for total pancreatectomy? Ann Surg 246(6):966–974; discussion 974–975

Poultsides GA, Reddy S, Cameron JL et al (2010) Histopathologic basis for the favorable survival after resection of intraductal papillary mucinous neoplasm associated invasive adenocarcinoma of the pancreas. Ann Surg 251:470–476

Reddy RP, Smyrk TC, Zapiach M, Levy MJ, Pearson RK, Clain JE, Farnell MB, Sarr MG, Chari ST (2004) Pancreatic mucinous cystic neoplasm defined by ovarian stroma: demographics, clinical features, and prevalence of cancer. Clin Gastroenterol Hepatol 2(11):1026–1031

Reid-Lombardo KM, Mathis KL, Wood CM et al (2010) Frequency of extrapancreatic neoplasms in intraductal papillary mucinous neoplasm of the pancreas: implications for management. Ann Surg 251(1):64–69

Schmidt CM, White PB, Waters JA, Yiannoutsos CT, Cummings OW, Baker M, Howard TJ, Zyromski NJ, Nakeeb A, DeWitt JM, Akisik FM, Sherman S, Pitt HA, Lillemoe KD (2007) Intraductal papillary mucinous neoplasms: predictors of malignant and invasive pathology. Ann Surg 246(4):644–651; discussion 651–654

Schmitz-Winnenthal FH, Z'graggen K, Volk C, Schmied BM, Büchler MW (2003) Intraductal papillary mucinous tumors of the pancreas. Curr Gastroenterol Rep 5:133–140

Sohn TA, Yeo CJ, Cameron JL, Hruban RH, Fukushima N, Campbell KA, Lillemoe KD (2004) Intraductal papillary mucinous neoplasms of the pancreas: an updated experience. Ann Surg 239(6):788–797; discussion 797–799

Tanaka M, Chari S, Adsay V, Fernandez-del Castillo C, Falconi M, Shimizu M, Yamaguchi K, Yamao K, Matsuno S, International Association of Pancreatology (2006) International consensus guidelines for management of intraductal papillary mucinous neoplasms and mucinous cystic neoplasms of the pancreas. Pancreatology 6(1–2):17–32. Review

Thompson LD, Becker RC, Przygodzki RM, Adair CF, Heffess CS (1999) Mucinous cystic neoplasm (mucinous cystadenocarcinoma of low-grade malignant potential) of the pancreas: a clinicopathologic study of 130 cases. Am J Surg Pathol 23(1):1–16

Tseng J, Tseng JF, Warshaw AL, Sahani DV, Lauwers GY, Rattner DW, Fernandez-del Castillo C (2005) Serous cystadenoma of the pancreas: tumor growth rates and recommendations for treatment. Ann Surg 242(3):413–419; discussion 419–421

Turrini O, Waters JA, Schnelldorfer T et al (2010) Invasive intraductal papillary mucinous neoplasm: predictors of survival and role of adjuvant therapy. HPB (Oxford) 12:447–455

Wasif N, Bentrem DJ, Farrell JJ et al (2010) Invasive intraductal papillary mucinous neoplasm versus sporadic pancreatic adenocarcinoma: a stage-matched comparison of outcomes. Cancer 116:3369–3377

Yoon WJ, Ryu JK, Lee JK et al (2008) Extrapancreatic malignancies in patients with intraductal papillary mucinous neoplasm of the pancreas: prevalence, associated factors, and comparison with patients with other pancreatic cystic neoplasms. Ann Surg Oncol 15:3193–3198

Yoon LS, Catalano OA, Fritz S, Ferrone CR, Hahn PF, Sahani DV (2009) Another dimension in magnetic resonance cholangiopancreatography: comparison of 2- and 3-dimensional magnetic resonance cholangiopancreatography for the evaluation of intraductal papillary mucinous neoplasm of the pancreas. J Comput Assist Tomogr 33(3):363–368

Z'graggen K, Rivera JA, Compton CC, Pins M, Werner J, Fernández del Castillo C, Rattner DW, Lewandrowski KB, Rustgi AK, Warshaw AL (1997) Prevalence of activating K-ras mutations in the evolutionary stages of neoplasia in intraductal papillary mucinous tumors of the pancreas. Ann Surg 226(4):491–498; discussion 498–500

Zamboni G, Scarpa A, Bogina G, Iacono C, Bassi C, Talamini G, Sessa F, Capella C, Solcia E, Rickaert F, Mariuzzi GM, Klöppel G (1999) Mucinous cystic tumors of the pancreas: clinicopathological features, prognosis, and relationship to other mucinous cystic tumors. Am J Surg Pathol 23(4):410–422

Commentary

16

Katherine A. Morgan and David B. Adams

16.1 Relevant Basic Information, Indications and Contradictions

Cystic neoplasms of the pancreas that are selected for operative resection are the tip of the iceberg of the near-epidemic proportion of incidental pancreatic "cysts" identified on modern imaging studies. CT and MRI are utilized with ever-increasing frequency for evaluation of all gastrointestinal symptoms, and the result is the identification of both symptomatic and asymptomatic pancreatic cysts. The stimulus to increasing pancreatic resection in the management of pancreatic cystic lesions is the hope that early recognition and resection of pre-malignant or early cancers will lead to decreased incidence of and mortality from pancreatic cancer. When cystic neoplasms are associated with symptoms, the indications for resection are clearer, though symptoms of pain, jaundice, and weight loss are present only infrequently with pre-malignant cystic disease. The incidental pancreatic cystic neoplasm is analogous to the benign adenomatous colonic polyp. Colonoscopic polypectomy decreases the rate of colon cancer mortality. Will resection of benign IPMN and MCN diminish the mortality rates of pancreatic cancer? The risk-benefit ratio of resecting pre-malignant pancreatic cystic lesions, most commonly IPMN, is complicated by the inherent and notable risks of pancreatic resection procedures. Thus, the decision to resect pancreatic cystic lesions underscores the four fundamental mistakes a surgeon can make: Operate too soon, operate too late, do too much, and do too little.

Although much is known, much remains to be known in the natural history of pancreatic cystic neoplasms. Prior to resection, the malignant potential of each individual lesion is unknown and uncertain. Many pancreatic cystic lesions have a low risk of malignant transformation, and the hazards of operative management must be weighed carefully, particularly in the elderly population and those with medical comorbidities. The most important decisions in managing these patients with presumed pancreatic cystic neoplasms are resection versus observation, extent of resection, and method and interval of surveillance.

Differentiating a pancreatic pseudocyst from a cystic neoplasm is relevant to the general discussion of cystic tumors of the pancreas. There are many cystic lesions of the pancreas. Rare cystic disorders include parasitic cysts and congenital cysts. Extrapancreatic cysts, including duplication, splenic, adrenal, and mesenteric cysts, may be difficult to identify as cysts of extrapancreatic origin on imaging studies. Cystic ductal adenocarcinoma, and the uncommon acinar cell cystadenocarcinoma, cystic choriocarcinoma, cystic teratoma, angiomatous cystic neoplasm, and

K.A. Morgan • D. B. Adams, M.D. (✉)
Division of Gastrointestinal and Laparoscopic Surgery, Department of Surgery,
Medical University of South Carolina,
25 Courtenay Drive, Suite 7100A – MSC 290,
Charleston, SC 29425, USA
e-mail: adamsdav@musc.edu

R. Mantke et al. (eds.), *International Practices in Pancreatic Surgery*,
DOI 10.1007/978-3-540-74506-8_16, © Springer-Verlag Berlin Heidelberg 2013

cystic lymphangioma can be difficult to identify pre-operatively based on imaging studies, FNA cytology, and serology. Solid pseudopapillary neoplasm and cystic endocrine neoplasms are not uncommon and are difficult frequently to differentiate preoperatively because of scant cellularity on FNA.

The first step in the assessment of a newly discovered pancreatic cystic lesion is to distinguish neoplasm from pancreatitis. Often the history will provide the greatest insight, because most bouts of pancreatitis that result in a pseudocyst are well-recounted. The distinction can be unclear, however, in some patients. For example, a patient with a history of episodic epigastric abdominal pain may have undiagnosed pancreatitis, or a patient without known risk factors may have a pancreatic neoplasm as the cause of pancreatitis. The clinical history is very helpful, because cystic neoplasms affect distinctive demographic groups. Though radiographic imaging can be distinctive and diagnostic, cystic neoplasms may be indistinguishable from a pseudocyst based on MRCP, CT, and EUS imaging. No imaging study has 100 % sensitivity and specificity. Even ERCP may be misleading inasmuch as ductal communication with a cyst is possible with pseudocysts, IPMN, and allegedly MCN. MRCP with secretin stimulation has become an integral modality in cyst evaluation. MRCP can demonstrate more specific morphology than CT and can help determine the relationship of the lesion to the main pancreatic duct. Though invasive and operator-dependent, EUS has great sensitivity in delineating septation and mural nodules and is both a blessing and a curse in cyst fluid analysis.

Analysis of cyst fluid is one of the most controversial but evolving area of our understanding of cystic neoplasms of the pancreas. On aspiration, an increased fluid viscosity can be suggestive of a mucinous versus a serous cyst. High cyst fluid amylase activity is suggestive of a connection of the lesion to the pancreatic duct. Various cell surface markers have been evaluated for their diagnostic ability. Currently, cyst fluid CEA seems to have the greatest clinical correlation in determining a mucinous from a SCN. Cyst fluid DNA analysis using commercially available kits has shown that mucinous lesions have a high correlation with increased K-ras, LOH mutations, and increased DNA amount. Thus far, however, there is a disappointing lack of correlation with CEA levels and pathologic results. Cytology has excellent specificity (94 %) but poor sensitivity (33 %) given the paucity of cells within the fluid. Mucin stains can be falsely positive and thus unreliable or non-available in many laboratories. Histology from fine needle biopsy is highly insensitive due to sampling error. At best, cyst fluid analysis can be useful currently only in distinguishing a mucinous cystic lesion with some corresponding risk for malignant transformation from a nonmucinous lesion with negligible malignant risk. It is not reliable in disproving the presence of invasive disease. Despite the imperfect nature of the present state of cyst fluid analysis, the future of our understanding and management of cystic neoplasms of the pancreas likely lies in the maturation of this field. Guidelines and recommendations continue to evolve. Because no cytologic or serologic analysis is diagnostic, the prudent surgeon carefully weighs the risk of falsely negative studies and considers the malignant and pre-malignant potential of pancreatic cysts.

16.2 Operative Management of Cystic Pancreatic Neoplasms

Once some combination of clinical history, imaging, and cyst fluid analysis has been undertaken, a reasonable differential diagnosis can determine the treatment plan: wait or operate. Findings on CT, MRCP, and EUS of duct communication, cyst septations, and mural nodules are evaluated in the decision-making tree. Pancreatic enzymes, viscosity, cytology and tumor markers in cyst fluid aspiration and analysis are also part of the general formula. The data from radiologic studies and cyst fluid analysis are added to patient history and physical examination to formulate the surgical gestalt that leads to operative management.

16.3 SCN

The typical patient with an SCN is an older woman with an asymptomatic lesion in the head or uncinate process of the pancreas. Cystic fluid obtained by FNA has a low CEA and is mucin negative. The male to female ratio is 2:1, and the typical CT findings of central starburst calcification or a honeycomb pattern may appear as an incidental CT finding. The mucin-filled, multiseptated MCN or branch chain IPMN may occasionally be confused with an SCN. SCNs are associated with mutations in Von Hipel-Lindau tumor suppressor gene (chromosome 3p25). SCNs lack mutations in K-ras, p53, or DPC4. Resection is undertaken if the tumor mass is symptomatic, grows substantially during observation, or most importantly if the diagnosis is uncertain. Although SCNs may grow to substantial size with displacement of structures adjacent to the pancreas, they are neither invasive nor prone to peri-tumoral inflammation. Thus, even large SCNs can be resected safely with standard techniques of pancreatic resection. Application of more extensive oncologic resection is applied if the diagnosis of SCN is uncertain at the time of resection. Because SCNs are so uncommonly malignant, the risk: benefit ratio of operative management is high and demands outcomes with near-zero mortality.

16.4 MCN

The typical patient with an MCN is a middle-aged woman with minimal symptoms. Upper abdominal pain or discomfort may be present, or commonly, the cyst is an incidental finding on CT. Mucin-producing columnar cells line the cyst. This dense neoplastic tissue, with underlying ovarian stroma, may involve only a small portion of the cyst wall and be invisible to the naked eye, seen only on microscopic examination of the cyst wall. This characteristic neoplastic lining is easy to miss on biopsy of the cyst wall when doing a cyst internal drainage procedure. Thick, mucinous fluid fills the MCN cavity, and though communication with the pancreatic duct is rare, the MCN may develop a pancreatic ductal communication and have amylase-rich fluid when aspiration is possible. Commonly, the aspirate is so mucin-rich that cellular aspirate is scant, and there is little assayable fluid for CEA or CA19-9 analysis. Patients with MCN who have been diagnosed erroneously with pseudocyst disease and have undergone cyst-jejunostomy or endoscopic cyst-gastrostomy, have persistent symptoms and a persistent "pseudocyst" which brings them to appropriate surgical attention. This diagnostic error can be avoided by following the dictim that women in the fourth and fifth decade of life with cysts in the pancreatic tail or body without a prior history of pancreatitis or pancreatopathy should undergo distal pancreatectomy. Because neither imaging studies nor cytologic analysis are diagnostic, patients who are fit can go directly to operation without further work-up. The uncommon MCN in the head of the pancreas is managed with standard pancreatoduodenectomy. Mid body lesions may be managed with mid segment "central pancreatectomy," weighing the relative risks of post-operative pancreatic fistula with long-term diabetes risk due to resection of the islet-rich pancreatic tail. MCNs in the tail lend themselves well to laparoscopic resection. In all cases the extent of resection is guided by the malignant potential and appearance of the neoplasm. Enucleation of the small, non-invasive MCN may prove to be a safe and effective strategy with a compelling rationale similar to the strategy proposed by some groups for local excision of the small branch-duct IPMN.

16.5 IPMN

The history of primary cystic neoplasms of the pancreas is one of the great surgical stories of this current generation, and nowhere is the story more dynamic than in the sector of IPMN. This pancreatic epithelial cell neoplasm which produces mucus and forms papillary projections within the pancreatic duct is not a new disease, but one that became prevalent due to clinical awareness, better and more radiologic imaging, improved pathologic identification, and careful scrutiny of cases of presumed chronic pancreatitis. Much information on the natural history of the disease as well as its diagnosis and treatment has led to the development of management guidelines and consensus statements. In evaluating the evidence and recommendations, it is important to remember the generic truth that dogmatic certainty is directly proportional to factual ignorance. Although much as been learned about IPMN, much remains to be learned, and the level of our understanding of this disease has not advanced that much since Kawarada and colleagues reported four cases of IPMN and classified the disease into four types (Kawarada et al. 1992).

Main-duct IPMN is most problematic because of the indication for total pancreatectomy when the disease involves the entire gland. In particular, the elderly, asthenic patient who undergoes total pancreatectomy will have substantial diminishment in quality-of-life related to the inevitable exocrine and endocrine insufficiency. Malabsorption and malnutrition are frequent despite oral enzyme replacement. Pancreatogenic diabetes is brittle and dangerous in a new-onset diabetic facing wide swings from hyperglycemia to symptomless hypoglycemia. Nevertheless, in selected compliant patients with a diffuse field defect of tumor induction in the main pancreatic duct, total pancreatectomy is indicated. Postoperative pancreatogenic diabetes frequently requires management with an insulin pump, and effective timing and dosing of oral pancreatic enzyme supplementation is a continuous challenge. An essential component of the specialty team caring for the patient with IPMN is a pathologist with formal interest and expertise in pancreatic disorders. Pathology, like surgery, is as much an art as a science; frozen section evaluation of the ductal margin requires the eyes of an experienced pathologist. The operating surgeon should be in the frozen section room to look into the microscope with the pathologist to confirm what the pathologist reports and to weigh the thoughts behind the words of the written report. Low grade PanIn-1 changes at the resection margin are not an indication for total pancreatectomy. When undertaking exploration for presumed main duct IPMN with dilation of the entire dominant ductal system, it is not necessary to undertake obligatory total pancreatectomy, as the diffuse ductal dilation may be related to chronic obstruction of the duct in the head of the pancreas due to the mucin obstruction of a localized neoplasm in the main duct or a side-branch papillary neoplasm. Frozen section evaluation of the resection margin in the body or neck of the gland may justify preservation of the caudal parenchyma. In any case, local or remote recurrent or "de novo" IPMN necessitates life-long surveillance after operative resection.

Management of branch-duct IPMN based on the "Sendai criteria" has trended to become more the exception than the rule. Environmental and genetic factors are at work always in progression from benign to malignant neoplasia, and guidelines applicable in Asia may not fit the disease observed in Europe or the Americas. The point is that nature and disorders of nature do not operate in discrete variables, and a continuum of transformation exists from benign to malignant disease. There are no reliable predictors of malignancy, and the decision for operation continues to depend on assessment and interpretation of all patient historic, radiologic imaging, laboratory data. Enucleation of small, branch-duct IPMNs is sound and safe in experienced hands. Frozen-section microscopic examinations require an experienced pancreatic pathologist. Laparoscopic resection can be undertaken with excellent exposure and magnification of smaller cysts in many instances. In both open and laparoscopic cases, identification of the relationship of the cystic lesion to the dominant pancreatic duct is critical. Occlusion of the branching duct with small metallic clips may grant more certainty of duct occlusion than suture ligation. When violation of the dominant pancreatic duct occurs, it is possible to repair the duct over an internal transpapillary stent, though pancreatic resection may be a more prudent course if dominant duct continuity cannot be secured. Post-operative infusion of octreotide after resection has intuitive merit, though direct clinical evidence of efficacy is lacking.

16.6 Conclusion

The imperative for health care in the United States is improving the quality of health care delivery and cutting costs. The Centers for Medicare and Medicaid Services have made major efforts to provide better individual care, better health for populations, and lower costs. Patient-centered care has focused on respect for individual patient preferences, needs, and values. Nowhere are these principles more applicable than in the management of patients with pancreatic cystic neoplasms. Traditional, condition-specific indicators of short-term outcome such as post-operative morbidity and long-term outcome, disease-free survival, and overall mortality, may not work for the elderly patient with medical comorbidities whose quality of care depends on more than disease-specific outcomes (Reuben and Tinetti 2012). Patient outcome goals may be different from traditional surgical outcomes. The patient with the 2-cm branch duct IPMN whose father died of pancreatic cancer may prefer excision to the daily worry of watchful waiting. The octogenarian with a 4 cm cyst in the head of the pancreas with a mural nodule may prefer to make plans to attend her granddaughters wedding than to face the uncertain outcomes of a major pancreatectomy. The pancreatic surgeon with a scientific understanding of pancreatic cystic neoplasms is the one best-suited to keep the patient's interest foremost and to ensure that patient values guide clinical decisions. The management of every pancreatic cystic neoplasm involves a doctor and patient relationship that should search for a decision that is best for each individual patient at that moment in time.

References

Kawarada Y, Yano T, Yamamoto T, Yokoi H, Imai T, Ogura Y, Mizumoto R (1992) Intraductal mucin-producing tumors of the pancreas. Am J Gastroenterol 87(5):634–638

Reuben DB, Tinetti ME (2012) Goal-Oriented patient care – an alternative health outcomes paradigm. N Engl J Med 366:777–779

Commentary

17

Roberto Salvia, Marco Dal Molin, and Claudio Bassi

Although considered uncommon historically, cystic neoplasms of the pancreas have been diagnosed with increasing frequency over the last two decades, due mainly to the widespread use (and availability) of advanced cross-sectional imaging techniques.

This "epidemic" in the diagnosis of pancreatic cystic neoplasms has been paralleled by an increasing number of studies focusing on the clinical behavior and management of these diseases. As a result, our knowledge of pancreatic cystic neoplasms has improved dramatically. Three main histologic types have been identified (SCNs, MCNs, IPMNs), and detailed pathologic as well as molecular and clinical data have been investigated for each one of these cystic neoplasms.

Current guidelines for the management of pancreatic cystic neoplasms are based on relatively distinctive features shown at cross-sectional imaging. One must be aware that a certain degree of morphologic overlap exists between different lesions, and the possibility of preoperative misdiagnosis should always be considered.

The most appropriate management of pancreatic cystic neoplasms still remains unclear and, for mucinous neoplasms in particular, the clinical and radiologic work-up is not always able to predict the likelihood of progression to invasive cancer in a given patient. This uncertainty has generated controversies on whether to offer resection or enroll patients in surveillance protocols with periodic check-ups. Several other unsettled aspects exist, including the appropriate timeframe for surveillance, the role of analysis and cytology of cystic fluid, the role of atypical, non-anatomic resections and of lymphadenectomy, the recurrence rate and association with ductal adenocarcinoma and other non-pancreatic neoplasms, in case of IPMNs.

Such dilemmas are encountered frequently in the everyday practice of physicians working in tertiary centers dealing with pancreatic surgery, in which pancreatic cystic neoplasms represent now a substantial group of diseases referred for treatment. Several questions often remain unanswered when dealing with a patient affected by a cystic lesion in the pancreas: is the lesion completely benign? Does it have malignant potential? And if so, how long does it take to become malignant? What is the best management, surveillance, or surgical resection? And if operative resection is advocated, what type of resection is most appropriate?

To address these questions, familiarity with the morphologic spectrum of these lesions, and

R. Salvia, M.D., Ph.D. • M.D. Molin, M.D.
Department of Surgery,
University of Verona, Verona, Italy

C. Bassi, M.D., FRCS, FACS (✉)
Department of Surgery, University of Verona,
Verona, Italy

General Surgery B – Pancreas Institute, 'G.B. Rossi'
Hospital, University of Verona Hospital Trust,
P.le L.A. Scuro 10, 37134 Verona, Italy
e-mail: claudio.bassi@univr.it

R. Mantke et al. (eds.), *International Practices in Pancreatic Surgery*,
DOI 10.1007/978-3-540-74506-8_17,

collaboration among surgeons, radiologists, gastroenterologists and pathologists is mandatory.

At our Institution, more than 6,000 patients with pancreatic diseases were managed between 1985 and 2011, 20 % of whom were affected by cystic lesions. In the same period, more than 2,200 pancreatic resections were carried out, 23 % of which were for cystic neoplasms.

SCAs occur more frequently in middle-aged women than men. Any portion of the pancreatic gland can be affected, but SCAs are detected more frequently in the pancreatic head. SCAs are usually asymptomatic and discovered incidentally on cross-sectional imaging performed for unrelated complaints. When present, the most common symptom is abdominal discomfort or low-grade pain. A correct clinical and radiologic diagnosis is of paramount importance, because these neoplasms, unlike other cystic neoplasms of the pancreas, are virtually always benign. Whenever possible, a conservative approach represents the treatment of choice.

On CT, these previously-called microcystic tumors appear as a non-enhancing mass deforming the profile of the gland. The density is homogeneous or slightly superior to that of water and isodense in respect to the parenchyma. When calcifications are present, the location is quite always central, punctate or globular, as opposed to the lamellar calcifications seen in mucinous cystic tumors. Usually a central fibrous scar is visible in the larger masses because the scar forms later on in the disease and may appear as the classic starburst radial calcification. Maximal visualization of septa occurs in the pancreatic parenchymal phase as well as the honeycomb appearance. The presence of central calcification in correspondence with scars or septa definitively characterizes a cystic mass as a SCA.

Magnetic Resonance Imaging (MRI), coupled with the MRCP technique, provides a precise evaluation of spatial relationship between the mass and the biliary or pancreatic duct, thereby discriminating SCAs from intraductal papillary mucinous neoplasms (IPMNs), especially when the lesion is located on the head or in the uncinate process of the gland.

A recent study from our institution (Malleo et al. 2012) of 145 patients with SCA enrolled in a surveillance protocol with serial MRI + MRCP showed that the overall mean growth rate was only 0.28 cm/year. There were two distinct phases of growth during follow-up, with the first 7 years growth at 0.1 cm/year, and after 7 years at 0.6 cm/year. The rare oligocystic/macrocystic variant, a history of other non-pancreatic malignancies, and patients' age were demonstrated to impact on tumor growth. Tumor size at the time of diagnosis was not a predictor of growth and should not be used for decisional purposes. A surveillance protocol with MR + MRCP was proposed for all well-characterized and asymptomatic SCN, but patients with factors that impact on tumor growth should be informed about an increased likelihood of a pancreatic resection in the long-term. A follow-up time frame of 2 years seems to be appropriate. In conclusion, we no longer consider a 4-cm diameter to be a sufficient criteria to pursue resection as suggested by others (Tseng et al. 2005).

Mucinous Cystic Neoplasms (MCNs) are cystic epithelial neoplasms occurring almost exclusively in women and are located preferentially in the body and tail of the pancreas. MCNs are formed by epithelial cells producing mucin, all of which are supported by ovarian-type stroma (a required finding for the diagnosis of MCN), showing no communication with the pancreatic ductal system. According to the grade of epithelial dysplasia they may be classified into mucinous cystic neoplasm with low-grade dysplasia, moderate dysplasia, or high-grade dysplasia (carcinoma in situ).

When our series was combined with the Massachusetts General Hospital experience (Crippa et al. 2008), the incidence of malignancy for MCN was 17.5 %. Early diagnosis of malignant transformation of mucinous cystic neoplasm is essential, because the prognosis, once the invasive malignant form occurs, is the same as ductal adenocarcinoma, while in the forms of non-invasive, carcinoma in situ, resection is cureative.

A thickened wall, presence of papillary proliferations arising from the wall or septa, evidence of peripheral "egg shell" calcifications as well as invasion of surrounding vascular structures are considered the best signs of malignancy at imaging. The diagnosis will be more evident if extracapsular extension of the lesion is detected on contrast-enhanced CT. When thick walls, thick septa and calcifications are present simultaneously, the probability of malignancy is 95 %. When fewer than three signs are present, the probability of malignancy decreases to almost zero when there are no calcifications or septae, and the wall is thin. Because calcifications cannot be detected by MRI, CT is the primary imaging modality for these patients.

All MCNs should be resected, both cystadenomas and cystadenocarcinomas, when possible. Current thinking is that all MCNs may progress to malignancy, and the life-expectancy of most of these patients, middle-aged women, will allow the development of mucinous cystadenocarcinoma; unfortunately, once established, cystadenocarcinoma has a very low rate of resectability and a very poor prognosis. Predictors of malignancy are large size (≥4 cm), the presence of nodules, septae and eggshell calcification. In these cases, a "standard," anatomic, oncologic pancreatic resection should be performed, avoiding middle pancreatectomies and spleen preservation during the left pancreatectomies. Interestingly, lymph node metastases were never found in our series, even in MCN with associated cancer (Crippa et al. 2008). Based on this finding, more limited resections could be considered, and a laparoscopic approach can be ideal in such cases.

Intraductal Papillary Mucinous Neoplasms (IPMNs) represent the most frequent cystic neoplasm of the pancreas, even in asymptomatic patients, in which they represent an incidental finding. In our experience, IPMNs are one of the most common indications for pancreatic resection, up to 25 % of all resections.

IPMNs may affect the main pancreatic duct (MD-IPMN), branch ducts (BD-IPMN) or both ("mixed duct" IPMN). The great majority of IPMNs are detected and then characterized with cross-sectional imaging study, such as CT and MRCP. The radiologic and endoscopic features of IPMNs vary with their morphologic type. The typical feature of MD-IPMNs is dilation of the main pancreatic duct >1 cm, eventually extending into the secondary branches that may appear as cysts. The dilation can affect the duct only in the distal pancreas or, if it is located in the head or in the uncinate process, can be present throughout because of obstructive effect. BD-IPMNs appear as cysts or a cluster of cysts without dilation of the main duct and are located more commonly in the head-uncinate region. It is estimated that 40–60 % of BD-IPMNs can be multifocal. Calcifications occur in 10 % of patients, and nodules and papillary projections, which are associated with the presence of a malignant neoplasms, usually appear as filling defects within the cystic lesions. The pancreatic gland may appear as enlarged with signs of pancreatitis or atrophic. CT and MRCP can localize the tumor and assess its relationship with vessels and other organs. MRCP is particularly useful in the characterization of single or multifocal BD- IPMNs, given its ability to demonstrate a communication between the main duct and the cyst.

At our Institution the initial assessment of patients with suspected IPMN usually involves contrast-enhanced ultrasonography (CEUS), which is able to identify and characterize the "cysts" in great detail.

In those patients in whom the diagnosis is uncertain, endoscopic ultrasonography (EUS) may be helpful. EUS can identify the dilated main pancreatic duct and provide morphologic detail of any solid component, nodules, or small projections, in the main duct and/or in the cyst communicating with it. Moreover, EUS represents a safer approach for sampling of fluid and targeted biopsies by fine needle aspiration or core biopsy.

Examination of fluid sampled from IPMNs provides information to help in diagnosis by analyzing viscosity, the presence of mucin or mucinous cells, and an increased value of Carcinoembryonic antigen (CEA).

The best management of IPMN is still debated. During a consensus conference held in Sendai (Tanaka et al. 2006), a group of surgeons, gastroenterologists, and pathologists produced the first guidelines in the management of IPMNs. A secondary, updated set of guidelines is being developed currently. Before 2006, all patients with a diagnosis of IPMN were considered potentially at risk for developing malignancy, and therefore resection was always proposed. After the Sendai meeting two different approaches have been defined when considering MD-IPMN (together with the mixed form) or BD-IPMN.

17.1 Main Duct-IPMN

Patients affected by IPMN involving the main duct or the mixed form, when medically fit, should always be candidates for resection because of the high prevalence of in situ and invasive carcinoma found in the resected specimens (40 % invasive, 30 % only in situ).

The operative management of MD- IPMNs represents a challenge for the surgeon. While in other pancreatic neoplasms the preoperative imaging can locate the tumor accurately and plan a pancreatic resection accordingly, this is not always the case in MD- IPMNs. The segmental dilation of the main pancreatic duct in the preoperative studies may occur both proximal and distal to the tumor, because of mucin overproduction, making the localization of the neoplasia more difficult.

A typical resection (pancreatoduodenectomy, left pancreatectomy, total pancreatectomy, according to the site and extension of the disease) with lymph node dissection must be performed. Limited resections, such as middle pancreatectomy, have been proposed for MD-IPMN, but we had too great a rate of positive resection margins and recurrences when central pancreatectomy was performed for what appeared to be MD-IPMN localized the proximal body of the gland, and similar results have been reported by other authors. For these reasons, we believe that standard resections should be performed in this setting. Because IPMN extends along the pancreatic duct and it can do so without a macroscopically-evident lesion, it is important to exclude residual tumor with frozen section.

Three different aspects of ductal mucosa can be detected by analyzing the operative margin: (1) normal ductal epithelium in the main duct means that radical resection is achieved; (2) de-epithelialized with denuded epithelium that should not be considered as a negative margin, because the abnormal epithelium may have sloughed off and local recurrence can occur; (3) adenoma, borderline, or carcinoma that requires an extension of the resection up to total pancreatectomy in selected individuals.

In cases of de-epithelialization, adenoma, or borderline tumor at the margin, the optimal strategy remains controversial: we usually extend the resection a few centimeters to obtain a new margin, trying to obtain a negative resection margin. In our experience with 140 patients affected by MD-IPMN who underwent resection, the rate of negative margins in the surgical specimen was 60 %, and the results of the intraoperative, frozen section analysis modified the operative plan, leading to an extension of the resection or to total pancreatectomy in 29 patients (20 %) (Salvia et al. 2004).

Recurrence in the pancreatic remnant may develop even if the transection margin is negative and even in patients with noninvasive disease. The presence of a "positive" resection margin, multicentric IPMNs with synchronous "skip" lesions along the main duct, still present (but not detectable) at the time of operation and metachronous lesions (given that IPMN may be a marker of a "field defect" associated with a propensity for tumor development) may be responsible for recurrence in the pancreatic remnant after resecting a MD-IPMN.

17.2 Branch-Duct IPMN

According to the Sendai criteria (Tanaka et al. 2006), a strict follow up is suggested for patients with BD-IPMN less than 3 cm, with no nodules nor duct dilation (which would imply a mixed IPMN), in which progression toward cancer is considered low.

Follow up can be performed MRCP repeated 6 months after the first diagnosis and then yearly together with following serum CA19.9 dosage, unless there is an increase in size, the development of nodules, or the onset of symptoms. We believe that non-operative management of patients affected by BD-IPMN should be carried out in experienced centers, because data from large series is needed to validate this approach.

In our earlier experience of 109 patients with BD-IPMN (Salvia et al. 2007), 20 patients (18 %) underwent immediate resection because of symptoms and/or parameters associated with malignancy; pathologic diagnosis of BD-IPMN was always confirmed, and 2 patients (10 %) had an invasive carcinoma, while 1 (5 %) had carcinoma in situ. Eighty-nine patients (82 %) were followed up for a median of 32 months. After a mean follow-up of 18 months, 5 patients (6 %) had an increase in size of the lesion and underwent resection. The pathologic diagnosis was branch-duct adenoma in three patients and borderline in two; no patient developed malignancy on follow-up. These findings have been substantiated by other studies. Tanno et al. (2008) reported a follow up study of IPMN, showing similar results compared with our study; the authors found that the presence of mural nodules was the only predictive factor of malignancy in BD-IPMNs.

In contrast, other Institutions have advocated prompt resection for BD-IPMN. As illustrated in a dedicated chapter of this book, the Heidelberg group suggests that the incidence of malignant BD-IPMN may be greater than what has been reported in other studies, and that currently used predictors of malignancy may be inadequate.

One may argue (and we would agree with their argument) that such results may be reflective of a selected population. More importantly, most studies about BD-IPMN have focused on patients who have undergone resection, but little is known about the real incidence of invasive cancer in patients under surveillance programs. Recently, Cauley et al. (2012) published results on primary surveillance of 292 patients with BD-IPMN. These patients were defined as low risk and high risk for malignancy, according to clinical, serologic, and radiographic criteria. Interestingly, among the low-risk patients, only 12 % developed criteria for resection during the surveillance period. Of these patients, only 4 % presented high-grade dysplasia and only 1 % invasive cancer, underscoring the low malignant potential of BD-IPMNs with no obvious worrisome signs or characteristics of their IPMN.

In conclusion, correct diagnosis and appropriate management of pancreatic cystic neoplams (especially BD-IPMN) is still hampered by our lack of knowledge of the biologic behavior of these diseases. As a result, there still is heterogeneity in the choice of which treatment to offer to patients. We believe that further studies and continuous discussion among different groups will soon shed some light on one of the most fascinating topics in Pancreatology.

References

Cauley CE, Waters JA, Dumas RP, Meyer JE, Al-Haddad MA, DeWitt JM, Lillemoe KD, Schmidt CM (2012) Outcomes of primary surveillance for intraductal papillary mucinous neoplasm. J Gastrointest Surg 16:258–267

Crippa S, Salvia R, Warshaw AL, Domìnguez I, Bassi C, Falconi M, Thayer SP, Zamboni G, Lauwers GY, Mino-Kenudson M, Capelli P, Pederzoli P, Castillo CF (2008) Mucinous cystic neoplasm of the pancreas is not an aggressive entity: lessons from 163 resected patients. Ann Surg 247(4):571–579

Malleo G, Bassi C, Rossini R, Manfredi R, Butturini G, Massignani M, Paini M, Pederzoli P, Salvia R (2012) Growth pattern of serous cystic neoplasms of the pancreas: observational study with long-term magnetic resonance surveillance and recommendations for treatment. Gut 61(5):746–751

Salvia R, Fernandez-del Castillo C, Bassi C, Thayer SP, Falconi M, Mantovani W, Pederzoli P, Warshaw AL (2004) Main-duct intraductal papillary mucinous neoplasms of the pancreas: clinical predictors of malignancy and long-term survival following resection. Ann Surg 239:678–685

Salvia R, Crippa S, Falconi M, Bassi C, Guarise A, Scarpa A, Pederzoli P (2007) Branch-duct intraductal papillary mucinous neoplasms of the pancreas: to operate or not to operate? Gut 56:1086–1090

Tanaka M, Chari S, Adsay V, Fernandez-del Castillo C, Falconi M, Shimizu M, Yamaguchi K, Yamao K, Matsuno S, International Association of Pancreatology (2006) International consensus guidelines for management of intraductal papillary mucinous neoplasms and mucinous cystic neoplasms of the pancreas. Pancreatology 6:17–32

Tanno S, Nakano Y, Nishikawa T, Nakamura K, Sasajima J, Minoguchi M, Mizukami Y, Yanagawa N, Fujii T, Obara T, Okumura T, Kohgo Y (2008) Natural history of branch duct intraductal papillary-mucinous neoplasms of the pancreas without mural nodules: long-term follow-up results. Gut 57:339–343

Tseng JF, Warshaw AL, Sahani DV, Lauwers GY, Rattner DW, Fernandez del Castillo C (2005) Serous cyst-adenoma of the pancreas: tumor growth rates and recommendations for treatment. Ann Surg 242:413–419

Commentary

18

C. Max Schmidt

This commentary serves to: (1) draw attention to the importance of the chapter by Professor Buechler's group; (2) reinforce the concept that identification and screening of patients with pancreatic cysts is a unique opportunity to prevent and cure pancreatic cancer through early detection and (3) review current management and anticipate future changes in management of these complex patients.

Pancreatic cancer is the deadliest cancer. Although the incidence of pancreatic cancer is only 45,000 cases per year, the mortality is substantial. The mortality from pancreatic cancer is on an upward trajectory to surpass the mortality from breast cancer in the US within the next few years.

Long term survival from pancreatic cancer is rare, and no cure for pancreatic cancer has been discovered. By identifying and screening patients at increased risk for harboring or developing pancreatic cancer (pancreatic cysts, hereditary pancreatic cancer, chronic pancreatitis, certain genomic-based disorders), there is hope of early detection and prevention of pancreatic cancer for a substantial number of individuals.

Assessment of clinical, radiographic, and cytopathologic features of pancreatic cystic lesions is the standard of care for identification of pancreatic cystic neoplasms, proper cancer risk stratification, and appropriate management of patients with pancreatic cystic lesions. Symptomatic patients have a greater incidence of pancreatic cancer development, especially with symptoms/signs of pancreatic exocrine or endocrine failure. In terms of radiographic parameters, arguably the most important indicator of malignancy is the presence of main pancreatic duct (MPD) dilation. The extent of MPD dilation is directly proportional to pancreatic cancer risk. Although the degree of MPD dilation predicts pancreatic cancer risk, branch duct or cyst size is no longer considered a reliable indicator of malignant potential. Another very specific radiographic indicator of malignancy is the presence of mural nodules within the cystic lesion. While quite specific, mural nodules are not, however, very sensitive, because they are present in only 30 % of pancreatic cystic neoplasms harboring invasive cancer. Mural nodules suspected on static imaging (MRI, CT) should be confirmed by dynamic imaging (EUS) to exclude mobility; if mobile, these "nodules" are likely to be debris/mucin and thus, not associated with the same cancer risk. High grade atypia on cytopathology is highly specific for the presence of malignant cells in the pancreatic cyst either as *carcinoma-in-situ* or invasive carcinoma; however, high

C.M. Schmidt, M.D., Ph.D., MBA, FACS (✉)
Department of Surgery, Biochemistry and Molecular Biology, IU Health Pancreatic Cyst and Cancer Early Detection Center,
Indianapolis, IN, USA
e-mail: maxschmi@iupui.edu

Department of Surgery, Biochemistry, and Molecular Biology, Indiana University School of Medicine,
980 W. Walnut Street, R3 Bldg, Room C522,
Indianapolis, IN 46202, USA

R. Mantke et al. (eds.), *International Practices in Pancreatic Surgery*,
DOI 10.1007/978-3-540-74506-8_18, © Springer-Verlag Berlin Heidelberg 2013

grade atypia is not very sensitive, because only 50 % of invasive mucinous cystic neoplasms have high grade atypia recognizable in the samples of the cyst fluid. Accordingly, we maintain that formal resection should be performed in fit patients with new or worsening symptoms, mural nodules, progressive MPD dilation, and high grade dysplasia on cytopathology. These parameters, however, by themselves are not sufficient to guide our management of these patients (Cauley et al. 2012; Miller et al. 2011). Patients without these parameters have developed invasive cancer in pancreatic cystic lesions. The only clues in these patients have often been subtle changes in serum tumor markers, such as alkaline phosphatase, amylase, lipase, CA19-9, and hemoglobin a1c. These serum markers alone are unlikely to insure early detection, but serial determination of these serum markers is reasonable and deserves further study. Clearly, we need better indicators to guide our management of these patients.

Most recently, the collective knowledge of patients with pancreatic cystic lesions is moving forward at a tremendous pace. Biochemical and more recently molecular marker discovery in pancreatic cystic fluid appears to be most promising. Such novel and exciting analyses may diagnose and/or assess malignant potential.

Two useful markers in pancreatic cyst fluid currently are CEA and Kras. CEA level >192 ng/ml is consistent with a mucinous cystic neoplasm (IPMN or MCN). CEA is a widely available diagnostic biochemical test. CEA level in the cyst fluid does not predict the presence of malignancy but does predict cystic lesions with malignant potential. Kras mutations when detected also indicate the presence of a mucinous pancreatic cyst. The combination of CEA and Kras in the cystic fluid is nearly 100 % predictive of a mucinous cystic neoplasm of the pancreas and discriminates between cystic neoplasms and pseudocysts or other benign cysts.

More recently, a molecular profile of DNA mutations (Pathfinder TG™, RedPath, Inc.) present at multiple pancreatic cancer relevant genetic loci (e.g., KRas, p53, DPC4, P16, PTEN, 17q, etc.) was developed." This profile is commercially available now to provide serial quantification of the malignant potential of pancreatic cystic lesions. When the mutation panel is tested on known pancreatic cancers, >3 of these mutations are typically detected.

A newly discovered molecular marker in pancreatic cyst fluid is GNAS (Wu et al. 2011a), which is the oncogene encoding guanine nucleotide regulatory protein S alpha (GSα). GNAS mutations (i.e., codon 201: R201H or R201C) are diagnostic of IPMN but are present in only 66 % of IPMNs. When combined with analysis of Kras mutations, either GNAS and/or Kras mutations are present in 95 % of IPMNs (Wu et al. 2011a). Another newly discovered molecular marker is RNF43 which is expressed in the cyst epithelium in 75 % of IPMNs and 38 % of MCNs examined (Wu et al. 2011b). RNF43 is a tumor suppressor gene which encodes for a protein with intrinsic E3 ubiquitin ligase activity on chromosome 17q. Interestingly, 17q is the location of one of the genetic loci examined currently with the Pathfinder TG™. The development of miRNA profiling of pancreatic cyst fluid holds promise as a predictor of malignant potential in pancreatic cystic lesions but awaits further validation (Ryu et al. 2011). Finally, a recently discovered diagnostic marker $VEGF_{B9}$™ (B9, Inc.) an isoform of VEGF A, when present in pancreatic cyst fluid at a threshold level, approaches 100% accuracy in diagnosing the uniformly benign serous cystic neoplasms thereby altering the necessity of surveillance and possibly pancreatectomy in patients with cystic lesions of uncertain diagnosis. In summary, biochemical (CEA) and molecular (Kras, Pathfinder TG™) profiling, including the newly discovered markers GNAS, RNF43, miRNA and $VEGF_{B9}$ offer the potential to transform how we manage patients with pancreatic cystic lesions.

While we are looking for a cure for pancreatic cancer, it is equally critical to identify and screen patients at increased risk of pancreatic malignancy (family history, pancreatic cysts) to promote both early detection and prevention of advanced pancreatic cancer.

References

Cauley CE et al (2012) Outcomes of primary surveillance for intraductal papillary mucinous neoplasm. J Gastrointest Surg 16(2):258–67

Miller JR et al (2011) Outcome of the pancreatic remnant following segmental pancreatectomy for non-invasive intraductal papillary mucinous neoplasm. HPB (Oxford) 13(11):759–66. doi:10.1111/j.1477-2574.2011.00354.x, Epub 2011 Sep 9

Ryu JK, Matthaei H, Dal Molin M, et al. (2011) Elevated microRNA miR-21 levels in pancreatic cyst fluid are predictive of mucinous precursor lesions of ductal adenocarcinoma. Pancreatology. 2011;11(3):343–50. doi:10.1159/000329183, Epub 2011 Jul 12

Wu J et al (2011a) Recurrent GNAS mutations define an unexpected pathway for pancreatic cyst development. Sci Transl Med 3(92):92ra66. doi:10.1126/scitranslmed.3002543

Wu J et al (2011b) Whole-exome sequencing of neoplastic cysts of the pancreas reveals recurrent mutations in components of ubiquitin-dependent pathways. Proc Natl Acad Sci USA 108(52):21188–21193

Commentary

19

Masao Tanaka

19.1 Commentary

Among the various types of cystic neoplasms of the pancreas, the management of solid pseudopapillary neoplasm (SPN) does not have any controversy. Mucinous cystic neoplasm (MCN) described in this chapter also poses little controversy to the clinician who happens to diagnose them by some imaging modalities. Most of the MCNs found incidentally are still benign and represent currently a very good indication for laparoscopic distal pancreatectomy or local resection (enucleation) when feasible. Serous cystic neoplasms (SCNs) also presented in this chapter do not need resection unless they are indistinguishable from other types of cystic neoplasm detailed in the chapter, such as intraductal papillary mucinous neoplasm (IPMN) or MCN, when SCN takes on a macrocystic or oligocystic appearance as opposed to its typical microcystic appearance.

In contrast to SPN, MCN, and SCN, IPMN of the pancreas, especially the branch duct type (BD-IPMN), excites a lot of controversies in regard to differentiation from other pancreatic cysts, diagnosis of malignancy, and need for and type of operative/non-operative management. BD-IPMNs must be differentiated from MCNs, macrocystic or oligocystic SCNs, epidermoid cysts, lymphoepithelial cysts, and cystic variants of other neoplasms. Even with complete understanding of the imaging characteristics of each entity (Tanaka et al. 2006), it is sometimes difficult to differentiate BD-IPMNs confidently from MCNs, macrocystic or oligocystic SCNs, and lymphoepithelial cysts preoperatively.

Because it is especially important to differentiate non-mucinous cysts from IPMNs and MCNs with malignant potential, endoscopic ultrasonography-guided fine-needle aspiration (EUS-FNA) is receiving enthusiastic interest lately. A high level of carcinoembryonic antigen (CEA) in the cystic fluid is characteristic of mucinous cysts. Although the cut-off concentration that provides a confident diagnosis of mucinous epithelium varies from report to report (>367 (Lewandrowski et al. 1993), >800 (van der Waaij et al. 2005), ≥480 (Linder et al. 2006), >800 (Attasaranya et al. 2007), and >192 ng/ml (Brugge et al. 2004)), an increased value of even >5 ng/ml is highly suggestive of a mucinous neoplasm. Although the CEA levels are not necessarily consistent with levels of other molecular markers, including a glycan variant of MUC-5AC (Haab et al. 2010), mucin-like carcinoma-associated antigen (Khalid et al. 2009), *KRAS* mutations (Bernard et al. 2002) and CA72-4 (Jang et al. 2005), the diagnostic sensitivity was reported to improve when combined (Haab et al. 2010; Sawhney et al. 2009).

The diagnosis of malignant transformation of BD-IPMN remains controversial at present.

M. Tanaka
Department of Surgery and Oncology, Graduate School of Medical Sciences, Kyushu University, Fukuoka, Japan
e-mail: masaotan@med.kyushu-u.ac.jp

R. Mantke et al. (eds.), *International Practices in Pancreatic Surgery*,
DOI 10.1007/978-3-540-74506-8_19, © Springer-Verlag Berlin Heidelberg 2013

The original Sendai guidelines recommend resection of BD-IPMN with one or more of five criteria for suspected malignancy, i.e., positive pancreatic juice cytology, the presence of mural nodules, cyst size >3 cm, dilation of the main pancreatic duct, and abdominal pain (Tanaka et al. 2006). Nevertheless, 80–85 % of all BD-IPMNs resected according to these guidelines are benign. Therefore, we need to identify other diagnostic aids that would avoid or at least minimize a "false positive" resection. Based on the understanding of histologic subtypes, i.e., gastric, intestinal, pancreatobiliary, and oncocytic, and the recent observation that the intestinal subtype is more likely to de-differentiate into malignancy, selection of the intestinal subtype may be helpful to distinguish BD-IPMNs with a greater tendency for malignant transformation. A few such attempts have been reported by immunohistochemical or molecular analysis of cells contained in the pancreatic juice (Hibi et al. 2007; Nakata et al. 2009).

On the contrary, the authors of this chapter have suggested that even small BD-IPMNs ≤3 cm without malignant stigmata ("Sendai-negative") have a relatively high risk of malignancy. Among their 69 patients with "Sendai-negative" BD-IPMNs, 25 % had in situ or invasive carcinoma. Lee et al. (2008) claimed that one of 30 BD-IPMNs resected with no Sendai criteria had carcinoma in situ; however, the absence of mural nodules was judged by CT, MR, or EUS in both of these studies. It is well accepted that EUS is the most sensitive modality to evaluate the presence or absence of a mural nodule and not CT or MR. In a collective series of 349 patients who underwent EUS initially to prove the absence of mural nodule, there were 7 patients who underwent resection without any of the Sendai criteria during a median follow-up of 3.5 years, and none of them had carcinoma (Maguchi et al. 2011). There have been four series describing clearly the relationship of malignancy to the size and the presence/absence of mural nodules. In 124 BD-IPMNs <3 cm without mural nodules, there was no single case of malignancy (Tanaka 2011).

If expertise in EUS-FNA and cytologic interpretation of "high grade atypia" in the cyst fluid are available, the cytologic analysis of the cyst fluid obtained by EUS-FNA might add diagnostic value, although the sensitivity is often limited by scant cellularity of the aspirate and contamination by gastrointestinal mucosal cells (van der Waaij et al. 2005; Pitman and Deshpande 2007; Pitman et al. 2010; Frossard et al. 2003; Belsley et al. 2008; Recine et al. 2004; Michaels et al. 2006; Layfield and Cramer 2005; Emerson et al. 2006; Maire et al. 2003, 2008). Cells with "high-grade atypia" in mucinous cyst fluid obtained by EUS-FNA indicated the presence of malignancy with a sensitivity of 72 % and an accuracy of 80 % (Pitman et al. 2010). The same group claimed that "high-grade atypia" was the most sensitive predictor of malignancy even in small (≤30 mm) BD-IPMNs (67 %), compared to mural nodules and a dilated main pancreatic duct which were highly specific (>90 %) but insensitive (39–44 %) (Genevay et al. 2011).

Follow-up surveillance of BD-IPMNs without malignant signs is an especially challenging problem in the management of IPMNs. EUS seems to be the best modality but has the drawbacks of increased cost, invasiveness, and intraobserver and interobserver variability. In reality, we cannot subject all patients to routine surveillance by EUS. How and how often to detect malignant changes of BD-IPMNs and to survey the development of distinct ductal adenocarcinoma remain very important controversies. Since we reported the occurrence of in situ or invasive ductal carcinoma concomitant with a benign BD-IPMN (Tanaka et al. 1997; Yamaguchi et al. 1997, 2002), this phenomenon has attracted increasing attention. Several reports have suggested that 3–9 % of patients with BD-IPMNs had or developed pancreatic ductal carcinoma distinct from IPMN-related invasive cancer (Tanaka 2011). During a median follow-up of 87 months, in 60 patients with BD-IPMNs, even when <1 cm in size, developed 5 ductal carcinomas (8 %) (Uehara et al. 2008). Worsening diabetes and high or increasing levels of serum CA19-9 predicted the presence of ductal carcinoma (Ingkakul et al. 2010; Kanno et al. 2010). Also, older age, smaller size of BD-IPMN, and smaller caliber of the main pancreatic duct were reported to be associated with the development of ductal carcinoma compared with the patients who did not develop ductal carcinoma (Tanno et al. 2010). The appropriate method and interval of surveillance of BD-IPMNs remain to be further investigated.

References

Attasaranya S, Pais S, LeBlanc J, McHenry L, Sherman S, DeWitt JM (2007) Endoscopic ultrasound-guided fine needle aspiration and cyst fluid analysis for pancreatic cysts. JOP 8:553–563

Belsley NA, Pitman MB, Lauwers GY, Brugge WR, Deshpande V (2008) Serous cystadenoma of the pancreas: limitations and pitfalls of endoscopic ultrasound-guided fine-needle aspiratio biopsy. Cancer 114:102–110

Bernard P, Scoazec JY, Joubert M, Kahn X, Le Borgne J, Berger F, Partensky C (2002) Intraductal papillary-mucinous tumors of the pancreas: predictive criteria of malignancy according to pathological examination of 53 cases. Arch Surg 137:1274–1278

Brugge WR, Lewandrowski K, Lee-Lewandrowski E, Centeno BA, Szydlo T, Regan S, del Castillo CF, Warshaw AL (2004) Diagnosis of pancreatic cystic neoplasms: a report of the cooperative pancreatic cyst study. Gastroenterology 126:1330–1336

Emerson RE, Randolph ML, Cramer HM (2006) Endoscopic ultrasound-guided fine-needle aspiration cytology diagnosis of intraductal papillary mucinous neoplasm of the pancreas is highly predictive of pancreatic neoplasia. Diagn Cytopathol 34:457–462

Frossard JL, Amouyal P, Amouyal G, Palazzo L, Amaris J, Soldan M, Giostra E, Spahr L, Hadengue A, Fabre M (2003) Performance of endosonography-guided fine needle aspiration and biopsy in the diagnosis of pancreatic cystic lesions. Am J Gastroenterol 98:1516–1524

Genevay M, Mino-Kenudson M, Yaeger K, Konstantinidis IT, Ferrone CR, Thayer S, Fernandez-del Castillo C, Sahani D, Bounds B, Forcione D, Brugge WR, Pitman MB (2011) Cytology adds value to imaging studies for risk assessment of malignancy in pancreatic mucinous cysts. Ann Surg 254(6):977–983

Haab BB, Porter A, Yue T, Li L, Scheiman J, Anderson MA, Barnes D, Schmidt CM, Feng Z, Simeone DM (2010) Glycosylation variants of mucins and CEACAMs as candidate biomarkers for the diagnosis of pancreatic cystic neoplasms. Ann Surg 251:937–945

Hibi Y, Fukushima N, Tsuchida A, Sofuni A, Itoi T, Moriyasu F, Mukai K, Aoki T (2007) Pancreatic juice cytology and subclassification of intraductal papillary mucinous neoplasms of the pancreas. Pancreas 34:197–204

Ingkakul T, Sadakari Y, Ienaga J, Satoh N, Takahata S, Tanaka M (2010) Predictors of the presence of concomitant invasive ductal carcinoma in intraductal papillary mucinous neoplasm of the pancreas. Ann Surg 251:70–75

Jang JY, Kim SW, Ahn YJ, Yoon YS, Choi MG, Lee KU, Han JK, Kim WH, Lee YJ, Kim SC, Han DJ, Kim YI, Choi SH, Cho BH, Yu HC, Yoon DS, Lee WJ, Lee KB, Kim YC, Lee KS, Kim MW, Kim HJ, Kim HJ, Park YH (2005) Multicenter analysis of clinicopathologic features of intraductal papillary mucinous tumor of the pancreas: is it possible to predict the malignancy before surgery? Ann Surg Oncol 12:124–132

Kanno A, Satoh K, Hirota M, Hamada S, Umino J, Itoh H, Masamune A, Asakura T, Shimosegawa T (2010) Prediction of invasive carcinoma in branch type intraductal papillary mucinous neoplasms of the pancreas. J Gastroenterol 45:952–959

Khalid A, Zahid M, Finkelstein SD, LeBlanc JK, Kaushik N, Ahmad N, Brugge WR, Edmundowicz SA, Hawes RH, McGrath KM (2009) Pancreatic cyst fluid DNA analysis in evaluating pancreatic cysts: a report of the PANDA study. Gastrointest Endosc 69:1095–1102

Layfield LJ, Cramer H (2005) Fine-needle aspiration cytology of intraductal papillary-mucinous tumors: a retrospective analysis. Diagn Cytopathol 32:16–20

Lee CJ, Scheiman J, Anderson MA, Hines OJ, Reber HA, Farrell J, Kochman ML, Foley PJ, Drebin J, Oh YS, Ginsberg G, Ahmad N, Merchant NB, Isbell J, Parikh AA, Stokes JB, Bauer T, Adams RB, Simeone DM (2008) Risk of malignancy in resected cystic tumors of the pancreas < or =3 cm in size: is it safe to observe asymptomatic patients? A multi-institutional report. J Gastrointest Surg 12:234–242

Lewandrowski KB, Southern JF, Pins MR, Compton CC, Warshaw AL (1993) Cyst fluid analysis in the differential diagnosis of pancreatic cysts. A comparison of pseudocysts, serous cystadenomas, mucinous cystic neoplasms, and mucinous cystadenocarcinoma. Ann Surg 217:41–47

Linder JD, Geenen JE, Catalano MF (2006) Cyst fluid analysis obtained by EUS-guided FNA in the evaluation of discrete cystic neoplasms of the pancreas: a prospective single-center experience. Gastrointest Endosc 64:697–702

Maguchi H, Tanno S, Mizuno N, Hanada K, Kobayashi G, Hatori T, Sadakari Y, Yamaguchi T, Tobita K, Doi R, Yanagisawa A, Tanaka M (2011) Natural history of branch duct intraductal papillary mucinous neoplasms of the pancreas: a multicenter study in Japan. Pancreas 40:364–370

Maire F, Couvelard A, Hammel P, Ponsot P, Palazzo L, Aubert A, Degott C, Dancour A, Felce-Dachez M, O'toole D, Lévy P, Ruszniewski P (2003) Intraductal papillary mucinous tumors of the pancreas: the preoperative value of cytologic and histopathologic diagnosis. Gastrointest Endosc 58:701–706

Maire F, Voitot H, Aubert A, Palazzo L, O'Toole D, Couvelard A, Levy P, Vidaud M, Sauvanet A, Ruszniewski P, Hammel P (2008) Intraductal papillary mucinous neoplasms of the pancreas: performance of pancreatic fluid analysis for positive diagnosis and the prediction of malignancy. Am J Gastroenterol 103:2871–2877

Michaels PJ, Brachtel EF, Bounds BC, Brugge WR, Pitman MB (2006) Intraductal papillary mucinous neoplasm of the pancreas: cytologic features predict histologic grade. Cancer 108:163–173

Nakata K, Nagai E, Ohuchida K, Aishima S, Hayashi A, Miyasaka Y, Yu J, Mizumoto K, Tanaka M, Tsuneyoshi M (2009) REG4 is associated with carcinogenesis in the 'intestinal' pathway of intraductal papillary mucinous neoplasms. Mod Pathol 22:460–468

Pitman MB, Deshpande V (2007) Endoscopic ultrasound-guided fine needle aspiration cytology of the pancreas: a morphological and multimodal approach to the diagnosis of solid and cystic mass lesions. Cytopathology 18:331–347

Pitman MB, Genevay M, Yaeger K, Chebib I, Turner BG, Mino-Kenudson M, Brugge WR (2010) High-grade atypical epithelial cells in pancreatic mucinous cysts are a more accurate predictor of malignancy than "positive" cytology. Cancer Cytopathol 118:434–440

Recine M, Kaw M, Evans DB, Krishnamurthy S (2004) Fine-needle aspiration cytology of mucinous tumors of the pancreas. Cancer 102:92–99

Sawhney MS, Devarajan S, O'Farrel P, Cury MS, Kundu R, Vollmer CM, Brown A, Chuttani R, Pleskow DK (2009) Comparison of carcinoembryonic antigen and molecular analysis in pancreatic cyst fluid. Gastrointest Endosc 69:1106–1110

Tanaka M (2011) Controversies in the management of pancreatic IPMN. Nat Rev Gastroenterol Hepatol 8:56–60

Tanaka M, Yokohata K, Konomi H, Yamaguchi K, Chijiiwa K, Ohta M (1997) Segmental balloon cytology for preoperative localization of in situ pancreatic cancer. Gastrointest Endosc 46:447–449

Tanaka M, Chari S, Adsay V, Castillo CF, Falconi M, Shimizu M, Yamaguchi K, Yamao K, Matsuno S (2006) International consensus guidelines for management of intraductal papillary mucinous neoplasms and mucinous cystic neoplasms of the pancreas. Pancreatology 6:17–32

Tanno S, Nakano Y, Sugiyama Y, Nakamura K, Sasajima J, Koizumi K, Yamazaki M, Nishikawa T, Mizukami Y, Yanagawa N, Fujii T, Obara T, Okumura T, Kohgo Y (2010) Incidence of synchronous and metachronous pancreatic carcinoma in 168 patients with branch duct intraductal papillary mucinous neoplasm. Pancreatology 10:173–178

Uehara H, Nakaizumi A, Ishikawa O, Iishi H, Tatsumi K, Takakura R, Ishida T, Takano Y, Tanaka S, Takenaka A (2008) Development of ductal carcinoma of the pancreas during follow-up of branch duct intraductal papillary mucinous neoplasm of the pancreas. Gut 57:1561–1565

van der Waaij LA, van Dullemen HM, Porte RJ (2005) Cyst fluid analysis in the differential diagnosis of pancreatic cystic lesions: a pooled analysis. Gastrointest Endosc 62:383–394

Yamaguchi K, Nakamura K, Yokohata K, Shimizu S, Chijiiwa K, Tanaka M (1997) Pancreatic cyst as a sentinel of in situ carcinoma of the pancreas. Report of two cases. Int J Pancreatol 22:227–231

Yamaguchi K, Ohuchida J, Ohtsuka T, Nakao K, Tanaka M (2002) Intraductal papillary-mucinous tumor of the pancreas concomitant with ductal carcinoma of the pancreas. Pancreatology 2:484–490

Part IV

Surgery of Acute Pancreatitis

Basic Chapter

20

René Mantke, Hans-Ulrich Schulz, and Hans Lippert

20.1 Relevant Basic Information, Indication, and Contraindication

Severe pancreatitis complicates about 15–20 % of all cases of acute pancreatitis.

The diagnosis of acute pancreatitis is based on the classic clinical features (abdominal pain, vomiting) and evaluation of lipase or pancreatic amylase in the plasma (Table 20.1). We prefer the use of lipase levels because of the longer half-life and slightly superior sensitivity and specificity. Ultrasonography may show pancreatic swelling, but bowel gas can prevent adequate visibility of the pancreas during the ultrasound procedure. Ultrasonography can also show gallbladder stones or dilation of the bile duct as a sign of stones in the bile duct. A plain abdominal x-ray should be obtained to exclude free abdominal air because the differential diagnosis of acute pancreatitis is broad and includes other abdominal emergencies such as a perforated peptic ulcer. Imaging by contrast-enhanced computed tomography (CT) provides

Table 20.1 Diagnostic in patients with suspicion of acute pancreatitis

Diagnostic methods	Questions
Clinic	Jaundice, pain, vomiting
Laboratory evaluation	Standard parameters, lipase, CRP, procalcitonin
Standard chest X-ray	Pulmonary lesions, pneumonia, pleural effusion
Plain abdominal x-ray	Exclusion of visceral perforation (free abdominal air), not needed if early CT is performed
Ultrasonography	Swelling of the pancreas if pancreas is visible, gallbladder stones, or dilation of the bile duct (gallstone history of the acute pancreatitis?), not needed if early CT is performed
CT (contrast-enhanced CT) initial assessment	Acute pancreatitis, bile duct obstruction, free intraperitoneal fluid, peripancreatic fat necrosis, indication of prophylactic antibiotics (early CT may underestimate the ultimate severity of pancreatitis)
CT (contrast-enhanced CT) follow up (not before 4 days after onset of pancreatitis	Determination and localization of necrosis, abscess, pseudocyst, change in the local situation
ERCP	*Verification and removing of bile duct stones*
MRI	*Optional in children or pregnant patients*

Italic – optional tests for specification of the diagnosis

R. Mantke (✉)
Professor of Surgery, Chair, Department of Surgery, City Hospital Brandenburg, 14770 Brandenburg, Germany
e-mail: mantke@klinikum-brandenburg.de

H.-U. Schulz
Department of Surgery, Otto von Guericke University, Magdeburg, Germany
e-mail: hans-ulrich.schulz@med.ovgu.de

H. Lippert, M.D.
Professor of Surgery, Chair, Department of Surgery, Otto von Guericke University of Magdeburg, 39129 Magdeburg, Germany
e-mail: hans.lippert@med.ovgu.de

R. Mantke et al. (eds.), *International Practices in Pancreatic Surgery*,
DOI 10.1007/978-3-540-74506-8_20, © Springer-Verlag Berlin Heidelberg 2013

the best evidence for the presence of acute pancreatitis and is better able to rule out other causes of the abdominal pain (initial CT assessment). C-Reactive Protein (CRP) levels over 150 mg/l, an APACHE II score greater than 8 in the first 24 h after admission, or persistent organ failure in the first 48 h after admission are established, clinically useful predictors of the severity of acute pancreatitis. Patients with severe acute pancreatitis should be admitted to an intensive care unit for optimal support. A determination of the amount of pancreatic necrosis by contrast-enhanced CT is usually possible 4 or 5 days after the onset of acute pancreatitis. Patients with sepsis, organ failure, or a worsening clinical status require urgent contrast-enhanced CT for determination of the local extent of necrosis or local complications. Both oral and intravenous administration of a contrast agent is necessary. If there is any evidence of a gallstone in the bile duct, urgent endoscopic retrograde cholangiography should be done with endoscopic sphincterotomy and stone removal.

After the diagnosis of necrosis is made based on CT, antibiotic prophylaxis is started.

The use of prophylactic antibiotics is still a matter of debate. Some guidelines have already rejected this recommendation, because several relevant prospective studies with high evidence failed to show a positive effect on mortality. The rationale for use of prophylactic antibiotics was suggested based on some older studies with a lower grade of evidence. A Cochrane meta-analysis in 2006 described a reduction in mortality using prophylactic antibiotics in necrotizing pancreatitis (5 studies, 294 randomized patients, 6 vs. 15 % mortality). For these reasons, the use of prophylactic antibiotics remains a viable option to us. We limit the use of antibiotic prophylaxis to a maximum of 14 days.

The management of acute necrotizing pancreatitis has changed substantially in the last several years. Early management is supportive and nonsurgical. Most patients with acute necrotizing pancreatitis survive the early phase of this disease (Systemic Inflammatory Response Syndrome, SIRS) due to improvements in intensive care medicine. Severe pancreatitis is usually associated with organ failure and local complications like infected necrosis or abscess formation and later sepsis. Early operative intervention (before the third to fourth week after the onset of illness) or the operative treatment of sterile necrosis should be reserved for select cases. Infection of the pancreatic necrosis is a well-accepted indication for operative intervention. Infected pancreatic necrosis can be the focus of a severe sepsis and is associated with a high mortality. The development of infected necrosis is the rationale of pancreatic surgery in acute necrotizing pancreatitis. In contrast, infected necrosis does not mandate operative treatment in every case. Focused antibiotic therapy combined with a local percutaneous drainage can cure some patients with stable, localized disease (Fig. 20.1).

Pancreatic necrosis is usually well demarked after about 3 weeks from the onset of acute pancreatitis. Removing only the well-demarked necrosis (focal necrosectomy) reduces the risk of bleeding and preserves the still vital pancreatic parenchyma. There is general agreement between surgeons that early operative intervention (necrosectomy) should be done only in select cases, for instance, when there are severe complications (bleeding, bowel perforation) or in severe critically ill patients with proven necrosis. Patients who present with signs of sepsis can undergo CT guided fine needle aspiration of pancreatic or peripancreatic necrosis to differentiate between sterile and infected necrosis. Furthermore, the CT findings of extraluminal gas within areas of necrosis is pathognomonic of infection. Persistent necrotic pancreatitis with a fulminate course can also, in selected cases, be an indication for operative intervention (necrosectomy). The surgeon will usually see only a select group of patients with acute pancreatitis (unstable patients with septic focus and multiple organ failure). For that reason, the indication for necrosectomy is often quite clear. The surgeon has now to determine the best time for operative intervention in concordance with the intensive care specialist.

20.2 Surgical Technique

Manual necrosectomy and continuous lavage is our preferred operating technique. The operation begins with a bilateral subcostal incision in the upper abdomen (Fig. 20.2). We use a self-retaining retraction system for the costal rim. This approach allows the greatest exposure to the area of interest. An inspection of the lower abdomen

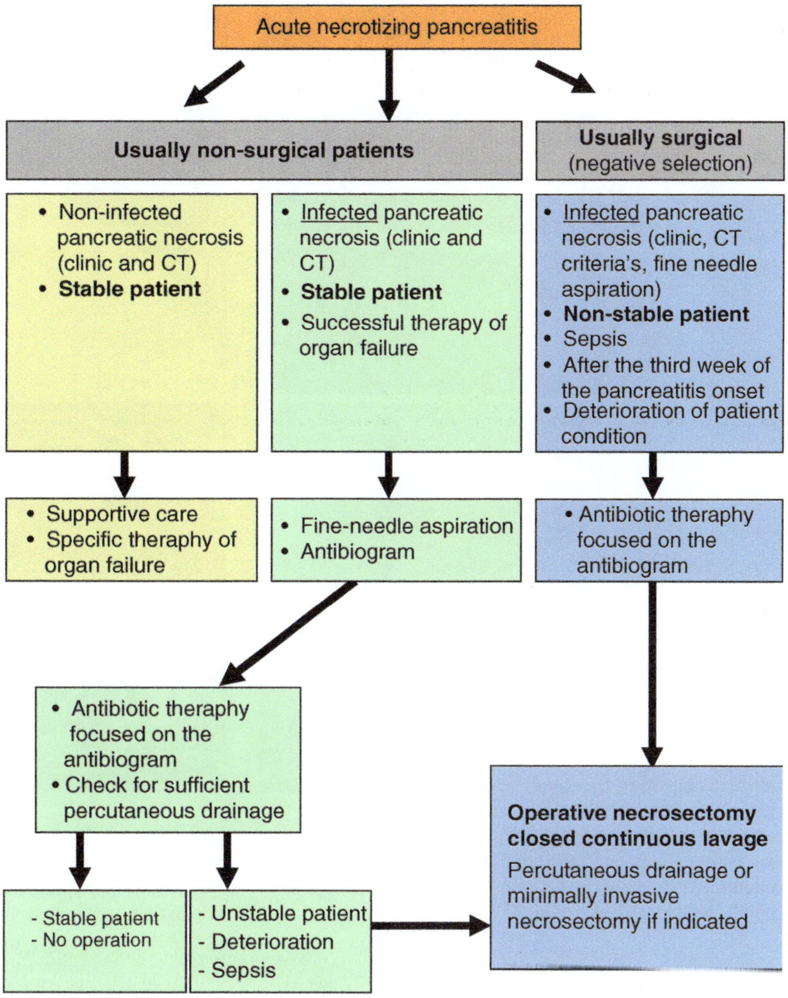

Fig. 20.1 Therapeutic flow in acute necrotizing pancreatitis

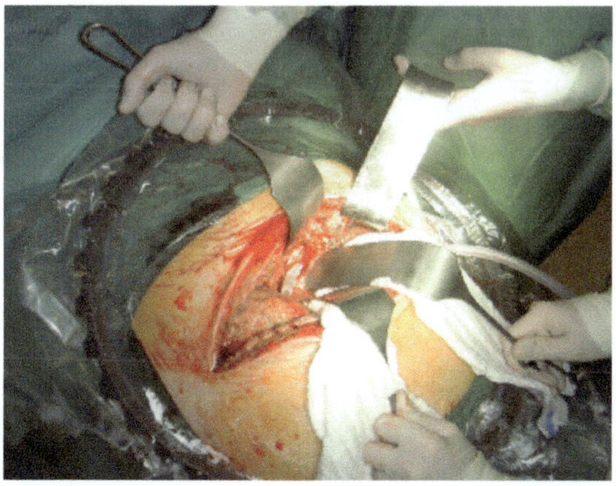

Fig. 20.2 A bilateral subcostal incision was done for a wide approach to the lesser sac. A special lavage fluid bag (Incise Pouch®, Moelnlycke Health Care AB, Göteborg, Sweden) is used for collecting the lavage and irrigation fluids

or a loop ileostomy is also possible if necessary using this approach.

The middle and the left half of the gastrocolic ligament is divided between sutures or using the harmonic scalpel (Generator 300, Ethicon Endo-Surgery, Johnson & Johnson, Somerville, USA). Edema and local fat necrosis with calcifications are often present in this region of the greater omentum at this step of the operation (Fig. 20.3). The greater omentum and transverse colon provide a natural barrier to the lower abdomen. Blunt dissection mobilizes the stomach off the transverse colon and off the anterior surface of the pancreatic body and tail (Figs. 20.3 and 20.4). The best way to avoid bleeding while removing viable pancreatic tissue is to use the fingers for preparation. The preparation is aided by repeated lavage of the lesser sac with warm isotonic saline

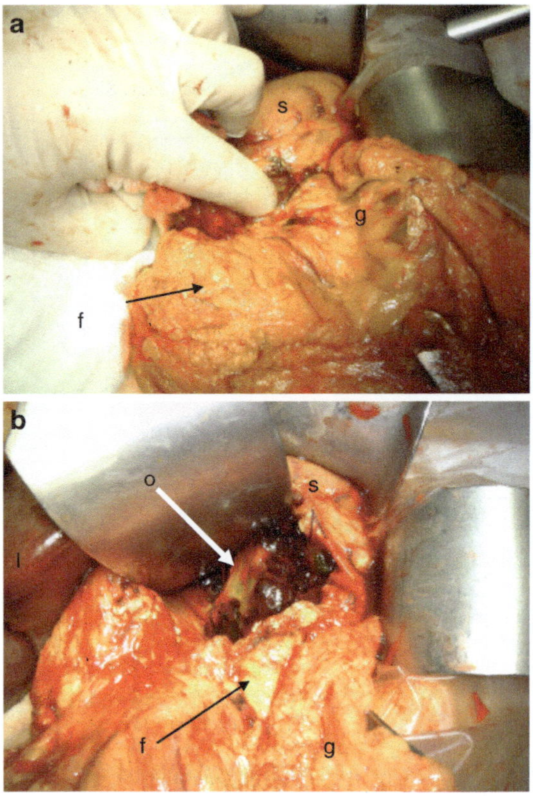

Fig. 20.3 (**a**, **b**) View into the incompletely opened lesser sac through the gastrocolic ligament (*s* stomach, *g* greater omentum, *f* fat necrosis, *o* open lesser sac with coagulated blood and necrotic material, *l* liver)

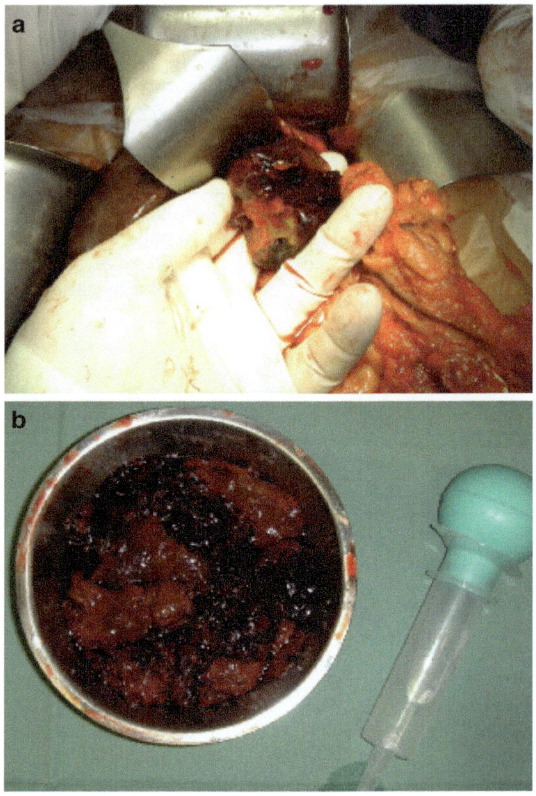

Fig. 20.4 (**a**, **b**) The character of necrotic pancreatic and peripancreatic tissue and coagulated blood removed. Necrosectomy is performed bluntly using the fingers (digitoclastic necrosectomy)

fluid. Coagulated blood, peripancreatic necrosis, and areas of pancreatic necrosis that have been separated from underlying viable pancreatic parenchyma or areas of necrosis are removed by this maneuver (Fig. 20.4). Necrotic debris that is adherent and cannot be teased free with gently exploring fingers should be left in place to avoid bleeding. Necrotic material needs to be sent to a laboratory for culture and sensitivity. Experience operating in this area in elective cases greatly helps one perform the necessary technical maneuvers and to understand the relevant anatomy to allow a safe necrosectomy. Computed tomography is used for guiding the procedure. Necrosis usually extends into the retroperitoneal area behind the splenic flexure and anterior to the left kidney. It is important to débride and drain this area, too.

Usually we prefer a continuous lavage of the lesser sac and retroperitoneum postoperatively via operatively placed drains. If areas of hemorrhage persist after the necrosectomy, temporary packing with operative dressings for 48 h is useful if control of the bleeding using bipolar forceps or sutures fail.

If no clinically significant bleeding is evident at the end of the necrosectomy, a large-bore silicon drain (30–36 French, Robinson Drainage System, Smith Medical, Kirchseeon, Germany) is placed in the pancreatic bed for the outflow of the continuous lavage. This drain tube is placed in the lesser sac and exits the abdomen by going posterior to the splenic flexure and anterior to the left kidney across the retroperitoneal perirenal space and exiting through a stab wound in the left lateral abdomen (Fig. 20.5). Dissecting this space behind the splenic flexure can be difficult; mobilization of the left colon in the area of the kidney and a bimanual digital technique can be useful in this situation. On the other hand, radiologic

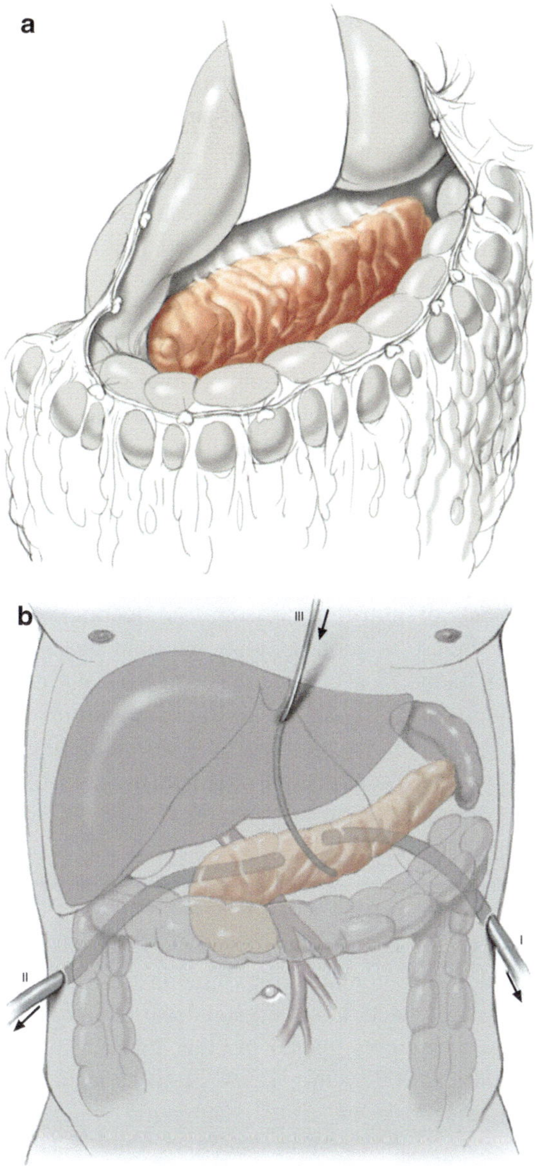

Fig. 20.5 (**a**) Exposure of the lesser sac by transecting the gastrocolic ligament and (**b**) position of drains for a continuous lavage. *I* left large silicone drain (36 French) behind the left colon splenic flexure, *II* optional right large silicone drain (36 French), *III* silicone inflow drain (12 French)

placement of a small percutaneous pigtail catheter preoperatively can make this procedure much easier.

Only in the case of extended necrosis in the pancreatic head, do we use a second large outflow drain placed subhepatically through the Foramen Winslowi into the lesser sac and brought

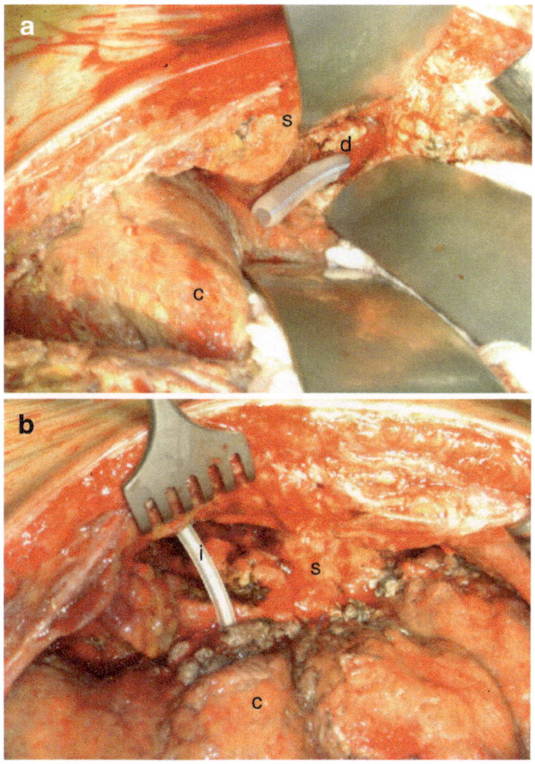

Fig. 20.6 (**a**, **b**) View into the lesser sac with large drainage tube with closure of the gastrocolic ligament with a silicone inflow drain (*d* outflow drain, *i* inflow drain, *s* stomach, *c* transverse colon)

out through a stab wound in the right lateral abdomen.

A smaller inflow catheter (12 French silicone gastric tube, VYGON, Ecouen France) is placed through the epigastric area into the opened lesser sac. The positioning of the drains for continuous lavage is very important (Fig. 20.5).

Function of the confirmed drains for continuous lavage should be confirmed before the abdomen is closed. If possible, the gastrocolic ligament is reapproximated with interrupted sutures (Vicryl® 2/0, Ethicon, Johnson & Johnson, Somerville, USA) (Fig. 20.6). If a gallstone etiology is evident, we remove the gallbladder during the procedure. The abdominal wound is closed with two continuous layers of an absorbable monofilament suture (PDS I® 2, Ethicon, Johnson & Johnson, Somerville, USA), one for the peritoneum and posterior rectus fascia and the other for the anterior rectus fascia. Postoperatively, a continuous lavage is performed with a standard peritoneal dialysis fluid (CAPD, Fresenius Medical Care AG & Co. KGaA, Bad Homburg, Germany) at a rate of 0.5 l/h. The lavage volume can be decreased depending on the appearance of the effluent and the clinical course. Usually drains can be removed within 2–3 weeks.

Some groups utilize radiologic percutaneous drainage or laparoscopic or endoscopic techniques to remove infected necrosis from the pancreatic area (minimally invasive necrosectomy). These methods seem to be most successful in cases with well-circumscribed necrosis containing a large fluid component. Repeated interventions form very talented and experienced surgeons are usually necessary in these cases to remove necrotic tissue. We believe that it is difficult to remove all infected pancreatic, peripancreatic, and retroperitoneal necrosis and associated inflammatory fluids by these techniques alone, but retroperitoneal endoscopic or endoscopic transgastric procedures are interesting methods and should be investigated further using randomized trials. At this time, minimally invasive necrosectomy is far from the standard practice in treating many patients requiring necrosectomy for acute necrotizing pancreatitis.

20.3 Additional Treatments and Procedures

- ICU admission with invasive monitoring and laboratory analysis are routine in patients with severe acute pancreatitis.
- Adequate fluid resuscitation monitored using the central venous pressure and urine output is standard therapy.
- Oxygen saturation (mask).
- All patients with severe necrotizing pancreatitis get prophylactic antibiotics (3×1 g Imipenem, Zienam®, MSD Sharp & Dohme GMBH, Haar, Germany) for 14 days.
- All patients get prophylaxis against deep vein thrombosis with low molecular weight heparin (0.3 ml Certoparin-Natrium, Mono-Embolex™, Novartis Pharma, Nuernberg, Germany) once daily started at admission until discharge. Prophylaxis against gastric stress ulcer is done with 40 mg pantoprazole daily intravenous (Pantozol®, Atlanta Pharma, Konstanz, Germany).
- If technically possible, all patients get an epidural catheter for pain management.
- All patients get a double lumen gastric/jejunal tube. The end of the tube is placed into the jejunum for enteral nutrition without direct passage of the stomach and duodenum. Oral water or tea are possible. Ileus or shock may limit the use of enteral nutrition. Nasogastric feeding may limit the use of enteral nutrition. Nasogastric feeding with limited volume is also possible in many patients. The continuous lavage usually continues for about 2 weeks, depending on the quality of the outflow fluid and the clinical course. Usually, drains can be removed within 2–3 weeks.

20.4 Results

Table 20.2 contains the relationship between patients treated in the surgical department in contrast to patients treated in other departments in 2006 and 2007. Only 1.3 % of all patients with the diagnosis of acute pancreatitis underwent operative intervention (necrosectomy). These data show impressively the decreased role of operative necrosectomy in the treatment of acute pancreatitis. The surgeons usually see a negative selection of patients who have failed conservative therapy.

The surgical results of our institution are contained in Table 20.3.

Table 20.2 Patients with acute pancreatitis treated at the university hospital in Magdeburg with acute pancreatitis in 2006 and 2007 (ICD 10 confirmed analysis)

Patients at the hospital	Patients in surgical department	Patients in surgical department and surgery of necrosis
461	49 (10.6 %)	6 (1.3 %)

Table 20.3 Patients with severe acute necrotizing pancreatitis from 2006 to 2007 surgically treated (surgical necrosectomy)

	Number
Patients	6
Hospital mortality	1
Hospital stay (median, days)	63 (16–378)
Biliary history	3
Alcoholic history	2
Other history	1
Microbiological proven infected necrosis	5
Closed continuous lavage	6
Open packing	–
Planned staged relaparotomy with repeated lavage	–
Closed packing (multiple drains + transcutaneous gauze)	–

Commentary

21

Hans G. Beger, B.M. Rau, and B. Poch

21.1 Multiorgan Insufficiency, Extent of Necroses and Infected Necroses Are the Risk Factors in Severe Acute Pancreatitis

The majority of patients with acute pancreatitis, particularly those with acute biliary pancreatitis suffer a mild disease; however 15–25 % develop severe acute pancreatitis, most of them in conjunction with a necrotizing course (Beger and Rau 2007). Abnormal intra-acinar calcium activity and premature activation of zymogens lead to autodigestion of the gland and local inflammation. Mild acute pancreatitis is dominated by intra-pancreatic oedema, spreading cell necrosis, accumulation of inflammatory cells, and local release of pro-inflammatory cytokines (Mayer et al. 2000; Poch et al. 1999). Using multi-slice contrast enhanced CT (CECT), necrotizing pancreatitis is defined by the presence of focal or extended necrosis; but even mild, acute oedematous-interstitial pancreatitis may be associated with some cell necrosis throughout the pancreas, despite the CECT showing only enlargement of the pancreas (Balthazar et al. 1990). Based on wet weight of the removed necrosis in patients undergoing debridement, extended necrosis (>180 g wet weight) is present in about 30 % of patients with necrotizing pancreatitis ultimately requiring operative intervention, respectively debridement. Infection of the necrosis occurs in about 20–35 % of all patients with necrotizing pancreatitis (Table 21.1). The necrotizing tissue process occurs in the first few days of the disease and does not appear to occur later on in the disease process.

Local production of inflammatory mediators, like interleukines and chemokines, and activation of neutrophils, macrophages, and lymphocytes contribute to the progression of the inflammatory process and the systemic amplification of the inflammatory response syndrome (SIRS) by the liver, the lungs, and the gut. The degree of SIRS during the first few days of disease provides important information in assessing severity of the disease and for decision making in terms of ICU treatment. Severe and persistent SIRS is considered to be the link between the inflammatory local process in the pancreatic tissue and the development of organ or multi organ dysfunction (Mole et al. 2009). Early and persistent multiple organ failure syndrome (MOFS)

H.G. Beger (✉)
Department of General and Visceral Surgery
Universitätsklinikum Ulm,
Albert-Einstein-Allee, 89081 Ulm, Germany
e-mail: hans@beger-ulm.de

B.M. Rau
Abteilung Allgemein-, Thorax-, Gefäß- und Transplantationschirurgie, Universitätsklinikum Rostock, Schillingallee 35 - Stat, B 18055 Rostock, Germany
e-mail: bettina.rau@med.uni-rostock.de

B. Poch
Zentrum für onkologische, endokrinologische und minimalinvasive Chirurgie,
Silcherstr., 36 89231 Neu-Ulm, Germany
e-mail: bertram.poch@eurosurgery.de

R. Mantke et al. (eds.), *International Practices in Pancreatic Surgery*,
DOI 10.1007/978-3-540-74506-8_21, © Springer-Verlag Berlin Heidelberg 2013

Table 21.1 Frequency of necrotizing pancreatitis: surgical and interventional versus conservative management of necrotizing pancreatitis

Severe Acute Pancreatitis – surgical and non-surgical treatment: Ulm experience: 1,568 patients[a], *n* (%)			
	Frequency	Treatment modality	
	Patients pats (*n*)	Conservative pats	Surg/drainage/intervent
Interstitial-oedematousp.	1,071/68.3%	1,056/98.6%	15/1.4%[b]
Necrotizing pancreatitis	359/22.9%	95/26.5%	264/73.5%
Sterile necrosis	227	85/37.5%	142/62.5%
Infected necrosis	132	10/7.6%	122/92.4%
Pancreatic abscess	42/2.7%	3/7.1%	39/92.9%
Postacute pseudocyst	96/6.1%	22/22.9%	74/77.1%

Beger and Rau (2007)

[a]5/1982 to 12/1999 Department of General Surgery, University of Ulm, Germany

[b]Biliary tract surgery not included

and infection of necrosis causing clinical sepsis are determinants of outcome of severe acute pancreatitis (Rau et al. 2006). A subgroup of about 5–8 % of patients with severe acute pancreatitis shows systemic organ dysfunction within the first 72 h after onset of acute pancreatitis with the risk of early MOFS (Isenmann et al. 2001). Fatalities within the first 2 weeks after onset of acute pancreatitis account for about 50 % of the in-hospital deaths due to MOFS (Beger and Rau 2007). About 5–10 % of patients die in the first days of fulminant acute pancreatitis with MOFS but without the clinical diagnosis of acute pancreatitis, but the diagnosis of acute pancreatitis is only established by autopsy (Lankisch et al. 1991). The mortality of severe acute pancreatitis due to persistent MOFS during the later course of severe acute pancreatitis appears to be related to super infection of the pancreatic necrosis secondary to bacteremia from translocation of gut bacteria into the lymphatic and systemic circulation (Beger et al. 1986). Infection of the pancreatic and peripancreatic necrosis appears to be a time-related mechanism; up to 70 % of patients with infected necrosis present in the third or fourth week of the disease with a dominance of gram-negative bacteria (Beger et al. 1986). Patients with extensive necrosis (>50 % of the pancreas) appear to have a greater predilection to developing infected necrosis approaching 70 % (Beger et al. 1986). Sepsis secondary to infected necrosis is the dominant risk factor for death in the late course (after the third week) of severe acute pancreatitis.

21.2 Conservative, Non-interventional Management of Severe Acute Pancreatitis

Patients with severe acute pancreatitis (based on the Atlanta classification (Bradley 1993)), particularly those with organ dysfunction at time of hospital admission, should be treated in the intensive care unit (Table 21.2). Patients with systemic organ dysfunction in the first days of the disease require early maximum intensive care treatment. Early vigorous intra-venous fluid replacement as advocated by the Magdeburg Report is of foremost importance. The goal is to decrease the hematocrit and restore normal cardio-circulatory function (Brown et al. 2002).

21.3 Antibiotic Prophylaxis Contrary to Evidence-Based Data?

Antibiotic prophylaxis using antibiotics with the greatest penetration into pancreatic tissue has not been shown to be an effective preventive treatment (Isenmann et al. 2004). Based on results of four, randomized, controlled, double-blind clinical trials, antibiotic prophylaxis was unable to decrease neither hospital mortality nor the frequency of infected necrosis (Brown et al. 2002; Isenmann et al. 2004; Dellinger et al. 2007; Garcia-Barrasa et al. 2009). Consequently, a meta-analysis based on these trials concluded that antibiotic prophylaxis in severe acute pancreatitis was not effective; several prospective, albeit poorly controlled clinical trials of lesser level of evidence, came to a contrary conclusion. Different from the Magdeburg group, our group does not consider antibiotic prophylaxis as a standard in the treatment of severe acute pancreatitis (Mazaki et al. 2006). For patients with a systemic infection, e.g. pneumonia, urogenital infection, and/or bacteriaemia, a rational antibiotic application is, however, used.

Early enteral nutrition in patients with severe acute pancreatitis is usually not possible in the first week of the disease because of ileus. Enteral nutrition has been shown convincingly to decrease the frequency of infected necrosis, shortens the ICU stay, and decreases systemic complications; in contrast, two meta-analyses of 6 randomized, controlled, clinical trials of enteral nutrition failed to show any decrease in hospital mortality (Oláh et al. 2002; Windsor et al. 1998).

For patients with biliary acute pancreatitis, early endoscopic intervention to clear the common bile duct from biliary stones by ERC with stone extraction has become a routine and successful treatment (Neoptolemos et al. 1988). Contrast-enhanced CT provides the greatest diagnostic accuracy for necrotizing pancreatitis when performed in the end of the first week of the disease. Several groups have shown convincingly a close correlation between extent (>50 % of pancreas) of necrosis and clinical severity (Bradley 1993; Rau et al. 2007).

To identify infection of pancreatic necrosis, fine needle aspiration of the area(s) of necrosis under contrast-enhanced, CT guidance has the greatest diagnostic accuracy; extraluminal gas in the pancreatic or peripancreatic area, as demonstrated by CECT, is also highly accurate.

21.4 Who Benefits from Conservative, Non-interventional and Non-surgical Treatment?

The first choice for treatment of patients with necrotizing pancreatitis and presence of organ failure is aggressive management in the ICU (Table 21.2). Patients with organ failure at admission are candidates for maximum ICU treatment to avoid MOFS. As shown in Table 21.2, patients with focal and extended sterile pancreatic necrosis without organ failure who respond to ICU treatment are not candidates for any intervention (Rau et al. 1995). Several groups have demonstrated like the authors' group that selected patients with infected necrosis established by FNA-positive aspiration but who lack signs of sepsis do not need any type of intervention other than focused parenteral antibiotics, provided clinical sepsis is absent (Rau et al. 2005).

Table 21.2 Who benefits from conservative treatment of acute pancreatitis?

First choice of treatment of Patients with NP+OF is ICU management
Patients with OF at admission are candidates for maximum ICU treatment to avoid MOFS
Benefit from ICU treatment:
NP: focal and extended sterile pancreatic necrosis without OF /MOF
Peripancreatic necrosis without OF/MOF
Infected necrosis: FNA positive necrosis without clinical signs of sepsis
Peripancreatic fluid collection (but EUS/CT-guided puncture/drainage may be indicated)

NP necrotizing pancreatitis, *OF* organ failure, *MOF* multiorgan failure, *FNP* CT-guided fine needle aspiration

Patients with sterile necrosis are considered candidates for conservative management; however, a substantial proportion of patients with extended (>50 %) sterile necroses develop organ or multi-organ dysfunction early in the course of their disease (Rau et al. 1995), and many will develop infection of the necrosis later in the course of the disease. In the authors' institution, patients with extended necrosis who do not respond to maximum ICU treatment (>50 %) are candidates for operative debridement (Rau et al. 1995).

21.5 Indications for Interventional and Operative Treatment of Pancreatic Necrosis

For patients with infected necrosis and organ or multi-organ dysfunction, an early intervention is indicated (Beger and Rau 2007) (Table 21.3).

Table 21.3 Surgical debridement of Necrotizing pancreatitis: necrosectomy and Bursa-Lavage and minimal invasive Debridement

	Period of public.	Pats.	Infect. necrosis	Postop. compl.	Reop.	Hospital mortality
Open debrid.	1990–2006[a]	814	64%	36%	25.1%	15.1%
Minimal invasive	1998–2006[a]	180	83%	70.6%	3–4/pat.	18.3%

Beger and Rau (2007)
[a]Pederzoli (1990), Farkas (1996), Beger (1998), Mai (2000), Hungness (2002), Farkas (2006)
[b]Freeny (1998), Gouzi (1999), Carter (2000), Horvath (2001), Castellanos (2002), Connor (2003), Zhou (2003), Connor (2005)

In our opinion, the recommendation of the Magdeburg group to delay operative debridement until after the 28th day of disease is not supported by convincing randomized trials, based on the demarcation hypothesis of necrosis. This concept has been propagated as a step up approach from a minimal invasive, radiologically guided drainage of the infected necrosis to a later open necrosectomy (Van Santvoort et al. 2010); however, no evidence-based data for the superiority of a minimal-invasive approach compared to early open necrosectomy have been published that document convincingly a decrease in hospital mortality (Van Santvoort et al. 2010).

21.6 Late Interventional Debridement Does Not Decrease the High Early Mortality

When comparing open versus the step-up approach in a prospective, randomized, multicentre trial, the final hospital mortality was the same in both groups, open necrosectomy versus the minimal invasive step-up approach (Van Santvoort et al. 2010). In contrast, the new onset of MOF was more frequent after open debridement as was the onset of post-operative diabetes and post-operative incisional hernias. The limitation of this randomized clinical trial as a guideline for all patients with severe acute pancreatitis with infected necrosis or extended sterile necrosis is the ability to delay intervention until after the third or fourth week of disease, because as many as 21–54 % of patients with early severe acute pancreatitis and persistent MOF die in the first or/and second week. The step-up approach is, thereby, limited by excluding those patients with early fatal necrotizing pancreatitis (Van Santvoort et al. 2010; Zerem et al. 2011).

As summarized in Table 21.3, the minimal invasive approach comprising a laparoscopic trans-abdominal and retroperitoneal approach has a similar level of hospital mortality as open debridement. For open debridement, we don't use a bilateral, subcostal incision, because this is an unnecessarily extensive access with an increased risk of wound infection; we prefer a small, mid-line incision of 10–15 cm length in the upper abdomen. The major advantage of radiologic intervention and minimal invasive debridement are the minimal invasive trauma (Zerem et al. 2011). In contrast, for radiologic drainage/intervention, drainage periods, frequency of re-access for multiple re-interventions for drain replacement and repositioning, recurrent episodes of sepsis, and a prolonged duration of hospitalisation are drawbacks of primary, radiologic drainage interventions (Table 21.4).

For the albeit rare patients who develop a true pancreatic "abscess" with a well localized collection of pus, radiologic drainage should be the first treatment option (Bittner et al. 1987). Comparing minimal invasive techniques with open necrosectomy, hospital costs are similar (Beenen et al. 2011). For drainage of infected necrosis, we believe strongly that the laparoscopic approach as well as the retroperitoneal minimal invasive necrosectomy should be combined with a continuous postoperative lavage of the infected cavity using a dialysis solution or physiologic NaCl solution (Rau and Beger 2008a).

Table 21.4 Necrotizing pancreatitis. Percutaneous catheter drainage (aPCD): results of seven clinical prospective trials

Time of Publications	Patients N	OF failure	Infected necrosis	Time to PCD	Successful	Need for additon surgery	Mortality	Hospital stay mean
1998–2009	305		207/305	17.6 day	197/305	92/305	55/305	27–89 day
		46–75%	68%		65%	30%	18%	

[a]Freeny, *Am J Roentgenol*, 1998; Fotoohi, *Radiology*, 1999; Navalho, *Clin Imaging*, 2006; Mortabé, *Am J Reontgenol*, 2009; Baril, *Ann Surg*, 2000; Bruennler, *World J Gastroenterol*, 2008; Rocha, *Arch Surg*, 2009

Table 21.5 Indication to minimal invasive and/or open surgical debridement for infected necrosis

The main goal of any intervention – interventional drainage of minimal invasive access or open debridement – is to interrupt the sepsis syndrome and to improve/eradicate organ failure/s
Infection of pancreatic/peripancreatic necrosis
+Clinical signs of sepsis
–Gas bubbles in CT
–FNA positivity with clinical persistence of sepsis
Infected necrosis: persistence of clinical sepsis + MOD after failure of repeated drainage or minimal-invasive interventions
Pancreatic abscess/Infected fluid collection
Clinical acute abdomen:
Colon transversum ischemia/perforation
Massive intrapancreatic hemorrhage
Abdominal compartment syndrome + OF/MOF

[a]Rau and Beger (2008a)

21.7 Indication for Open Necrosectomy (Table 21.5)

Patients with extended necrosis (>50 % of the pancreas) causing persistent clinical sepsis or MOF who do not respond to ICU treatment have been treated in the authors' institution with open debridement (Rau and Beger 2008a; Petrov et al. 2010) early after the diagnosis (Figs. 21.1 and 21.2) (Table 21.5). A minimally invasive or open necrosectomy is recommended for patients who have necrosis in the pancreatic head as well as other multicentric foci in the body and/or tail of the pancreas, because percutaneous drains have a limited role in these cases. The greatest risk of a complicated course and mortality involve patients with extended sterile necrosis extending to more than 50 % of the pancreas (Rau et al. 2006). Operative intervention for sterile necrosis is not considered in many institutions. Debridement has been performed in specialized institutions with low hospital mortality (Table 21.3) (Rau and Beger 2008b). Patients with an acute abdomen caused by intestinal perforation and patients with abdominal compartment syndrome and intra-cavitary bleeding respond immediately to an open operative treatment with improvement in their clinical course

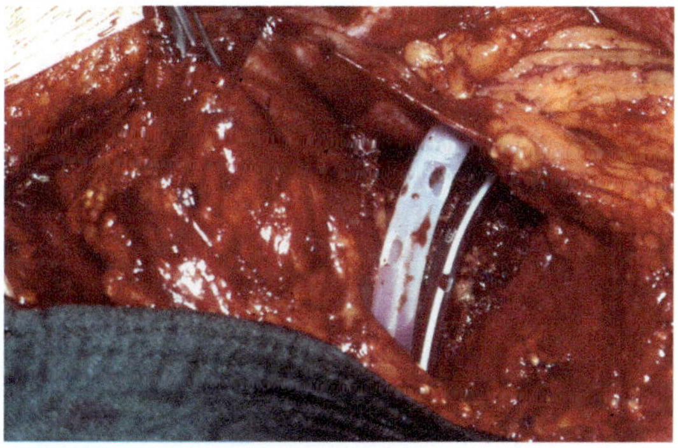

Fig. 21.1 Situs open debridement of extended sterile necrosis on the end of the first week of disease after small midline incision and small incision of the ligamentum gastrocolicum, exposition of the necrotic gravity 2 weeks after

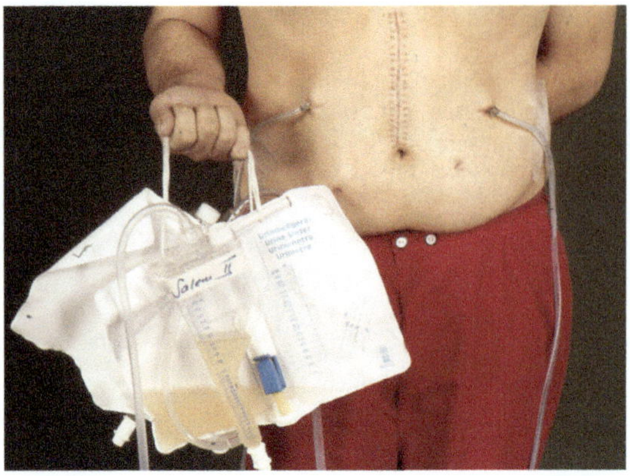

Fig. 21.2 Open debridement of infected necrosis after finishing the debridement two large catheters are placed in situ. The two catheters have a small inflow tube for institution of a continuous lavage with outflow through the large drains. The lavage catheters are channelled through incisions on both sides subcostally on the level of the axilliar line

(Wysocki et al. 2010; Remes-Troche et al. 2006). The randomized, prospective, controlled Dutch trial comparing minimal invasive drainage using the step up approach from a radiologically guided drainage to open necrosectomy to a primary open necrosectomy did not show any decrease in mortality for the minimal invasive approach compared to open necrosectomy. This study did, however, show that post-operative onset of MOF and new post-operative diabetes (after 6 months) was decreased significantly in the group with the minimal invasive step-up approach (Van Santvoort et al. 2010) compared to open debridement.

References

Balthazar EJ, Robinson DL, Megibow AJ, Ranson JH (1990) Acute pancreatitis: value of CT in establishing prognosis. Radiology 174:331–336

Baril NB, Ralls PW, Wren SM, Selby RR, Radin R, Parekh D, Jabbour N, Stain SC (2000) Does an infected peripancreatic fluid collection or abscess mandate operation? Ann Surg 231:361–367

Beenen E, Brown L, Connor S (2011) A comparison of the hospital costs of open vs. minimally invasive surgical management of necrotizing pancreatitis. HPB 13:178–184

Beger HG, Rau B (2007) Severe acute pancreatitis. Clinical course and management. World J Gastroenterol 13:5043–5051

Beger HG, Bittner R, Block S et al (1986) Bacterial contamination of pancreatic necrosis. Gastroenterology 49:433–440

Beger HG, Rau B, Isenmann R, Mayer J (1998) Surgical treatment of acute pancreatitis. Ann Chir Gynaecol 87:183–189

Bittner R, Block S, Büchler M, Beger HG (1987) Pancreatic abscess and infected pancreatic necrosis. Different local septic complications in acute pancreatitis. Dig Dis Sci 32:1082–1087

Bradley EL III (1993) A clinically based classification system for acute pancreatitis: summary of the international symposium on acute pancreatitis. Arch Surg 128:586–590

Brown A, Baillargeon JD, Hughes MD, Banks PA (2002) Can fluid resuscitation prevent pancreatic necrosis in severe acute pancreatitis? Pancreatology 2:104–107

Bruennler T, Langgartner J, Lang S et al (2008) Outcome of patients with acute, necrotizing pancreatitis requiring drainage-does drainage size matter? World J Gastroenterol 14:725–730

Carter CR, McKay CJ, Imrie CW (2000) Percutaneous necrosectomy and sinus tract endoscopy in the management of infected pancreatic necrosis: an initial experience. Ann Surg 232:175–180

Castellanos G, Pinero A, Serrano A et al (2005) Translumbar retroperitoneal endoscopy: an alternative in the follow up and management of drained infected pancreatic necrosis. Arch Surg 140:952–955

Connor S, Ghaneh P, Raraty M et al (2003) Increasing age and APACHE II scores are the main determinants of outcome following pancreatic necrosectomy. Br J Surg 90:1542–1548

Connor S, Raraty MGT, Howes N et al (2005) Surgery in the treatment of acute pancreatitis – minimal access pancreatic necrosectomy. Scand J Surg 94:135–142

Dellinger EP, Tellado JM, Soto NE et al (2007) Early antibiotic treatment for severe acute necrotizing pancreatitis. Ann Surg 245:674–683

Farkas G, Márton J, Mándi Y et al (1996) Surgical strategy and management of infected pancreatic necrosis. Br J Surg 83:930–933

Farkas G, Márton J, Maindi Y et al (2006) Surgical management and complex treatment of infected pancreatic necrosis: 18-year experience at a single center. J Gastrointest Surg 10:278–285

Fotoohi M, D'Agostino HB, Wollman B, Chon K, Shahrokni S, van Sonnenberg E (1999) Persistent pancreatocutaneous fistula after percutaneous drainage of pancreatic fluid collections: role of cause and severity of pancreatitis. Radiology 213:573–578

Freeny PC, Hauptmann E, Althaus SJ et al (1998) Percutaneous CT-guided catheter drainage of infected acute necrotizing pancreatitis: techniques and results. AJR Am J Roentgenol 170:969–975

Garcia-Barrasa A, Borobia F, Pallares R et al (2009) A double-blind, placebo-controlled trial fo ciprofloxacin prphylaxis in patients with acute necrotizing pancreatitis. J Gastrointest Surg 13:768–774

Gouzi JL, Bloom E, Julio C et al (1999) Percutaneous drainage of infected pancreatic necrosis: an alternative to surgery. Chirurgie 124:31–37

Horvath KD, Kao LS, Wherry KL et al (2001) A technique for laparoscopic-assisted percutaneous drainage of infected pancreatic necrosis and pancreatic abscess. Surg Endosc 15:1221–1225

Hungness ES, Robb BW, Seeskin C et al (2002) Early debridement for necrotizing pancreatitis: is it worthwhile? J Am Coll Surg 194:740–744

Isenmann R, Rau BM, Beger HG (2001) Early severe acute pancreatitis – characteristics of a new subgroup. Pancreas 22:274–278

Isenmann R, Rünzi M, Kron M et al (2004) Prophylactic antibiotic treatment in patients with predicted severe acute pancreatitis: a placebo-controlled, double-blind trial. Gastroenterology 126:997–1004

Lankisch PG, Schirren CA, Kunze E (1991) Undetected fatal acute pancreatitis: why is the disease so frequently overlooked? Am J Gastroenterol 86:322–326

Mai G, Uhl W, Muller C et al (1999) The conservative surgical management of severe acute pancreatitis: the bernese approach. In: Buechler MW, Uhl W, Friess H et al (eds) Acute pancreatitis: newer concepts in biology and therapy. Blackwell Science, Oxford, pp 475–486

Mayer J, Rau B, Gansauge F, Beger HG (2000) Inflammatory mediators in human acute pancreatitis: clinical and pathophysiological implications. Gut 47:546–552

Mazaki T, Ishii Y, Takayama T (2006) Meta-analysis of prophylactic antibiotic use in acute necrotizing pancreatitis. Br J Surg 93:674–684

Mole DJ, Olabi B, Robinson V et al (2009) Incidence of individual organ dysfunction in fatal acute pancreatitis: analysis of 1024 death records. HPB 11: 166–170

Mortelé KJ, Girshman J, Szejnfeld D et al (2009) CT-guided percutaneous catheter drainage of acute necrotizing pancreatitis: clinical experience and observations in patients with sterile and infected necrosis. AJR Am J Roentgenol 192:110–116

Navalho M, Pires F, Duarte A et al (2006) Percutaneous drainage of infected pancreatic fluid collections in critically ill patients: correlation with C-reactive protein values. Clin Imaging 30:114–119

Neoptolemos JP, Carr-Locke DL, London NJ et al (1988) Controlled trial of urgent endoscopic retrograde cholangiopancreatography and endoscopic sphincterotomy versus conservative treatment for acute pancreatitis due to gallstones. Lancet 2:979–983

Oláh A, Pardavi G, Belágyi T et al (2002) Early nasojejunal feeding in acute pancreatitis is associated with a lower complication rate. Nutrition 18:259–262

Pederzoli P, Bassi C, Vesentini S et al (1990) Retroperitoneal and peritoneal drainage and lavage in the treatment of severe necrotizing pancreatitis. Surg Gynecol Obstet 170:197–202

Petrov MS, Shanbhag S, Chakraborty M et al (2010) Organ failure and infection of pancreatic necrosis as determinants of mortality in patients with acute pancreatitis. Gastroenterology 139:813–820

Poch B, Gansauge F, Rau B et al (1999) The role of polymorphonuclear leukocytes and oxygen-derived free radicals in experimental acute pancreatitis: mediators of local destruction and activators of inflammation. FEBS Lett 461:268–272

Rau BM, Beger HG (2008a) Surgical management of necrotizing pancreatitis – debridement and continuous lavage. The pancreas, 2nd edn. Blackwell Publishing, Malden, pp 308–313

Rau BM, Beger HG (2008b) Necrosectomy and closed lavage. In: Beger HG, Matsuno S, Cameron JL (eds) Diseases of the pancreas. Current surgical therapy. Springer, Heidelberg, pp 231–240

Rau B, Pralle U, Uhl W et al (1995) Management of sterile necrosis in instances of severe acute pancreatitis. J Am Coll Surg 181:279–288

Rau B, Bothe A, Beger HG (2005) Surgical treatment of necrotizing pancreatitis by necrosectomy and closed lavage: changing patient characteristics and outcome in a 19-year, single-center series. Surgery 138:28–39

Rau BM, Bothe A, Kron M, Beger HG (2006) Role of early multisystem organ failure as major risk factor for pancreatic infections and death in severe acute pancreatitis. Clin Gastroenterol Hepatol 4:1053–1061

Rau BM, Kemppainen EA, Gumbs AA et al (2007) Early assessment of pancreatic infections and overall prognosis in severe acute pancreatitis by procalcitonin (PCT): a prospective international multicenter study. Ann Surg 245:745–754

Remes-Troche JM, Uscanga LF, Peláez-Luna M et al (2006) When should we be concerned about pancreatic necrosis? Analysis from a single institution in Mexico City. World J Surg 30.2227–2233; discussion 2234–5

Rocha FG, Benoit E, Zinner MJ et al (2009) Impact of radiologic intervention on mortality in necrotizing pancreatitis: the role of organ failure. Arch Surg 144:261–265

Van Santvoort HC, Besselink MG, Bakker OJ et al (2010) A step up approach or open necrosectomy for necrotizing pancreatitis. N Engl J Med 362:1491–1502

Windsor AC, Kanwar S, Li AG, Barnes E et al (1998) Compared with parenteral nutrition, enteral feeding attenuates the acute phase response and improves disease severity in acute pancreatitis. Gut 42:431–435

Wysocki AP, McKay CJ, Carter CR (2010) Infected pancreatic necrosis: minimizing the cut. ANZ J Surg 80:58–70

Zerem E, Imamovi G, Suši A, Hara i B (2011) Step-up approach to infected necrotising pancreatitis: a 20-year experience of percutaneous drainage in a single centre. Dig Liver Dis 43:478–483

Zhou ZG, Zheng YC, Shu Y et al (2003) Laparoscopic management of severe acute pancreatitis. Pancreas 27:46–50

Commentary

22

Peter Fagenholz and Carlos Fernández-del Castillo

22.1 Relevant Basic Information, Indications, and Contraindications

The diagnosis of acute pancreatitis is generally straightforward. The pillars of diagnostic evaluation are the clinical history (abdominal pain, nausea, vomiting) and serum amylase and lipase determination. We perform ultrasonography primarily to assess for gallstones as the cause of the episode of pancreatitis, and to look for bile duct dilation as a possible sign of ongoing choledocholithiasis – however, ultrasonography is of limited utility in evaluating the pancreas itself.

We agree that contrast-enhanced computed tomography (CT) is the most specific imaging modality available for diagnosing acute pancreatitis. CT is rarely necessary for diagnosis, though CT may be valuable for excluding other potential sources of abdominal pain, assessing biliary obstruction, identifying necrosis at an early stage, and for prognostication. We do not, however, perform routine "initial CT assessment" of patients in whom we confidently diagnose acute pancreatitis for several reasons. First, patients with severe pancreatitis often present with acute kidney injury which may be worsened by the administration of intravenous contrast agents. Second, there is some experimental and clinical evidence that intravenous contrast may contribute to the worsening of pancreatic necrosis. Finally, in our experience, many patients who will go on to develop extensive necrosis may lack obvious non-enhancement of the pancreatic parenchyma and have only edema evident on a CT performed at the time of presentation, as the authors allude to in Table 22.1 where they state, "early CT may underestimate the ultimate severity of pancreatitis." Most of these patients will require a repeat CT early in their course (such as at 4–5 days, as the authors suggest) to determine the extent of necrosis. We find that an initial CT evaluation rarely alters our management during this initial period, while carrying some risk of possible harm. Recent studies have stressed the overuse of CT in necrotizing pancreatitis and outlined the very real dangers with regard to radiation exposure and financial impact.

As the authors point out, antibiotic prophylaxis remains a matter of debate. Historically, the vast majority of our patients have received antibiotic prophylaxis, usually with a carbepenem. Nevertheless, more recently we have trended away from the routine use of antibiotics because of the lack of proven efficacy in Level 1, randomized studies. We agree that endoscopic retrograde cholangiography (ERC) should not be used routinely in cases of gallstone pancreatitis, but ERC is indicated if there is evidence of biliary obstruction due to a retained gallstone in the common bile duct.

Management throughout the early phase of the systemic inflammatory response syndrome (SIRS) that accompanies acute pancreatitis so frequently

P. Fagenholz, M.D. (✉) • C.F.-del Castillo, M.D.
Department of Surgery, Massachusetts General Hospital, Harvard Medical School, Boston, MA, USA
e-mail: pfagenholz@partners.org

R. Mantke et al. (eds.), *International Practices in Pancreatic Surgery*,
DOI 10.1007/978-3-540-74506-8_22,

Table 22.1 Pancreatic débridements for acute necrotizing pancreatitis performed from 2006 to 2010

	Number (%)
Patients	67
Etiology	Alcoholic 23 (34 %)
	Biliary 20 (30 %)
	Unknown 9 (13 %)
	Hypertrigyceridemia 5 (8 %)
	Post-ERCP 4 (6 %)
	Post-operative 4 (6 %)
	Other 2 (3 %)
Indications	Infection 47 (71 %)
	SIRS 9 (13 %)
	Persistently unwell 6 (9 %)
	Persistent pancreatitis 4 (6 %)
	Hemorrhage 1 (1 %)
Microbiology	Infected necrosis 52 (77 %)
	Sterile necrosis 15 (23 %)
Reoperation	11 (16 %)
Mortality	6 (9 %)

ERCP endoscopic retrograde cholangiopancreatography, *SIRS* systemic inflammatory response syndrome
Indications: All patients had demonstrated necrosis. If infection was proven or strongly suspected, that was considered the primary indication for débridement. SIRS was considered the indication in cases where the decision to operate was based on the presence of necrosis without demonstrable infection in a patient with escalating, life-threatening SIRS. Persistent pancreatitis denotes repeated episodes of acute pain with increases in serum amylase and lipase after the primary episode of necrotizing pancreatitis. The persistently unwell patient usually has chronic, low grade, but unresolving symptoms (e.g. intolerance of oral feeds, nausea, weight loss, abdominal pain, or fever) after an episode of necrotizing pancreatitis

is generally non-operative. We attempt to use enteral nutrition whenever possible because its use has been associated with decreased rates of infected pancreatic necrosis. If nutritional needs cannot be met enterally, then parenteral nutritional support is utilized. The surgeon must remain involved closely throughout this phase of the illness because infected necrosis or abscess may intervene, and plans for treatment need to be made with an eye toward possible eventual operative intervention should a less invasive approach not be indicated.

Proven infected necrosis remains the one consensus indication for some formal necrosectomy in acute pancreatitis. Infected necrosis is demonstrated typically by either CT findings of extraluminal gas within areas of pancreatic necrosis or by staining and culture of specimens from CT-guided fine needle aspiration (FNA) of areas of pancreatic or peripancreatic necrosis. It is important to note, however, that CT-guided FNA may have a 20–25 % false negative rate and even occasional false positives. We cannot overemphasize the clinical observation that when faced with a patient with known pancreatic necrosis who is failing to improve, either in the critically ill phase (persistent organ failure, SIRS) or even as an outpatient (low grade fever, failure to tolerate oral feeding, the so-called "persistent unwell") the diagnosis of infected necrosis must be entertained and necrosectomy considered strongly, even after a negative FNA. Many of these patients will have infection demonstrated from the operative samples; in addition, we have found that many with sterile necrosis will nonetheless improve clinically. As the authors point out, localized areas of infected necrosis can be treated sometimes with a combination of endoscopic and percutaneous drainage. More commonly, however, with extensive peripancreatic necrosis, we maintain that operative necrosectomy is required.

Even in patients who have documented infected necrosis early in their course, we prefer to wait 4 weeks if possible from the onset of pancreatitis until operation. This delay in necrosectomy allows the necrotic tissue to completely demarcate from viable pancreatic and retroperitoneal tissue, minimizing the risks of incomplete débridement, bleeding, and post-operative pancreatic insufficiency. We developed this general policy after a review of our own data demonstrated an optimal composite outcome score (including death, intensive care utilization, need for further operative or percutaneous procedures, and other major complications) if débridement was performed at 27 days. Waiting for a greater period of time did not confer added advantage.

22.2 Operative Technique

It is critical that a recent CT, preferably with oral and intravenous contrast, be available in the operating room to ensure that all areas with necrosis

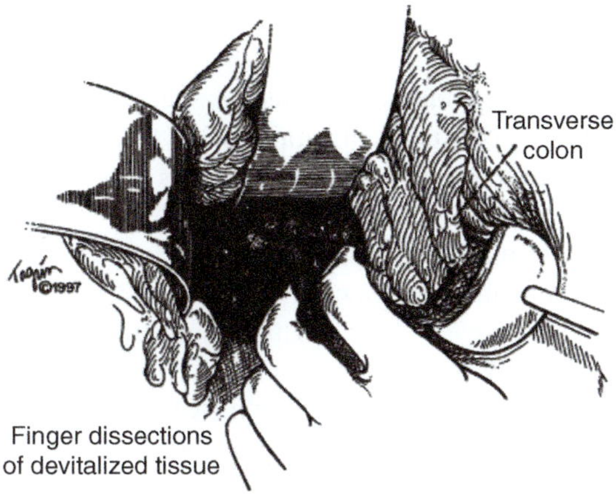

Fig. 22.1 Blunt débridement of the lesser sac through the transverse mesocolon (Reproduced with permission from: Fernández-del Castillo et al. (1998))

or fluid recognized preoperatively are recognized and addressed intraoperatively. Manual blunt necrosectomy with closed packing is our preferred technique. We usually begin with a midline incision.

Our primary approach to the lesser sac is through the transverse mesocolon (Fig. 22.1). We believe this approach offers a number of advantages over an anterior approach into the lesser sac:

1. It avoids a difficult and time-consuming dissection of the stomach and omentum off the transverse colon, which is often densely adherent due to inflammation in the lesser sac.
2. By avoiding the risk of even small serosal tears to the transverse colon in a setting of infection and possible pancreatic fistula, this approach may decrease the risk of colo-cutaneous fistula.
3. Entry through the base of the mesocolon allows drains to be placed in a dependent position posterior in the lesser sac.

Commonly, the mesocolon to the left of the ligament of Treitz is thinned, allowing easy entry through this usually avascular region into the area of necrosis and fluid collection. The middle colic vessels are often thrombosed, but if they are patent and present an impediment, they can be divided, usually without sequelae. If left-sided collections in the retrocolic or pararenal spaces cannot be reached by this approach, they may require medial mobilization of the splenic flexure of the colon. If collections or necrosis surrounding the head of the pancreas cannot be reached via this left-sided approach, a second opening may be made in the right side of the transverse mesocolon. Care should be taken to remain oriented to the position of the superior mesenteric vessels relative to the areas of necrosis when this approach is used. Right sided collections that cannot be reached via the transmesocolic approach can be exposed by mobilizing the hepatic flexure of the colon medially with the second and third portions of the duodenum as necessary.

While this anterior, transperitoneal, transmesocolic approach is our primary technique, it is worth noting that in selected patients with a localized retroperitoneal area of necrosis or fluid collection, a primary retroperitoneal approach can be simpler and yield excellent results. In cases fitting this description, we prefer, if possible, to have a percutaneous drain placed by a totally retroperitoneal access route. If this does not resolve the infection and débridement is required, a more limited incision can be made over the skin access point of the drainage catheter, and the catheter can then be followed into the area of necrosis. This operative approach to necrosectomy can also be done videoscopically.

Once areas of fluid and necrosis are exposed by any approach, fluid should be drained and devitalized tissue débrided bluntly. Dissection with fingers combined with use of blunt, circular sponge clamps and vigorous irrigation allows separation of necrotic tissue from still viable tissue. All necrotic tissue should be removed and sent for microbiologic analysis. Sharp dissection should be avoided. Bleeding from cavity walls may be from granulation tissue or from major vascular structures. Bleeding from major vessels should be controlled with sutures if possible, but if exposure is difficult, packing may be required.

Once all areas of necrosis have been drained and débrided thoroughly, we pack any resulting cavities with ¾ in. Penrose drains stuffed with gauze, and then place soft, silicone-rubber closed-suction drains into each major extension of the cavity (Fig. 22.2). Each drain, Penrose or closed

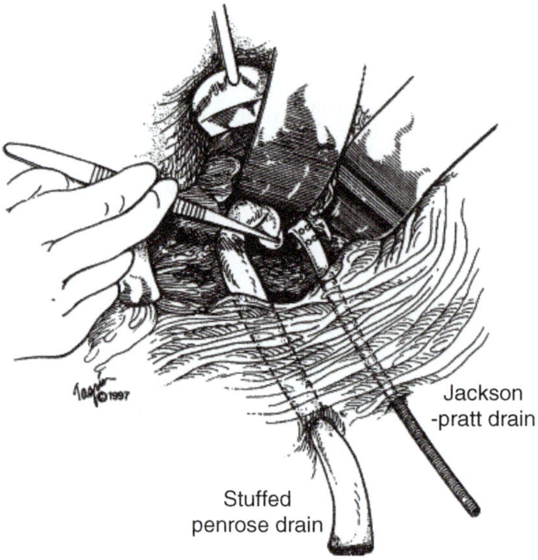

Fig. 22.2 Packing of the cavity with stuffed Penrose and Jackson-Pratt drains (Reproduced with permission from: Fernández-del Castillo et al. (1998))

suction, is brought out through a separate stab incision in the abdominal wall and sutured to the skin.

If indicated, cholecystectomy is performed at the time of débridement. Bowel resection or diversion may be required if enteric fistula or perforation is present. Occasionally involvement of the splenic vessels may result in splenic infarction necessitating splenectomy. Rarely, decompressive gastrostomy or feeding jejunostomy is also performed.

22.3 Additional Treatments and Procedures

Postoperative antibiotics are tailored to the culture results as they become available. We continue antibiotics usually for 10–14 days after débridement. Enteral feeding is preferred. Many patients can tolerate an oral diet. In those who cannot, nasogastric or nasojejunal tubes are placed as needed, or gastrostomy or jejunostomy feeding can be instituted.

The stuffed Penrose drains are left in place for 1 week and then removed, usually at the rate of one drain every other day. Removal of these drains allows the packed cavity to close gradually and allows large particulate matter a route of egress. Closed suction drains are left in place until output is minimal, and there is no evidence of ongoing pancreatic fistula. Low output (<100 mL/day) fistulas may be managed by sequentially withdrawing the closed suction drain by 2 cm every week. This lengthening of the fistulous tract encourages closure of the fistula. If fever, abdominal pain, or inability to tolerate oral intake occurs during the process of sequential drain withdraw, abdominal CT is performed seeking an intraabdominal collection. Regardless of the presence of a fistula, any patient who does not continue to improve after débridement should undergo abdominal CT scanning. In our experience, 30 % of patients will require subsequent percutaneous drain placement after débridement, so residual fluid collections should be sought actively if clinical progress is poor.

22.4 Results

Results from 2006 to 2010 are included in Table 22.1. We have reported our results previously for 1990–2005 using the technique described above Rodriguez et al. (2008). For that longer time period, our overall mortality in 167 patients undergoing operative débridement was 11 % (20 % in patients operated before 28 days vs. 5 % in patients operated after 28 days, $P=0.002$). The reoperation rate was 13 % and the rate of post-operative percutaneous intervention was 30 %. The median post-operative duration of hospital stay was 19 days (range 4–195 days).

22.5 Summary

A comparison of our method for operative treatment of necrotizing pancreatitis with that of the authors both demonstrates areas of growing consensus, but also illustrates points of divergence in contemporary management of this disease. CT imaging for the identification of necrosis and planning of operative therapy, infected necrosis as the primary indication for débridement, and delaying débridement to 4 weeks after the onset of symptoms whenever possible have taken hold as accepted principles of management. Nonetheless, considerable variability in practice likely persists regarding the role of débridement in the persistently unwell patient without preoperatively proven infected necrosis, the role of minimally invasive drainage or débridement techniques, and the technical approaches to open débridement. These areas require further research to optimize patient care in the interesting and challenging disease.

References

Fernández-del Castillo C, Rattner DW, Makary MA et al (1998) Débridement and closed packing for the treatment of necrotizing pancreatitis. Ann Surg 228(5):676–684

Rodriguez JR, Razo AO, Targarona J et al (2008) Débridement and closed packing for sterile or infected necrotizing pancreatitis: insights into indications and outcomes in 167 patients. Ann Surg 247(2):294–299

Commentary

23

H.G. Gooszen

23.1 Introduction

Acute pancreatitis is a relatively common, potentially life-threatening disease, with annual costs exceeding $2 billion in the United States alone where more accurate estimates are available (Fagenholz et al. 2007; Shaheen et al. 2006). Approximately 20 % of patients develop severe acute pancreatitis, defined by organ failure or necrotizing pancreatitis (Banks and Freeman 2006). Mild pancreatitis is associated with a mortality of 0–1 %, whereas the mortality of severe pancreatitis ranges from 15 % for the severe form without infection to as great as 30 % for those patients who develop infected necrosis (Besselink et al. 2009). Sterile pancreatic necrosis and sterile peripancreatic collections can usually be treated conservatively. In contrast, secondary infection of necrosis – usually presenting clinically 3–4 weeks after the onset of disease – requires some form of active intervention in most cases (Besselink et al. 2009); if left untreated, mortality of infected necrosis approaches 100 % (Banks and Freeman 2006).

H.G. Gooszen
Department of Operating Theatres/Evidence Based Surgery, Radboud University Medical Centre, Nijmegen, The Netherlands
e-mail: h.gooszen@ok.umcn.nl

23.2 Clinical Presentation

It is widely accepted to base the diagnosis of acute pancreatitis on two of the following criteria: (a) severe abdominal pain, (b) serum amylase or lipase activity more than three times greater than the institution's upper limit, and findings of acute pancreatitis on (c) contrast-enhanced computed tomography (CECT) or magnetic resonance imaging (MRI). Usually, the first two criteria are present for confirmation of the diagnosis, and CECT is required only in those patients who present after several days of abdominal pain, when the serum amylase and lipase levels have normalized or in patients with organ failure of unknown origin. CECT will often fail to demonstrate the presence pancreatic necrosis and peripancreatic collections in the first 72–96 h of disease. For confirmation of the presence of necrosis, intravenous, not oral, contrast administration is required.

Ultrasonography may show pancreatic swelling, but bowel gas can prevent adequate visibility of the pancreas.

In this early stage, abdominal ultrasonography is essentially inadequate and unreliable in visualizing the pancreas. Detection of gallstones in search of the cause of the disease represents the only potential indication for abdominal ultrasonography at this time point in the course of

R. Mantke et al. (eds.), *International Practices in Pancreatic Surgery*,
DOI 10.1007/978-3-540-74506-8_23, © Springer-Verlag Berlin Heidelberg 2013

acute pancreatitis. In order to detect necrosis, CECT or MRI are far superior.

Recent insights in pathophysiology have proven very helpful, not only for understanding the disease but also to serve as a justification for new forms of treatment.

Severe acute pancreatitis normally runs a biphasic course. The first phase is characterized by a systemic inflammatory response syndrome (SIRS) and lasts about 2 weeks. Infection of necrosis is rare in this phase, but other systemic infections needing antibiotic treatment do occur during this phase of SIRS. In a recent study on 731 acute pancreatitis patients focusing on the timing of infection and the time frame available for prevention of infection, bacteriaemia and pneumonia (ventilator associated) were diagnosed most often in the first week of admission, whereas infection of the pancreatic and/or peripancreatic necrosis became manifest clinically in about the fourth week of disease (Besselink et al. 2009). Organ failure in this first phase of the disease is considered, therefore, not to be related to infection but rather to the effect of severe systemic inflammatory response.

The second phase of severe acute pancreatitis is characterized by a counteractive anti-inflammatory response syndrome (CARS), a phase wherein the patient becomes (highly) susceptible to infection. Organ failure in the second phase of severe acute pancreatitis (the CARS phase) is related to infections, such as infected necrosis. During this second phase, the necrosis becomes encapsulated, most likely by a similar sort of process as the formation of an abscess.

The impact on treatment of this pathophysiological concept is that in the SIRS phase there is essentially no place for surgery for the removal of (infected) necrosis, whereas in the second phase timing and type of intervention dominate treatment. The crucial elements in timing are: the moment of clinical manifestation of infection and the completion of encapsulation.

23.3 Predicting Severity

> C-reactive protein levels over 150 mg/l, an APACHE II score greater than 8 in the first 24 hours, or persistent organ failure in the first 24 hours, are established, clinically useful predictors of severity….

The clinical course of acute pancreatitis is highly unpredictable and may vary from full recovery within a single day to multi-organ failure and mortality within the first day or two. There is considerable confusion on how these "predictive scoring" systems can be or should be used in clinical practice, for several reasons: (1) there is no form of conservative or operative method to prevent the disease from progressing from a mild to the severe form, other than aggressive fluid administration to prevent dehydration or a "low flow state." This approach may prevent development of multiple organ failure or small bowel ischemia, but controlled studies are not available.

The most frequently used scores and cut-off points are listed in Table 23.1. If a patient meets one of the cut-off values for "predicted severe pancreatitis," this only means that such a patient is at greater risk of developing the severe form of the disease. The clinical value of the stigma "predicted severe pancreatitis" is limited, because the positive predictive value (the chance of truly developing severe pancreatitis) is around 50–70 %. With a negative predictive value of 85–90 %, patients with predicted mild pancreatitis run a 10–15 % risk of developing the severe form of disease.

"Predictive scoring" and Classifications Systems like the Atlanta Classification are indispensable in clinical studies to inform the reader about the characteristics of the population under study, but these scores do not help the clinician in their difficult task of taking care of the individual patient with severe acute pancreatitis.

> … and persistent organ failure in the first 24 hours, are established, clinically useful predictors of severity….

The same study on the timing of infection and the time frame available for prevention of infec-

Table 23.1 Most used predictive laboratory scoring systems in acute pancreatitis and their cut-off for predicted severe pancreatitis

Predictive score	Cut-off
APACHEII[a] score	≥8 in first 24 h
BISAP[b] score	≥3 in first 24 h
Modified Glasgow (or Imrie) score	≥3 in fist 48 h
Ranson score	≥3 in fist 48 h
Urea at admission	>60 mmol/L
C-reactive protein	>150 U/L in first 72 h

[a]*APACHE* Acute physiology and chronic health evaluation
[b]*BISAP* bedside index for severity in acute pancreatitis

tion, showed that organ failure is not so much a predictor of severity, but it turned out to be the most important determinant for mortality in acute pancreatitis (Besselink et al. 2009).

23.4 Classification of Severity

The updated Atlanta classification of acute pancreatitis continues to be developed. This classification may include a clinical subdivision into either *mild* or *severe* disease.

In the early phase, this subdivision is based on clinical parameters only, whereas in the weeks that follow, the development of complications prolonging hospitalization, either requiring active intervention (operative, endoscopic, laparoscopic, or percutaneous) or other supportive measures (such as need for respiratory ventilation, renal dialysis, or nasojejunal feeding) and morphologic changes on CECT, dominate the clinical picture. In this phase, classification relies on radiologic findings and is dominated by the presence or absence of intra- and/or extrapancreatic collections and necrosis and whether these collections are infected or not.

23.5 Conservative Management

In the first phase of severe pancreatitis, adequate fluid resuscitation represents the mainstay of treatment (Mao et al. 2009). A fluid regime guided by urine output (goal 1 ml/kg h urine production) is sufficient in the initial phase, as long as organ failure is not present yet. In this phase of the disease, we maintain that there is no room for necrosectomy, radiologically, endoscopically, or operatively in an attempt to "turn the tide." Intra-abdominal bleeding not able to be controlled by arterial coiling or development of the intra-abdominal compartment syndrome are the only reasons for operative intervention in the SIRS phase.

23.5.1 Management in the CARS Phase and Thereafter (2–12 Weeks)

When there has been no improvement or actual clinical deterioration after initial improvement, infection of the pancreatic and/or peripancreatic collections must be sought, excluded, or treated. In an attempt to anticipate on further deterioration, some groups have advocated weekly fine needle aspiration (FNA) of the collection to confirm or exclude infection. Our group does not support this strategy. There is a risk of a false-negative results, and infection may be introduced by FNA. Moreover, clinical deterioration, accompanied by a negative result of the FNA should not withhold the clinician from intervention. Based on a recent randomized controlled trial (RCT) on treatment of infected necrosis, we refrain from routine FNA, because 92 % of patients proved to have infected necrosis at the initial intervention, while only a small minority had infection discovered only on FNA (Van Santvoort et al. 2010). Gas in peripancreatic collections are, however, pathognomonic for infected necrosis.

Once the necrosis becomes infected, mortality increases dramatically from about 15 % to around 30 %, so the prevention of infection is an ultimate goal of treatment in the early phase of the disease (Besselink et al. 2009).

Systemic intravenous antibiotics, selective bowel decontamination, enteral probiotics and enteral nutrition all have been proposed to lessen the rate of infection.

23.5.2 Systemic Intravenous Antibiotics

Many studies have addressed the effect of systemic antibiotic prophylaxis in lessening the rate of infectious complications in (predicted) severe acute pancreatitis (De Vries et al. 2005, Wittau et al. 2011). The initial, non-blinded, non-placebo controlled, randomised trials suggested rather dramatic positive effects.

> …A Cochrane meta-analysis in 2006 described a decrease in mortality using prophylactic antibiotics in necrotizing pancreatitis. For these reasons, the use of prophylactic antibiotics remains a viable option to us….

Enteral nutrition is hypothesized to decrease small bowel bacterial overgrowth by a positive effect on small bowel motility, which limits intraluminal bacterial overgrowth and by a positive effect on intestinal mucosal barrier function which decreases bacterial translocation. This cascade of events could lead to a decrease in infectious complications (super infection by bacteria entering the systemic circulation) (Eckerwall et al. 2007; Petrov and Zagainov 2007; Petrov et al. 2009, Petrov et al. 2010). In predicted severe pancreatitis, we now start enteral nutrition by nasojejunal feeding if the patient is not expected to resume a normal diet within approximately 3 days.

The optimal route for the administration of enteral feeding – through a nasojejunal or a nasogastric feeding tube – has yet to be established. Two small, randomized trials involving 80 patients found no difference in tolerance for feeding and complications rates by either route of delivery. The overall mortality was rather high, and the studies may have missed relevant differences in complications, such as aspiration, due to their small size. Results of ongoing larger studies should be awaited before using nasogastric feeding routinely in patients with severe acute pancreatitis.

23.5.3 Selective Bowel Decontamination (SBD)

Only one RCT studied the value of SBD in acute pancreatitis (Luiten et al. 1995). The study demonstrated a decrease in mortality in the SBD group. Nevertheless, this therapy has not gained wide acceptance, but the data suggest that the concept of early intervention in the cascade of events – small bowel bacterial overgrowth, mucosal barrier failure, bacterial translocation, systemic infection – deserves further exploration.

23.5.4 Probiotics

Several studies including two small RCTs from Hungary suggested a beneficial effect of prophylactic probiotics in predicted severe pancreatitis (Van Santvoort et al. 2008). In the large Dutch probiotics trial (PROPATRIA) in patients with predicted severe acute pancreatitis, no effect on infectious complications was found; more worrisome, however, was a more than twofold greater mortality rate in the probiotics group. Although there is no satisfactory answer yet to this puzzling outcome, at this stage it seems that the prophylactic probiotics as administered in this study should no longer be given to patients with "predicted severe acute pancreatitis."

23.6 The Role and Timing of Intervention

The large differences in outcome of series from the last decades illustrate a wide variation in the indication for intervention, technique, timing, and selection of patients included in the different studies. Most of the studies published are retrospective in nature and only two RCT's have been conducted (Van Santvoort et al. 2010; Mier et al. 1997):

- Differences in the indications for intervention: this chapter shows clearly that the Magdeburg group also struggles with a clear description of the indications for intervention, illustrated by "early intervention (<3–4 weeks) or the operative treatment of sterile necrosis, should be reserved for select cases." These are two different indications for intervention "early intervention (<3–4 weeks)" and "the operative treatment of sterile necrosis." Early intervention for the treatment of necrosis without documented or highly suspected infection has no place in our opinion in the treatment of necrotizing pancreatitis early in the disease, even if the patient's clinical condition is deteriorating. A small RCT on operative necrosectomy in this phase was performed in 1989. In this study, intervention within 72 h ("early") was compared with operation after 12 ("late") days (Mier et al. 1997). The authors terminated the study prematurely because of a much greater, though not yet statistically significant, mortality for operative intervention within 72 h (58 vs. 27 %). After this study, operative necrosectomy as the primary therapy for acute pancreatitis in the absence of infection was essentially abandoned. Currently uncontrollable bleeding and abdominal compartment syndrome represent what we believe to be the only indications for operative intervention in the first 2–3 weeks of the disease.

- "The operative treatment of sterile necrosis, should be reserved for select cases," raises the question about patient selection. In our practice, sterile necrosis is treated by some form of interventional necrosectomy when causing persistent mechanical obstruction of the duodenum or the common bile duct, or when it's leading to "failure to thrive" or what others have called "the persistent unwell." There are no controlled series on this controversial topic, and many operative and endoscopic series reporting on technical success are a mixture of infected and sterile pancreatic and peripancreatic collections.
- Other topics of debate are: "infection of pancreatic necrosis is a well-accepted indication for operative intervention" and "in contrast, infected necrosis does not mandate operative treatment." We regard both of the statements as true in the sense that infection of necrosis is a well-accepted indication, but, indeed, not all infected cases need aggressive operative necrosectomy and some may not even require a more minimal access necrosectomy by percutaneous, endoscopic or laparoscopic type interventions.
- In the Dutch RCT on intervention in infected necrosis, infection with signs of sepsis was the only indication for intervention and all attempts were made to delay intervention for 30 days after onset of the disease. This approach led to an overall mortality of 17 %; the patients had a mean APACHE score of 15 and an infection rate of 92 %. Several patients developed infected necrosis with signs of sepsis before 30 days of onset of the pancreatitis, but because the protocol called for delay of necrosectomy until at least 30 days after onset, operative intervention was successfully postponed to 30 days, with intravenous antibiotic support. There is also uncontrolled data showing that necrosis with gas on CECT, can disappear on occasion without any form of intervention.
- The experience of the Magdeburg group in 2006 and 2007 is listed in Tables 3.2 and 3.3. These tables highlight another important feature of severe necrotizing pancreatitis; the Magdeburg group is a well-respected, experienced center, yet still only about five cases are managed operatively each year. Many other centers have similar numbers and, consequently, controlled studies from other expert centers are difficult to conduct and need many years to be built up, thus the need for organized multicenter trials.
- Differences in the techniques applied: the Magdeburg group describes their experience with open necrosectomy, the "therapeutic flow" (in Fig. 3.1) and the advantages of this approach. Their approach ("finger fracture") to open the necrotic collection is very similar to ours. When only a limited entrance to the collection is made, the cavity created after the necrosectomy can be closed adequately by suturing the opening closed using the greater omentum and the backside of the stomach, in order to create a closed system for continuous postoperative lavage; the drains can be guided out the right and left flank. We prefer a limited opening to the lesser sac collection rather than a large opening as shown on Fig. 3.5a, because we feel that adequate lavage with large amounts of fluid is more important than attempts at complete removal of all small remnants of necrosis in the far extremes of the often widely extending cavities. Creating a really closed compartment for lavage of the lesser sac, with infracolic extensions behind the right and left

colon – is crucial for successful long term lavage. The use of multiple drains is advisable for collections extending infracolically behind the right and left colon; non-productive drains can easily be removed early. We stop the lavage when the cavity has collapsed and not "when the draining fluid has become clear." When the sinogram demonstrates collapse of the cavity, we stop the lavage and remove the drains step-by-step over a period of 7–10 days.

- The statements of the Magdeburg of "some groups utilize radiologic percutaneous drainage or laparoscopic or endoscopic techniques" and "at this time, minimally invasive necrosectomy is far from the standard practice in treating many patients requiring necrosectomy" are important, because their approach to this disease illustrates that any operative or nonoperative approach and any operative technique, once adopted with clinical results apparently accepted by experienced clinicians like the Magdeburg group, can only be "attacked" successfully and replaced new techniques, when successfully tested in controlled studies. Recent studies, however, do show that "minimally invasive necrosectomy is" not all "that far from the standard practice." The RCT from the Netherlands (Van Santvoort et al. 2010) and a recently published systematic review (Van Baal et al. 2011) show that about 30–55 % of patients may need no further treatment after successful percutaneous catheter drainage. So, percutaneous or transgastric catheter drainage (PCD or TCD), has now become our accepted first step of interventional treatment for patients with infected pancreatic necrosis. If PCD/TCD is not successful, operative or endoscopic (Seifert et al. 2009) necrosectomy is the next step. Controlled studies have to show which operative approach or technique is the best option, the videoscopic-assisted retroperitoneal debridement (Horvath et al. 2001, Van Santvoort et al. 2007, Horvath et al. 2010), a laparoscopic approach (Raraty et al. 2010), endoscopic (Papachristou et al. 2007) or open necrosectomy (this chapter). Probably a tailored approach depending on patient condition and the extent and location of the necrosis after failure of PCD/TCD will be the future approach.
- Differences in timing of operative intervention: in the Dutch RCT (Van Santvoort et al. 2010), delay of necrosectomy until at least 4 weeks after onset of disease was adhered to rigidly, because this time interval was based on a study showing that waiting for 4 weeks improved outcome in terms of mortality (…). In the Dutch RCT, it was found that at 2–3 weeks encapsulation was often incomplete and that after waiting another 10 days or 2 weeks, encapsulation of the necrotic collection matured, thereby allowing a safe necrosectomy. Therefore, based on this experience, we maintain that planning some form of necrosectomy at 3 weeks, because "pancreatic necrosis is usually well demarked after about 3 weeks from onset of acute pancreatitis…" may not be the best strategy. We fully agree with the statement "demarcation is of paramount importance" and that indeed "removing the well-demarked necrosis reduces the risk of bleeding and preserves still vital parenchyma." If, in some cases, in the RCT, demarcation or encapsulation was completed at 2 weeks, we still waited for another 2 weeks, under antibiotic coverage to protect against bacteriaemia and sepsis. Currently, a strategy of "wait and encapsulate" has well-documented advantages, but the exact and optimal interval needs further determination.

References

Banks PA, Freeman ML (2006) Practice guidelines in acute pancreatitis. Am J Gastroenterol 101(10): 2379–2400

Besselink MG, Van Santvoort HC, Boermeester MA, Nieuwenhuijs VB, van Goor H, Dejong CH et al (2009) Timing and impact of infections in acute pancreatitis. Br J Surg 96(3):267–273

De Vries AC, Besselink MGH, Van der Kraats CIB, Buskens E, van Erpecum KJ, Gooszen HG (2005) Antibiotic prophylaxis in acute necrotising pancreatitis: methodological quality of randomised controlled trials in relation to outcome. Gut 54(Suppl VII):A38–A39

Eckerwall GE, Tingstedt BB, Bergenzaun PE, Andersson RG (2007) Immediate oral feeding in patients with mild acute pancreatitis is safe and may accelerate recovery – a randomized clinical study. Clin Nutr 26(6):758–763

Fagenholz PJ, Fernandez-del Castillo C, Harris NS, Pelletier AJ, Camargo CA (2007) Direct medical costs of acute pancreatitis hospitalizations in the United States. Pancreas 35(4):302–307

Horvath KD, Kao LS, Wherry KL, Pellegrini CA, Sinanan MN (2001) A technique for laparoscopic-assisted percutaneous drainage of infected pancreatic necrosis and pancreatic abscess. Surg Endosc 15(10):1221–1225

Horvath K, Freeny P, Escallon J, Heagerty P, Comstock B, Glickerman DJ et al (2010) Safety and efficacy of video-assisted retroperitoneal debridement for infected pancreatic collections: a multicenter, prospective, single-arm phase 2 study. Arch Surg 145(9):817–825

Luiten EJ, Hop WC, Lange JF, Bruining HA (1995) Controlled clinical trial of selective decontamination for the treatment of severe acute pancreatitis. Ann Surg 222(1):57–65

Mao EQ, Tang YQ, Fei J, Qin S, Wu J, Li L et al (2009) Fluid therapy for severe acute pancreatitis in acute response stage. Chin Med J (Engl) 122(2):169–173

Mier J, Luque-de León E, Castillo A, Robledo F, Blanco R (1997) Early versus late necrosectomy in severe necrotizing pancreatitis. Am J Surg 173(2):71–75

Papachristou GI, Takahashi N, Chahal P, Sarr MG, Baron TH (2007) Peroral endoscopic drainage/debridement of walled-off pancreatic necrosis. Ann Surg 245(6): 943–951

Petrov MS, Zagainov VE (2007) Influence of enteral versus parenteral nutrition on blood glucose control in acute pancreatitis: a systematic review. Clin Nutr 26(5):514–523

Petrov MS, Loveday BP, Pylypchuk RD, McIlroy K, Phillips AR, Windsor JA (2009) Systematic review and meta-analysis of enteral nutrition formulations in acute pancreatitis. Br J Surg 96(11):1243–1252

Petrov MS, Shanbhag S, Chakraborty M, Phillips AR, Windsor JA (2010) Organ failure and infection of pancreatic necrosis as determinants of mortality in patients with acute pancreatitis. Gastroenterology 139(3): 813–820

Raraty MG, Halloran CM, Dodd S, Ghaneh P, Connor S, Evans J et al (2010) Minimal access retroperitoneal pancreatic necrosectomy: improvement in morbidity and mortality with a less invasive approach. Ann Surg 251(5):787–793

Seifert H, Biermer M, Schmitt W, Jurgensen C, Will U, Gerlach R et al (2009) Transluminal endoscopic necrosectomy after acute pancreatitis: a multicentre study with long-term follow-up (the GEPARD Study). Gut 58(9):1260–1266

Shaheen NJ, Hansen RA, Morgan DR, Gangarosa LM, Ringel Y, Thiny MT et al (2006) The burden of gastrointestinal and liver diseases, 2006. Am J Gastroenterol 101(9):2128–2138

Van Baal MC, Van Santvoort HC, Bollen TL, Bakker OJ, Besselink MG, Gooszen HG et al (2011) Systematic review of percutaneous catheter drainage as primary treatment for necrotizing pancreatitis. Br J Surg 98(1):18–27

Van Santvoort HC, Besselink MGH, Horvath KD, Sinanan M, Bollen TL, Ramshorst B et al (2007) Videoscopic assisted retroperitoneal debridement in infected necrotizing pancreatitis. HPB(Oxford) 9(2): 156–159

Van Santvoort HC, Besselink MG, Timmerman HM, van Minnen LP, Akkermans LM, Gooszen HG (2008) Probiotics in surgery. Surgery 143(1):1–7

Van Santvoort HC, Besselink MG, Bakker OJ, Hofker HS, Boermeester MA, Dejong CH et al (2010) A step-up approach or open necrosectomy for necrotizing pancreatitis. N Engl J Med 362(16):1491–1502

Wittau M, Mayer B, Scheele J, Henne-Bruns D, Dellinger EP, Isenmann R (2011) Systematic review and meta-analysis of antibiotic prophylaxis in severe acute pancreatitis. Scand J Gastroenterol 46(3): 261–270

Commentary

24

C.W. Imrie and C.R. Carter

After many years in the learning process, our therapeutic guiding principle has become that interventional procedures in patients with severe acute pancreatitis (AP) should be directed specifically at treating or ameliorating complications and the risk of recurrent AP. Open operations have now little place in this approach.

Once the diagnosis of acute pancreatitis (AP) has been established, usually by the combination of clinical presentation and increased blood amylase >3 times the upper limit of normal, efforts should focus on treating the pain, hypovolaemia, and hypoxaemia. Patients with evidence of organ dysfunction (based on the modified Marshall Score which omits the hepatic index) are admitted to our surgical high dependency care unit or the respiratory intensive care unit as appropriate.

Checks to identify etiology by ultrasonography for gallstones and biochemical checks for hyperlipidemia and hypercalcemia are routine. Lipase measurements are done rarely.

CT is performed very early in the admission only when there is real diagnostic doubt regarding the diagnosis of AP and to exclude vascular or visceral complications. We place less emphasis on obtaining a staging CT to determine location and extent of pancreatic necrosis, because this does not affect early management. Patients with major renal compromise have contrast enhanced CT delayed or occasionally performed with no contrast.

Magnetic resonance imaging (MRI) has little role in the early management but does provide additional accurate information on the presence of common bile duct stones and the content and location of post acute fluid collections more precisely than CT scan.

Nutritional support is routine in patients with severe AP, preferably by the nasoenteric route. We showed in a prospective, randomized study of patients with objectively graded severe AP that nasogastric (NG) feeding was as effective and safe as nasojejunal (NJ) feeding. Therefore, we initiate NG feeding switching to NJ feeding or occasionally intravenous parenteral nutritional support for the small proportion of patients who do not tolerate proximal or distal enteric feeding.

Prophylactic antibiotics are not used routinely in patients who are admitted directly to our care, based on the outcome of the largest two multicentre studies which showed no distinct benefit to the patients. In contrast, tertiary referral patients from other hospitals who have already been prescribed antibiotics prior to transfer will have the course completed (target total treatment of 7 days) after their transfer to Glasgow Royal Infirmary. Antibiotics would then be stopped and only prescribed thereafter for specific indications based on microbiologic culture results.

There is little role for early endoscopic retrograde cholangiopancreatography (ERCP) and sphincterotomy in patients with gallstones and

C.W. Imrie (✉) • C.R. Carter
Pancreato-Biliary Unit, Department of Surgery,
Glasgow Royal Infirmary, Glasgow, G31 2ER, UK
e-mail: clemimrie@gmail.com

R. Mantke et al. (eds.), *International Practices in Pancreatic Surgery*,
DOI 10.1007/978-3-540-74506-8_24,

mild pancreatitis. The exceptions are patients rated too unfit to have a laparoscopic cholecystectomy. Emergency endoscopic sphincterotomy can be required in patients with an impacted stone in the ampulla of Vater and those with accompanying cholangitis.

Definitive management of cholelithiasis to minimize the risk of recurrent AP either by laparoscopic cholecystectomy or endoscopic sphincterotomy (with common duct stone clearance) will usually be scheduled during the same admission to hospital.

In severe AP with acute fluid collections ± pancreatic and peripancreatic necrosis, the timing of the clearance of the gallstone hazard will be determined by the intention of combining laparoscopic cholecystectomy with any other indicated operative intervention under the same general anaesthetic.

In our international clinical practice, we have for many years had 3–4 senior surgeons within our own team who are expert in therapeutic endoscopic procedures via the sphincter of Oddi. We do not use emergency endoscopic retrograde cholangiopancreatography (ERCP) with sphincterotomy in AP, except for the small number of patients with an impacted ampullary stone and those with accompanying cholangitis.

Patients who are systemically the most ill present with early (<48 h) SIRS driven multiple organ failure with a mortality in the 30–50 % range, or later (7–28 days) with sepsis-associated organ failure. Both groups are very poor candidates for open surgery.

We consider early operation to be avoided in the most severely ill patients with AP; in particular, there is little evidence to support the use of decompressive laparotomy for abdominal compartment syndrome. Such operations may produce transient improvements in cardio-vascular and biochemical parameters, but no associated improvement in mortality and often lead to difficult abdominal wall hernias.

Within the sepsis group, the guiding principle for us since 1998 has been to strive primarily to downgrade this later septic process associated with severe AP by means of a multi-modality approach utilising:

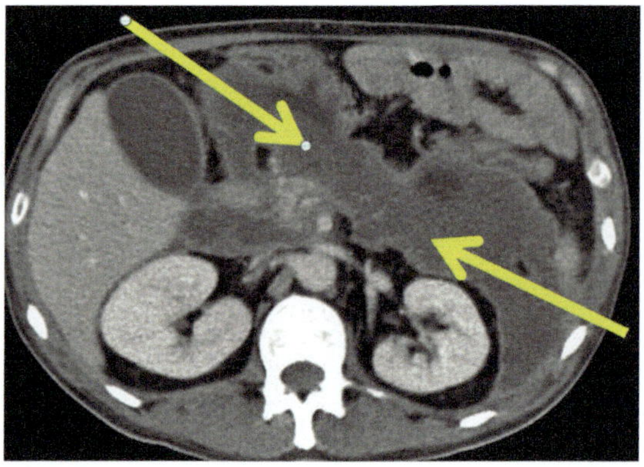

Fig. 24.1 CT of patient with infected pancreatic and peripancreatic necrosis with *yellow arrows* indicating the commonly used left side percutaneous and less frequently used right oblique drainage routes

(a) CT-guided catheter drainage alone or
(b) Percutaneous minimally invasive operative drainage or
(c) Endoscopic ultrasonography-guided transgastric drainage.

Immediate gram stain and speedy culture of organisms will guide further antibiotic therapy.

(a) *Repeated CT catheter drainage of pus* can, on occasion, prove to be effective therapy in some patients with infected peripancreatic necrosis.
(b) More frequently our experience is that percutaneous catheter drainage alone, whilst resulting in immediate improvement, is insufficient to obtain long-term control of the sepsis and, in these patients, the drain tract (most often in the left mid axillary line, Fig 24.1) is dilated to 10 mm diameter, allowing a formal, percutaneous necrosectomy using a rigid nephroscope. A large, soft, polyethylene outflow drain is left in the peripancreatic area with an attached 8 FG inflow umbilical catheter to permit continuous post operative closed lavage.
(c) More recently, patients with centrally placed infected collections adjacent to the posterior wall of the stomach have undergone EUS-guided cyst gastrostomy with the tract and drainage being maintained by the use of multiple pigtail stents and a nasocystic lavage catheter. Tract dilation and formal transmural exploration and debridement of the necrotic cavity may be performed later.

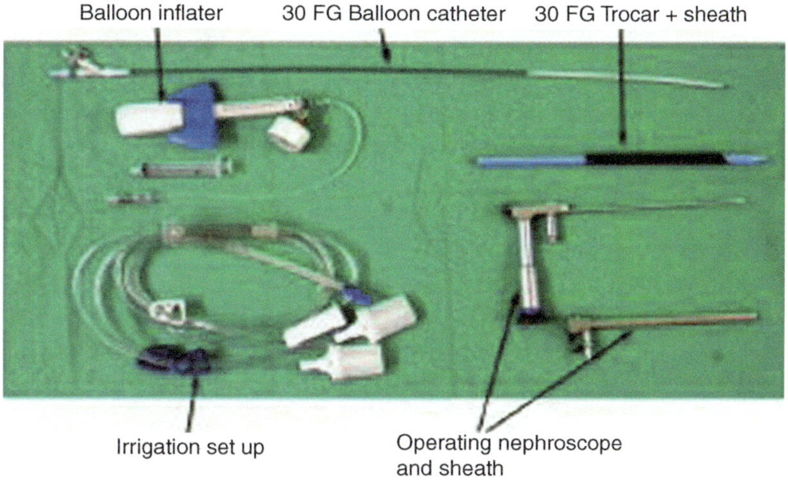

Fig. 24.2 PN – dilatation system, rigid dilator equipment plus dilator (Cook Medical) utilised for minimally invasive necrosectomy

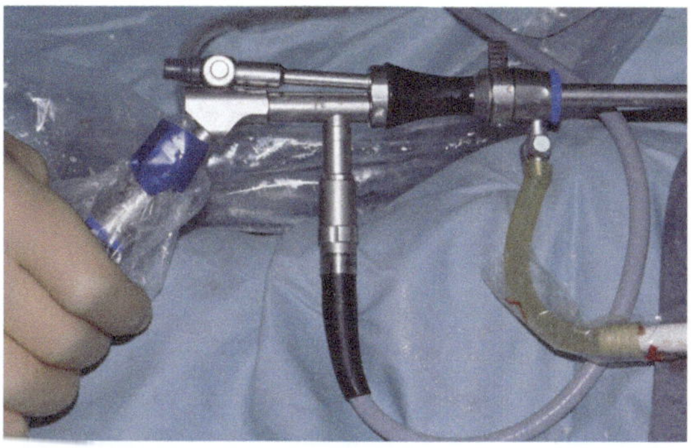

Fig. 24.3 PN – nephroscope, view from the left shoulder area of a patient with nephroscope inserted through the left flank

In both the approaches outlined in (b) and (c) above, the major focus at the initial procedure is to obtain effective drainage of pus in order to downgrade severity of illness. Some friable necrotic tissue may be removed easily; however, post procedural continuous lavage with body temperature isotonic fluids is an important aspect of both these techniques. This approach enables easier removal of necrotic infected tissue at second and subsequent procedures.

In approximately 10 % of patients treated using the nephroscopic, left lateral abdominal retroperitoneal technique, an additional more anterior, right-sided percutaneous approach may be indicated by CT imaging to access infected pockets around the head of pancreas (Fig. 24.1). Since the original technique, we first described in the Annals of Surgery in 2000 in a small number of patients, the standard nephroscopes are no longer used, because wider (12-mm diameter) modified nephroscopes (made by Olympus) have

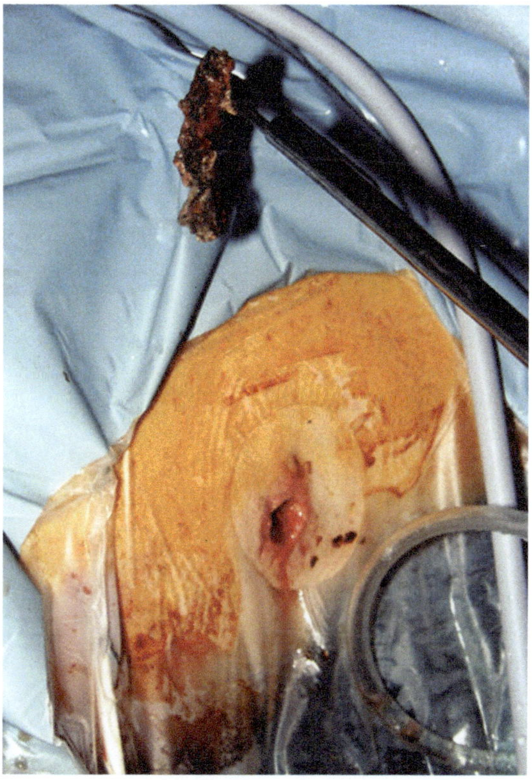

Fig. 24.4 PN – necrosis in grasper, peri-pancreatic necrotic tissue extracted by grasper via left flank approach and viewed from the patient's left hip area

been our choice (Figs. 24.2, 24.3, and 24.4). These nephroscopes permit easier employment of the more standard, minimally invasive surgical instruments to remove infected necrotic tissue as well as to introduce the vascular clip applicators when needed.

Pancreatic fistula may occur associated with percutaneous necrosectomy and usually close eventually and spontaneously or aided by the placement of an endoscopic transpapillary pancreatic duct stent. Enteric fistulas are managed by a variety of means, including parenteral nutrition, NJ feeding, and a defunctioning ileostomy contingent on the site of the fistula.

Both intra-operative and spontaneous intracavity hemorrhage associated with severe AP are best treated by an interventional radiology approach.

In order to illustrate the extent of the transformation of our approach in the therapy of over 100 patients with infected pancreatic and peripancreatic necrosis since 2003–2011, we have resorted to an open operative necrosectomy in only one patient.

Commentary 25

Åke Andrén-Sandberg

25.1 Diagnosis and Severity Assessment

The diagnosis of those cases of acute pancreatitis that need treatment is seldom a problem. Almost all patients in our Swedish practice that have the severe form is very obvious: ill already when they arrive in the emergency ward, lying flat on the back with little movements, shallow breathing, paleness, low blood pressure, almost somnolent, and with difficulties speaking and giving a proper medical history. These patients all have a short (some hours to almost a full day) history of illness, and the symptoms have very rapidly worsened. After half a day, many of the patients are desperately ill, and for those not arriving at hospital, there is a substantial risk of dying (Andersson and Andrén-Sandbder 2003). The diagnosis in the emergency room is seldom difficult for an experienced physician, whereas for the younger colleges it might be a problem to consider the diagnosis in the broad category of abdominal catastrophes. The only real differential diagnoses are perforation of the upper intestinal tract (ischemia of the small bowel, perforated ulcer etc.) or atypical myocardial infarction. In these cases, the difference in accuracy of amylase and lipase measurements are not important, but it may be noted that there are cases without any increases in these enzyme activities. It should also be noted that a high severity grade of pain is not a sign of severe pancreatitis, rather the other way around; for the patients with severe acute pancreatitis, most of the pain has faded away or the patients cannot express the feeling of pain due to their overwhelming illness when they arrive in hospital or are transferred from a smaller, less acute hospital or emergency room.

It is unusual that patients arrive to hospital with symptoms that indicate mild acute pancreatitis that only later develops into the severe form. In a few patients, aggressive fluid therapy may prevent a borderline pancreatitis from developing into a severe form of pancreatitis, and thus the importance of rapid diagnosis and treatment/resuscitation (Gardner et al. 2009).

The only patients with severe acute pancreatitis who present differently are those induced with ERCP. From a scientific point of view, ERCP-induced pancreatitis is an interesting model for study of the pathogenesis of the pancreatic process. These patients usually have pain beginning in a few hours after the ERCP, and then rather rapidly increasing (Badalov et al. 2009). Some patients have pain immediately after the ERCP due to the large volume of air insufflated during the procedure which might result in bowel distention and painful spasm. In addition to pain, asymptomatic increases in the amylase and/or lipase often occur after ERCP, with no clinical sequelae. Post-ERCP pancreatitis may, however, be suspected in any patient who develops increasing pain within 6 h of the procedure, and

Å. Andrén-Sandberg
Department of Surgery, Karolinska University Hospital, Huddinge, Stockholm, Sweden
e-mail: ake.andren-sandberg@karolinska.se

R. Mantke et al. (eds.), *International Practices in Pancreatic Surgery*,
DOI 10.1007/978-3-540-74506-8_25, © Springer-Verlag Berlin Heidelberg 2013

especially when the symptoms escalate progressively and become full-blown at 12 or 18 h after the ERCP. Symptoms are much less likely to begin after 12 h from the procedure – if the patient is well 12 h after the ERCP, the risk of an post-ERCP-pancreatitis is negligible.

Taken together the diagnosis and severity assessment in severe forms of acute pancreatitis seldom is a problem.

25.2 Aspects on Non-medical Treatment of Patients with Severe Acute Pancreatitis

It must be understood upfront that there is really no specific treatment of severe acute pancreatitis. There is, however, a need for sharp surveillance for early recognition and treatment of complications. These are partly unpredictable and partly predictable. In almost all patients, severe acute pancreatitis has some impact on the lungs (decreased space due to the distended abdomen, atelectasis due to insufficient breathing and surfactant, pleural fluid, and pneumonia), the kidneys (oliguria or anuria), the intestines (adynamic ileus), the cardiovascular system (depression of myocardial function due to cytokines negative influence and displacement of intravascular fluid into cellular interstitium leading to hypovolemia), and systemic metabolism (hyperglucosuria, hypocalcemia etc.). All these effects need to be anticipated with tight monitoring of physiological and laboratory parameters.

Despite the origin from the pancreas and he injury to the pancreatic parenchymal cells containing the enzymes, there is no need to follow the amylase or lipase levels, and CRP is almost always too closely followed. From an imaging point of view, CT is seldom needed to make the diagnosis, and as initially the kidneys often challenged, intravenous radiologic contrast agents should not be given if not necessarily needed. Also the initial hypotension may lead to an image of hypoperfusion of the pancreas that may be mistaken for necrosis. Thus, CT should be postponed until a complication potentially requiring active intervention is suspected, usually after the first week. We do not use prophylactic antibiotics – but of course we treat pneumonias, urinary tract infections etc. with antibiotics.

In a small portion of patients with severe acute pancreatitis, prolonged hypoperfusion may be the difference between the development and/or progression of necrosis or not. It is well documented that volume depletion and increased hematocrit are associated with poor prognosis in acute pancreatitis. Therefore, we focus on aggressive fluid treatment as soon as possible when a patient with predicted acute pancreatitis arrives in the emergency room. Patients with severe acute pancreatitis who do not receive at least one third of their initial 72-h cumulative intravenous fluid volume during the first 24 h are at risk for greater mortality than those who are resuscitated more aggressively. Changes in stroke volume, radial pulse pressure, and peak velocity of femoral artery flow induced by passive leg raising are accurate indices for predicting fluid responsiveness in nonintubated patients with severe acute pancreatitis (Préau et al. 2010).

25.3 Comments on the Operative Technique of Necrosectomy

Traditional open operative necrosectomy for treatment of infected pancreatic necrosis is associated with high morbidity and mortality, leading to a shift during the last decade toward minimally invasive endoscopic, radiologic, and laparoscopic approaches. Percutaneous drainage may be useful as a temporizing method to control sepsis and as an adjunctive treatment to later operative intervention; solely percutaneous techniques without some form of necrosectomy are limited, however, because of the requirement for frequent catheter care and the need for repeated procedures – these approaches seldom lead to cure. Endoscopic transgastric or transduodenal therapies with endoscopic debridement/necrosectomy have been described recently, are highly successful in selected patients, avoid the need for open necrosectomy, and can be used in poor operative candidates. Laparoscopic necrosectomy is also promising for treatment of pancreatic necrosis, but the need for inducing a pneumoperitoneum and the potential risk of infection limit the usefulness of a truly "laparoscopic" transabdominal approach in patients with critical illness. In contrast, the retroperitoneal access with a nephroscope or a "modified" laparoscope is used to approach the necrosis directly with complete removal of the necrosis. Retroperitoneal drainage using the delay-until-liquefaction strategy also appears to be successful to treat pancreatic necrosis. The anatomic location of the necrosis, clinical comorbidities, and operator experience determine the best approach for a particular patient (Navaneethan et al. 2009; Babu et al. 2010). We have, however, used minimally invasive procedures to manage pancreatic necrosis only in special cases due to good results of utterly conservative treatment policy (though including repeated percutaneous drainages) and open surgery.

For open surgery, which we postpone as long as possible to be able to remove all the necrotic tissue during one session when the fibrotic wall has matured, a recent CT for a "road map" of the necrosis is always required. For this kind of operation, we always use two experienced surgeons; all hands and brains may be required. Because our elective pancreatduodenectomies through a midline incision, we prefer this incision for the necrosectomies to be as familiar as possible with the view of the anatomy (Fig. 25.1). In these cases, there is never an option to perform small incisions; the operation may be difficult enough through large incisions, and we believe it wise to have as many options as possible should bleeding occur. Access to the lesser sac is chosen with regard to the CT picture and is usually obtained through the transverse mesocolon and into the retrogastric retroperitoneum. First a small entry, often using blunt fracture, is made into the most bulging place. After the first drainage of pus or "dirty" fluid, a finger is put gently into the necrotic cavity to evaluate the extent of the necrosis and the quality of the fibrotic wall. It should be understood that in most cases, a considerable part of the necrosis is peripancreatic – it is not only the pancreatic tissue that is dead. If there has been a sufficient time since the necrotic process started the necrosis is well demarcated

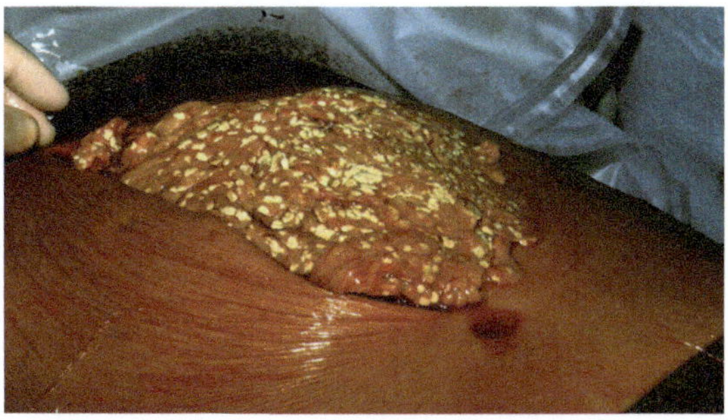

Fig. 25.1 Calcification in omenum majus at opening of the abdomen in a patient with severe pancreatitis

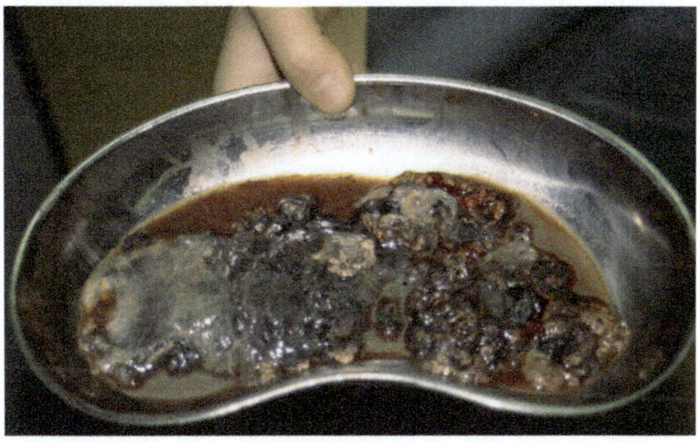

Fig. 25.2 Necrotic material 6 weeks after a necrotic acute pancreatitis

and leaves the wall of the cavity/collection after gentle traction. Much of the necrosis can be peeled or dissected bluntly by the finger and almost all of the rest can be removed with the suction device used judiciously (Fig. 25.2). The point of open surgery is to explore and debride all necrotic collections in total. That means that after removing the first 50–100 g of necrosis, it is obvious where more is to be found. The front wall of the necrotic cavity can then be opened up with diathermy with little risk of unexpected bleeding. Most often that means a transverse incision through the transverse mesocolon for 20 cm or more, exposing the whole pancreatic compartment. Care is taken to try to avoid injuring the middle colic artery. Commonly, the necrosis extends down on both psoas' muscles, and the paracolic gutters should be opened and explored. In the majority of cases, it will end up with a retroperitoneal incision of 40–50 cm. All necrotic tissue can then be removed with limited bleeding, and usually with a need for a later revi sion. Drains are put in the cavity (usually four or more), and a feeding jejunostomy is placed. Pancreatic necrosectomy may be combined with cholecystectomy when the etiology is gallstone-related if access and mobilization are thought to be safe. Postoperative closed irrigation has been performed with wide bore drains placed in the lesser sac through separate small incisions in some cases. Necrotic material is sent to a laboratory for culture.

These patients are always in a septic condition at the end of the operation, but this will fade away during a few days together with a gradually diminishing CRP.

At the Karolinska University, the aim of the open necrosectomy is to remove *all* necrotic tissue during *one* surgical session; i.e. we do not necessarily support the approach of staged necrosectomy proposed by Bradley (Bradley 1993). Our statement means that there is always an attempt to postponethenecrosectomyforatleast6weeks–preferably 8 weeks – to allow the development of a clear demarcation line between the necrotic and the viable tissue. These weeks are not always easy for the patient or the surgeons, but because earlier operative intervention almost always leads to repeated laparotomies considerable efforts must be made get the patient through this difficult time-period.

Although the surgeon usually thinks that a substantial part – or almost all – of pancreas has been removed, it is surprising how often that patients end up without endocrine or exocrine insufficiency.

25.4 Adjuvant Treatment to Surgery

It is important to understand that all kinds of surgical approaches to the treatment of necrotizing pancreatitis are only one part of the wider picture of treatment. That means that both before and after necrosectomy, all possible pathophysiologic aspects should be monitored and if necessary corrected appropriately.

Antibiotics should be given only after thorough consideration – at Karolinska after consultation with experts on antibiotic treatment, we maintain that sooner or later almost all patients will eventually develop some form of an overt infection, and then there must still be available effective antibiotics according to the results of cultures. We do not search actively for evidence of infection using fine needle aspiration to get material for culture but rather prefer to wait until the need for operative intervention or until there are clinical signs of sepsis. No prophylactic antibiotic treatment is used. In some cases, there will be fungemia after some weeks of antibiotics treatment, and cultures for fungus are therefore taken regularly after therapy with broad-spectrum antibiotics have been instituted (Trikudanathan et al. 2011).

Of course the fluid balance must be monitored and corrected continuously. Also, renal and pulmonary functions are evaluated and supported if necessary.

These patients always have a negative energy balance, and their degree of injury is comparable to the huge deficits of burn injuries. The patients need vitamins and trace elements (which are given routinely without measuring the actual deficiencies), and they need energy (i.e. calories *and* extra protein). Parenteral nutrition is instituted intravenously as soon as the patient arrives at the intensive care unit. The patient will then also have a nasogastric tube inserted to prevent vomiting, and as soon as there are no problems with gastric retention of fluids, enteral nutrition is started. Sometimes it can be started somewhat earlier if a nasojejunal tube can be inserted, but it has been shown that in most cases, enteral feeding through the stomach functions just as well (Eatock et al. 2005). We use a step-up protocol with 25 mL/h the first day, and than 25 mL/h more each day until 100 mL/h is reached. When the patient can deal with that without stomach retention (with risk for aspiration if not on a ventilator) or severe diarrhea (Petrov and Whelan 2010), the total energy demand is given over fewer hours, i.e. the stomach and small intestine should “rest” at night time.

References

Andersson R, Andrén-Sandbder A (2003) Fatal acute pancreatitis. Characteristics of patients never reaching hospital. Pancreatology 3:64–66

Babu BI, Sheen AJ, Lee SH, O'Shea S, Eddleston JM, Siriwardena AK (2010) Open pancreatic necrosectomy in the multidisciplinary management of postinflammatory necrosis. Ann Surg 251:783–786

Badalov N, Tenner S, Baillie J (2009) The prevention, recognition and treatment of post-ERCP pancreatitis. JOP 10:88–97

Bradley EL 3rd (1993) A fifteen year experience with open drainage for infected pancreatic necrosis. Surg Gynecol Obstet 177:215–222

Eatock FC, Chong P, Menezes N, Murray L, McKay CJ, Carter CR, Imrie CW (2005) A randomized study of early nasogastric versus nasojejunal feeding in severe acute pancreatitis. Am J Gastroenterol 100: 432–439

Gardner TB, Vege SS, Chari ST, Petersen BT, Topazian MD, Clain JE, Pearson RK, Levy MJ, Sarr MG (2009) Faster rate of initial fluid resuscitation in severe acute pancreatitis diminishes in-hospital mortality. Pancreatology 9:770–776

Navaneethan U, Vege SS, Chari ST, Baron TH (2009) Minimally invasive techniques in pancreatic necrosis. Pancreatology 9:867–875

Petrov MS, Whelan K (2010) Comparison of complications attributable to enteral and parenteral nutrition in predicted severe acute pancreatitis: a systematic review and meta-analysis. Br J Nutr 103: 1287–1295

Préau S, Saulnier F, Dewavrin F, Durocher A, Chagnon JL (2010) Passive leg raising is predictive of fluid responsiveness in spontaneously breathing patients with severe sepsis or acute pancreatitis. Crit Care Med 28:819–825

Trikudanathan G, Navaneethan U, Vege SS (2011) Intra-abdominal fungal infections complicating acute pancreatitis: a review. Am J Gastroenterol 106:1188–1192

26 Commentary

Michael G. Sarr

As discussed by Drs. Mantke and Lippert, the management of severe acute pancreatitis has changed markedly over the last several decades as we have come to understand more about the development and progression of necrotizing pancreatitis. Probably the biggest change/advance has been the move from an initial early and aggressive operative intervention/necrosectomy (Beger et al. 1982; Farrugia et al. 1993) to one of a more supportive, observational attempt at avoiding, if possible, any operative or interventional procedure in patients with sterile necrosis and delaying the timing of operative intervention to 3–4 weeks after onset of the disease, even in those with infected necrosis (Kendrick and Sarr 2005). This latter approach involves the use of targeted antibiotic treatment in patients with documented infected necrosis to prevent the systemic bacteremia and overwhelming sepsis and thereby to allow the local area(s) of infected necrosis to become "walled off" by the host response. By doing so, the eventual operative approach allows again a targeted necrosectomy in a contained area with much less postoperative morbidity and mortality. In addition, some patients avoid any operative or even radiologic intervention, because the disease process resolves spontaneously; how often such a phenomenon occurs, however, is unknown despite anecdotal reported experience (Runzi et al. 2005; Garg et al. 2010; Sarr and Seewald 2010).

Nevertheless, in our institution, the need for the classic, transabdominal, open necrosectomy has diminished tremendously, related in large part to a more aggressive policy of delay, possibly allowing a percutaneous approach to drainage/irrigation/necrosectomy or more commonly, to an endoscopic, transgastric/transduodenal necrosectomy in selected patients(Papachristou et al. 2007). We are lucky to have a group of extremely talented and aggressive interventional endoscopists who access the area of "walled off necrosis", whether infected or sterile, usually transgastrically, "drive" the endoscope into the necrosis, and attempt an actual necrosectomy using baskets, wires, etc., to pull the necrotic material back into the stomach. This approach does not require a general anesthetic and avoids the morbidity of a celiotomy, but this approach may require 2–4 subsequent re-interventions to obtain a satisfactory necrosectomy. This true NOTES procedure (*N*atural *O*rifice *T*rans *E*ndoscopic *S*urgery) has proven to be about 75–80 % successful, and may, on occasion, also involve the joint involvement of our interventional radiologists as well.

M.G. Sarr, M.D.
Division of Gastroenterologic and General Surgery, Mayo Clinic, College of Medicine, Rochester, MN 55902, USA
e-mail: sarr.michael@mayo.edu; frank.deborah@mayo.edu

R. Mantke et al. (eds.), *International Practices in Pancreatic Surgery*,
DOI 10.1007/978-3-540-74506-8_26,

26.1 Diagnosis of Acute Necrotizing Pancreatitis

At our institution, unlike at Magdeburg, we prefer serum amylase over lipase. Although lipase assays should in theory be universal, amylase activity has always been more sensitive and especially more specific for us in our institution. For imaging, we have favored contrast-enhanced computed tomography (CECT) over magnetic resonance imaging (MRI). Our preference involves cost, ready availability, and better integration with all treating disciplines. While several European centers argue that MR not only provides all the same information as does CECT *and* additional data such as the differentiation of solid from liquid material in peripancreatic collections, our group maintains that most all (if not *all*!) peripancreatic collections in patients with acute necrotizing pancreatitis are areas of necrosis and not areas of peripancreatic fluid or pseudocysts; and, therefore, imaging by CECT is adequate, easier to obtain, cheaper, and most every clinician can read a CT as opposed to a MRI.

26.2 Use of Prophylactic Antibiotics

Prior to the two most recent prospective studies (Isenmann et al. 2004; Dellinger et al. 2007), we had used prophylactic antibiotics routinely in most all patients with severe acute pancreatitis. But more recently, our infectious disease colleagues have been less convinced of the efficacy of routine prophylaxis. Moreover, the bacteriology of infection in patients treated with prophylactic carbapenems has changed from largely coliforms (*Klebsiella* and *E. coli* species) to *Staphylococcus* and *Candida* species (Grewe et al. 1999); these organisms can be more difficult to eradicate. More recently, we have not been convinced that any evidence-based guidelines for the selective use of prophylactic antibiotics have been proven; therefore, we tend to treat only patients with ERCP-induced pancreatitis and patients with gallstone-induced pancreatitis and evidence of biliary obstruction (and thus bacteriobilia) with prophylactic imipenem for 2–4 weeks depending on their clinical course. Not only do we obtain frequent surveillance blood cultures, but we are also not hesitant to perform FNA (fine needle aspiration) to determine the organisms involved in the infected necrosis; this approach allows us to focus the antibiotic treatment/suppression in an attempt to delay the timing of operative or endoscopic intervention. Moreover, we will use percutaneous catheters to "drain" any areas that have a more liquid-based collection, again in an attempt, not as definitive therapy, but rather to delay the timing of a definitive necrosectomy.

26.3 Operative Management of Necrotizing Pancreatitis

There are four basic operative techniques for the necrosectomy and the postoperative management of the bed of the pancreas and retroperitoneum: open marsupialization (Davidson and Bradley 1981), closed drainage (Warshaw and Gongliang 1985), postoperative lavage (Beger et al. 1988) as used by Mantke and Lippert in their chapter, and the staged reoperative approach with eventual abdominal wall closure over closed suction drains as used by our group (Tsiotos et al. 1998). There are advantages and disadvantages of each approach. In our practice, we have used all four approaches, depending on the clinical situation and patient comorbidities.

Early Necrosectomy ≤3 weeks after onset of Pancreatitis: When operative necrosectomy is required before the necrosis becomes walled off, we prefer a planned, staged reoperative approach. This operative approach has been adopted by us, because we recognized early on that we were almost never able to accomplish a satisfactory, complete necrosectomy at the initial necrosectomy when operative intervention was required early in the course of the disease. Tongues of necrosis insinuate along the blood vessels and become much more obvious and defined 2–4 days later. Moreover, as mentioned by Mantke and Lippert, areas of questionable necrosis that are still strongly adherent to variable tissue may not be evident visually and grossly early in the course of the disease (first 2–3 weeks), and, too aggressive of a "necrosectomy" can lead to rather impressive bleeding. By re-inspecting these areas 2 and 4 days later at the time of the re-exploration, the interface between the necrosis and the viable tissue will become evident. We learned these lessons after our initial experience with open marsupialization, because at the time of "repacking", multiple areas of persistent necrosis were virtually always evident. While the open marsupialization allowed these areas to slough off eventually, the morbidity of repeated, wet-to-dry dressings near or directly on exposed bowel and the open "peritoneostomy" led to bleeding, fluid and electrolyte abnormalities, and loss of tissue protein. Moreover, the open abdomen with loss of domain disrupted abdominal wall stability and pulmonary mechanics and, of course, led to a high rate of incisional hernias. With these considerations, our technique involved a temporary closure of the fascia over packing and drains (on top of the packing) utilizing cloth zippers sewn to the fascia. This technique not only allowed an easy and rapid re-opening of the wound on an every-other-day schedule but also maintained the abdominal domain. The average number of re-laparotomies is about 2.5 operative re-interventions. When we are satisfied with the necrosectomy, multiple closed suction drains are left in the bed of the necrosectomy, and the fascia is then closed in a delayed primary fashion over the drains, preserving the abdominal domain. We usually place a gastrostomy tube for patient comfort and either a needle catheter jejunostomy (Sarr 1999) or, if the necrosis involves the periduodenal area (head/uncinate process of the pancreas) and right retroperitoneal gutter where we would expect a marked delay in gastric emptying, then a formal tube jejunostomy. The tube jejunostomy allows safer and more effective nutritional support. Because of the temporary closure, gastrostomy and jejunostomy, and multiple drains, we prefer a midline celiotomy over a bilateral subcostal incision. We specifically avoid use of an epidural catheter for postoperative analgesia as used by Mantke and Lippert because of the potential risk of epidural infection.

One point we stress during the first necrosectomy is to use the preoperative CT as the road map for the necrosectomy. *All* areas of necrosis need to be exposed and explored, especially the areas in the retroperitoneum. Often these areas feel firm, but no external necrosis is evident to the inexperienced eye. These areas need to be incised and exposed. Other areas not immediately evident include the base of the small bowel mesentery where the superior mesenteric artery courses caudal to the transverse mesocolon; the necrotic process from the pancreatic body often tends to extend through the mesocolon and out into the small bowel mesentery – again, if indurated or involved on the CT, this area should be incised and exposed.

Several situations, however, deserve further discussion. First, selected patients are treated by the closed, postoperative lavage method. For instance, when the necrosis is limited to the distal gland and the peripancreatic area without extension too far down the left retroperitoneum and the patient has multiple comorbidities arguing against re-laparotomy (e.g. need for anticoagulation, such as mechanical heart valves, renal failure, or severe ischemic heart disease), then we will utilize a postoperative lavage similar to the method of Mantke and Lippert, but we perfuse at 2 l/h and avoid use of any thick, rigid, sump-type drains. Second, if the pancreatic and peripancreatic bed remains suppurative during the repeat laparotomies and sepsis persists, we will consider strongly converting to the open marsupialization technique of laparostomy; although this technique adds the above described morbidity, it assures optimal "drainage" under these conditions.

Delayed necrosectomy after development of walled-off necrosis: As discussed above, our goal from the onset in patients with infected necrosis is to delay the necrosectomy for at least 4 weeks to allow walling off of the necrosis by suppressing the systemic effects of the infected necrosis. Under these circumstances, a single, more definitive operative necrosectomy becomes possible. If the necrosis is relatively limited to the peripancreatic area and is accessible via the stomach (or rarely the duodenum), then we chose endoscopic necrosectomy (Papachristou et al. 2007). This technique assumes that there is no necrosis extending distant to the peripancreatic area and that all areas communicate and are continuous. If, however, the necrosis involves both paracolic, retroperitoneal gutters and/or extends caudally behind the small bowel mesentery, then an open operative necrosectomy is chosen. Attempts at treatment with percutaneous drain placement will require multiple trips to the interventional radiology department and may prove less effective.

We have had limited experience to date with minimal access, videoscopic necrosectomy (van Santvoort et al. 2010). Our initial experience with a minimal access approach using a perfused nephroscope was suboptimal; problems include the inability to perform the necrosectomy adequately through the nephroscope due to the limitations of in-line visualization and access to the necrosis, and the lack of good technology for the necrosectomy (forceps, scoops, wire baskets, etc.). Currently, the approach described by Horvath and colleagues (2001) is very attractive for selected patients with localized and accessible necrosis who are not candidates for a primary endoscopic necrosectomy (Papachristou et al. 2007).

When an open necrosectomy is required, again we usually chose a midline incision but plan on need for only a single, definitive necrosectomy. Under these conditions, a complete necrosectomy is usually possible, again using the CT as a crucial and important road map. All areas of suspected necrosis are exposed, explored aggressively, and débrided. Multiple soft, closed suction drains are placed, gastrostomy and/or feeding jejunostomy tubes are used, and the abdomen is closed primarily. We do not believe that postoperative lavage is necessary for further debridement under these conditions. Multiple drains, however, are necessary, because 30–50 % of patients with pancreatic parenchyma necrosis will develop a pancreatic fistula. If the necrosis is only peripancreatic, then one can anticipate the operative results to be superb (Sakorafas et al. 1999).

References

Beger HG, Block S, Krautzberger W et al (1982) Necrotizing pancreatitis. Surgical indications and results in 118 patients. Chirurg 53:784–789

Beger HG, Buchler M, Bittner R et al (1988) Necrosectomy and postoperative local lavage in necrotizing pancreatitis. Br J Surg 75:207–212

Davidson ED, Bradley EL III (1981) "Marsupialization" in the treatment of pancreatic abscess. Surgery 89:252–256

Dellinger EP, Tellado JM, Soto NE et al (2007) Early antibiotic treatment for severe acute necrotizing pancreatitis: a randomized, double-blind, placebo-controlled study. Ann Surg 245:674–683

Farrugia G, Rae JL, Sarr MG, Szurszewski JH (1993) Activation of a potassium current in human circular smooth muscle cells by carbon monoxide. Biophys J 64:A387

Garg PK, Sharma M, Mandank K et al (2010) Primary conservative treatment results in mortality comparable to surgery in patients with infected necrosis. Clin Gastroenterol Hepatol 8(12):1089–1094

Grewe M, Tsiotos GG, Luque-de Leon E, Sarr MG (1999) Fungal infection in acute necrotizing pancreatitis. J Am Coll Surg 188:408–414

Horvath KD, Kao LS, Wherry KL et al (2001) A technique for laparoscopic-assisted percutaneous drainage of infected pancreatic necrosis and pancreatic abscess. Surg Endosc 15:1221–1225

Isenmann R, Runzi M, Kron M et al (2004) Prophylactic antibiotic treatment in patients with predicted severe acute pancreatitis: a placebo-controlled double-blind trial. Gastroenterology 126:997–1004

Kendrick ML, Sarr MG (2005) Pancreatic necrosis and infections in patients with acute pancreatitis. In: Forsmark CE (ed) Pancreatitis and complications. Humana Press, Inc., Totowa, pp 99–112

Papachristou GI, Takahashi N, Chahal P, Sarr MG, Baron TH (2007) Peroral endoscopic drainage/debridement of walled-off pancreatic necrosis. Ann Surg 245:943–951

Runzi M, Niebel W, Goebell H et al (2005) Severe acute pancreatitis: nonsurgical treatment of infected necroses. Pancreas 30:195–199

Sakorafas GH, Tsiotos GG, Sarr MG (1999) Extrapancreatic necrotizing pancreatitis with viable pancreas: a previously under appreciated entity. J Am Coll Surg 188: 643–648

Sarr MG (1999) Appropriate use, complications and advantages demonstrated in 500 consecutive needle catheter jejunostomies. Br J Surg 86:557–561

Sarr MG, Seewald S (2010) Do all patients with documented infected necrosis require necrosectomy/drainage? Clin Gastroenterol Hepatol 8(12):1000–1001

Tsiotos GG, Luque-de Leon E, Soreide JA et al (1998) Management of necrotizing pancreatitis by repeated operative necrosectomy using a Zipper technique. Am J Surg 175:91–98

van Santvoort HC, Besselink MG, Bakker OJ et al (2010) A step-up approach or open necrosectomy for necrotizing pancreatitis. N Engl J Med 362:1491–1502

Warshaw AL, Gongliang J (1985) Improved survival in 45 patients with pancreatic abscess. Ann Surg 202: 408–415

Index

R. Mantke et al. (eds.), *International Practices in Pancreatic Surgery*,
DOI 10.1007/978-3-540-74506-8, © Springer-Verlag Berlin Heidelberg 2013

S

GPSR Compliance

The European Union's (EU) General Product Safety Regulation (GPSR) is a set of rules that requires consumer products to be safe and our obligations to ensure this.

If you have any concerns about our products, you can contact us on ProductSafety@springernature.com

In case Publisher is established outside the EU, the EU authorized representative is:

Springer Nature Customer Service Center GmbH
Europaplatz 3
69115 Heidelberg, Germany

Batch number: 10683152

Printed by Printforce, the Netherlands